AF454466

Multiple Sclerosis: Diagnosis and Treatment

Multiple Sclerosis: Diagnosis and Treatment

Editor

Víctor M. Rivera

MDPI • Basel • Beijing • Wuhan • Barcelona • Belgrade • Manchester • Tokyo • Cluj • Tianjin

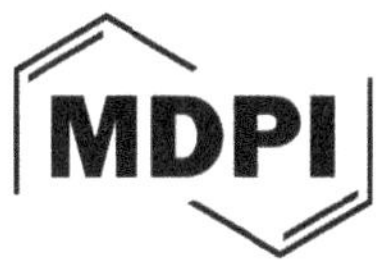

Editor
Víctor M. Rivera
Baylor College of Medicine
USA

Editorial Office
MDPI
St. Alban-Anlage 66
4052 Basel, Switzerland

This is a reprint of articles from the Special Issue published online in the open access journal *Biomedicines* (ISSN 2227-9059) (available at: https://www.mdpi.com/journal/biomedicines/special_issues/multiple_sclerosis).

For citation purposes, cite each article independently as indicated on the article page online and as indicated below:

LastName, A.A.; LastName, B.B.; LastName, C.C. Article Title. *Journal Name* **Year**, *Volume Number*, Page Range.

ISBN 978-3-0365-3096-3 (Hbk)
ISBN 978-3-0365-3097-0 (PDF)

Contents

About the Editor

Víctor M. Rivera, MD, FAAN, is a Distinguished Emeritus Professor at Baylor College of Medicine in Houston, Texas, US, and an Honorary Neurologist at Houston Methodist Hospital. Prof. Rivera is the founder and inaugural director of the Maxine Mesinger MS Comprehensive Care Center in Houston. He has trained and mentored numerous international MS and neuroimmunology specialists. He serves as an advisor on MS issues, including socioeconomic aspects affecting Latin American populations and access to care, and contributed to planning initiatives to support people with MS in the United Arab Emirates for the Abu Dhabi Crown Prince Court. Prof. Rivera received the Life Achievement Awards from the National MS Society (US) and the Consortium of MS Centers.

Preface to "Multiple Sclerosis: Diagnosis and Treatment"

Multiple Sclerosis (MS), a major inflammatory, demyelinating disease of the central nervous system (CNS), has become one of the most common causes of disability in young adults and constitutes an important socioeconomic challenge around the world. The MS International Federation estimates about 2.5 million people are affected by this disorder worldwide. While MS presents with an enormous variety of clinical facets, substantial progress in biological and sophisticated therapies has occurred [1]. The complex challenges posed by MS encouraged Biomedicines to emit a Special Issue on diagnosis and treatment.

Since its inception, MS has been a polygenic disease, but genetics also play a determining mechanistic role. Cardamone et al. [2] elegantly describe the influence of the alteration of the gene expression of the protein cytochrome b-245 (CYBB), essential in diverse aspects of immunological function, including the regulation of the phagocytic system and its interactions with reactive oxygen systems (ROS). Progressive forms of MS are characterized by increasing axonal dysfunction and neuronal degeneration, leading to increased clinical disability. This theme is addressed and clearly illustrated in a review by Correale et al. [3]. Emphasizing the clinical aspects of progressive MS, its diagnostic challenges and modern management are comprehensibly discussed by Macaron and Ontaneda [4]. The most common differential diagnoses with MS are Neuromyelitis Optica Spectrum Disorders (NMOSDs) and anti-Myelin Oligodendrocyte Glycoprotein antibody disease (MOGAD). These two entities are increasingly identified and indeed constitute real clinical challenges since their diagnostic process and therapies are entirely different from MS management. The most recent advances in this respect are discussed by Lana-Peixoto and Talim [5] utilizing excellent magnetic resonance imaging illustrations.

MS affects women in at least a 3:1 ratio compared to men; hence, women's issues are prominent in the clinical characterization of the disease. Tisovic and Amezcua [6] address the contemporary management in pregnancy and post-partum, both situations significantly affecting the clinical behavior of the disease, protectively or negatively. More than half of all patients with MS will experience some degree of cognitive problems, regardless of the duration or clinical form of the disease. Cognitive dysfunction constitutes the most common cause of work disability for people with MS. Macias Islas and Ciampi [7] discuss the assessment techniques and the societal impact of cognitive impairment in MS.

The Biomedicines Special Issue includes important therapeutic studies and reviews. Vogue and Alvarez [8] present the state of the art of relapsing and progressive treatment of MS utilizing monoclonal antibodies and the foreseen future of these therapeutic molecules in the management of the disease. A sophisticated report on the immunology and pharmacology involved in Daclizumab, a humanized alpha subunit binding to CD25, is provided by Cohan et al. [9]. The current perspectives utilizing cell-based therapies are analyzed by Cuascut and Hutton [10].

This Biomedicines Special Issue offers a comprehensive collection of scientific advances addressing diagnostic identification and the complex management of MS.

Víctor M. Rivera
Editor

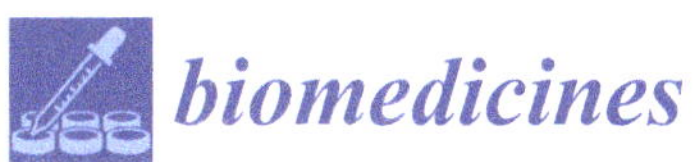 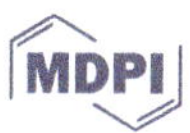

Commentary

Multiple Sclerosis: A Global Concern with Multiple Challenges in an Era of Advanced Therapeutic Complex Molecules and Biological Medicines

Victor M. Rivera

Department of Neurology, Baylor College of Medicine, Houston, TX 77030, USA; vrivera@bcm.edu; Tel.: +1-832-407-0668

Received: 11 November 2018; Accepted: 28 November 2018; Published: 30 November 2018

Abstract: Multiple sclerosis (MS) has become a common neurological disorder involving populations previously considered to be infrequently affected. Genetic dissemination from high- to low-risk groups is a determining influence interacting with environmental and epigenetic factors, mostly unidentified. Disease modifying therapies (DMT) are effective in treating relapsing MS in variable degrees; one agent is approved for primary progressive disease, and several are in development. In the era of high-efficacy medications, complex molecules, and monoclonal antibodies (MAB), including anti-VLA4 (natalizumab), anti-CD52 (alemtuzumab), and anti-CD20 (ocrelizumab), obtaining NEDA (no evidence of disease activity) becomes an elusive accomplishment in areas of the world where access to MS therapies and care are generally limited. Countries' income and access to public MS care appear to be a shared socioeconomic challenge. This disparity is also notable in the utilization of diagnostic tools to adhere to the proposed elements of the McDonald Criteria. The impact of follow-on medications ("generics"); injectable non-biological complex drugs (NBCD), oral sphingosine-1-phosphate receptor modulators, and biosimilars (interferon 1-a and 1-b), utilized in many areas of the world, is disconcerting considering these products generally lack data documenting their efficacy and safety. Potential strategies addressing these concerns are discussed from an international point of view.

Keywords: multiple sclerosis; genetics; disease modifying therapies; generic medicines

---

1. Introduction

Multiple sclerosis (MS) is an inflammatory and demyelinating disease that manifests pathologically and clinically after the disruption of the dynamic equilibrium of brain plasticity enables the development of a chronic process affecting the central nervous system (CNS). Common association with comorbidities impacts the course of disease and quality of life of the individual. MS derives from a complex multifactorial etiological process where genetic and environmental agents decisively interact. Neuroinflammation associated to MS results in a constellation of clinical manifestations as well as mood disorders, depression, and anxiety in a large proportion of patients [1]. Persistent inflammation is also one of the causes of chronicity of disease and phenotype definition [2]. The disease may become neurodegenerative, progressive, and incapacitating in almost of half of the untreated population [3]. This outcome has been improved by early and effective use of disease modifying therapies (DMT [4]. The disease commonly affects white Caucasians, particularly people of Northern European ancestry and their descendants living in recognized high-risk areas of the world: Scandinavia and the British Islands, Canada, the U.S., Australia, and New Zealand. Nevertheless, MS is increasingly identified among populations who were considered uncommonly affected by the disease. This phenomenon is generally attributed to genetic dissemination from high- to low-risk groups owing to historical and political events favoring racial intermixing. This situation has apparently contributed to the increasing frequency of the disease among Latin American Mestizos and African Americans [5]. Similar observations apply to Māori people in New Zealand, whose present genetic make-up is described as of both European and aboriginal descent [6]. Higher MS frequency rates have been reported recently in Middle Eastern and North African countries [7,8], while in other areas of the world (Asia, South America), serial epidemiologic studies reveal a true augmentation in regional rates occurring over short periods of time [9,10]. Other factors contributing to the globalization of MS are exposure to changing environmental factors, improved medical education on the disease, increasing availability of neurologists in most areas the world, as well as magnetic resonance imaging (MRI) machines, and widespread public awareness, including locally developed patient support groups and coordinated international advocacy groups like the MS International Federation (MSIF, London).

The increasing presence of MS has resulted in serious challenges to providing adequate care and accessibility to therapies. The socioeconomic challenges posed by MS as a universal disease are emphasized in countries with economies in development, but it is also an important consideration in industrialized countries that theoretically have more advanced health systems.

From initial diagnosis to long-term management, MS is a very onerous and complicated medical condition. The disease exerts a substantial economic impact on health systems, particularly where therapeutic availability is compromised by technological limitations to fulfilling all necessary elements for diagnosis proposed by modern criteria. The impact of follow-on "generic" and biosimilar medications in some areas of the world deserves discussion in view of the lack of data substantiating their efficacy and safety profiles. These preoccupations are enhanced in many areas of the world where limited capabilities exist affecting their local licensing agencies in their ability to provide an objective, analytical, and educated approval process for complex therapeutic molecules.

This commentary addresses the concerns derived from the expanding global presence of MS, the unexpected consequences of the socioeconomic burden to MS communities, and the impact exerted in the different aspects of the disease, from adequate application of the elements of the current diagnostic criteria to access to care. Potential alleviating strategies are discussed.

2. The Global Emergence of MS

Following Jean Martin Charcot's papers on his lessons on "La Sclèrose en Plaque Disseminées" in 1868 [11], scholars in France and Europe utilized the modified denomination "Insular sclerosis of the Brain and Spinal Cord". The term "The Multiple Scleroses (as utilized in the paper) was first employed by the Philadelphia botanist Horatio Curtis Wood in 1878 [12] and adopted internationally since then as multiple sclerosis. For decades, European and American clinicians considered it as a "new" but rare neurological disease studied merely in the U.S. and Western Europe. The perception that MS was minimally or non-existent in places with non-Caucasian populations was reinforced by the 1970 observation from Alter and Olivares [13] on the prevalence in Mexico as "one of the lowest in the world" (1.6/100,000). During the last part of the 20th century and the first decades of the current epoch, epidemiologic studies have shown a notable increase in prevalence in Latin American countries [14], including Mexico [15], and the Middle East [16], while frequencies remain elevated in North America and some European countries. On the American continent, the increasing presence of the disease is now evident in populations that were hypothetically "resistant" to the disease. For five centuries, historical, sociopolitical, and migratory events favored the introduction of the European genetic risk into Native Americans (or Amerindians) and into Central and West African groups brought to the continent between the 16th and 19th centuries, resulting in the modern emergence of MS among the Latin American populations [17]. Mestizo groups constitute the most representative ethnic group in Latin America and form the largest minority in the U.S. ("Hispanics"). Studies consistently show these groups carry the inherited MS genetic European signature: HLA-DRB1*1501 [18,19]. On the other hand, the disease is rare, or practically non-existent, among non-mixed Amerindians [20]. The most plausible explanation for this phenomenon lies in the fact that Native Americans (across the continent) possess a predominantly Asian genetic makeup probably owed to the early peopling of the Americas.

Low prevalence continues to be reported among Chinese communities (5.2/100,000) [21], in Japan (3.9/100,000), and in Korea (3.5/100,000) [22,23]. Contrarily, Western Siberian populations have increased their prevalence in the last thirty years from 24 to 54/100,000 [24]. It is noted the Western Siberian MS patients are practically of European origin (white Caucasians). The disease however remains unreported among Yakuts and smaller Asiatic tribes [25]. At present, the MS prevalence in the Russian Federation is at a medium risk level (30–70/100,000) [26].

Despite epidemiologic methodological inconsistencies in acquiring data in the Middle East and nearby areas, current information shows frequencies fluctuating from low to high prevalence in this region [27]. Substantial MS prevalence has been noted in some countries, i.e., the United Arab Emirates 64.4/100,000 [28] and Iran 101.13/100,000 [29]. Observations in Kuwait show Palestinian emigres have a higher prevalence (23.8/100,000) in comparison to local Kuwaitis (9.5/100,000) [30]. Qatar reports a high MS concentration (64.57/100,000), also contributed in part by a large immigrant working force [31].

The highest prevalence rates are reported from the Scottish Northern Isles: the Orkney (402/100,000) and Shetland Islands (295/100,000) [32]. Prevalence in mainland Scotland is very high as well: 229/100,000 [33]. Canada claims the highest national prevalence at 290/100,000 [34]. The prevalence in U.S. has been reported with varying rates: 110 to 192.1/100,000, from the Eastern and Western census, respectively [35]. The majority of global MS epidemiologic studies address prevalence whilst international incidence studies are scarce. Nevertheless, the MS world map exhibits frequent and dynamic changes as more epidemiologic data accumulates from the different regions of the globe.

3. Ubiquitous Application of MS Diagnostic Criteria

The criteria for diagnosing MS have evolved along with advances in knowledge of the disease. The process of diagnosing MS following an initial clinical event, or clinically isolated syndrome (CIS) suggestive of an inflammatory/demyelinating lesion, or lesions, in the CNS, has become more sophisticated, while concomitantly, the international panel authorizing the criteria strive for simplicity and general accessibility of the proposed guidelines. The 2017 McDonald Criteria [36] was designed to serve as a more accessible tool for practitioners and researchers for reaching a faster and more definite MS diagnosis. The criteria aim to increase sensitivity without affecting specificity, reducing the possibility of misdiagnosis, and adding novel aspects in its structure, like the inclusion of symptomatic and asymptomatic lesions, as well as cortical signals detected by MRI, to comply with the concepts of lesions disseminated in space (DIS). Another original addition introduced by the 2017 McDonald international panel is utilizing the presence of unique cerebrospinal fluid (CSF) oligoclonal bands substituting for dissemination in time (DIT) in cases lacking MRI asymptomatic post-gadolinium T1 enhancing images. Assessment of optic pathology, although important, is not included within the current stipulations of the 2017 McDonald Criteria.

Factors affecting realistic applicability of the criteria in all areas of the world are related to limited access to diagnostic technology or to economic constraints. The MSIF reports an increasing trend in the number of MRI machines in emerging countries, almost doubling in a five-year period. Still, 87% of low-income countries [37] do not use the McDonald Criteria reporting criteria, instead utilizing the outdated Poser criteria (1983) [38] which does not require MR imaging for the clinical diagnosis of MS. Another aspect determining effective universal applicability of the criteria is the fact that the most sensitive and recommended methodology for CSF oligoclonal bands analysis, isoelectric focusing immunoblotting [36], is not readily available through local clinical laboratories in countries with developing economies. This technique requires special equipment and expertise to perform the analysis. The older techniques, i.e., agarose gel electrophoresis, are less sensitive and carry substantial risk of providing false-positive results. Many neurological communities in regions facing this dilemma have opted to omit CSF analysis in the diagnostic workup of suspected MS.

The McDonald Criteria panel recognizes that the proposed elements for diagnosis have been acquired from large populations of Western European genetic origins presenting with typical CIS (the initial MS clinical event). The panel emphasizes the need to validate the criteria, either prospectively or retrospectively, in diverse populations, namely in patients from Asia, Latin America, the Middle East, Africa, and other relatively less studied geographical locations. Recent discussions at the Foro Centroamericano y del Caribe para Esclerosis Múltiple (FOCEM) [39] addressed the difficulties in fulfilling the diagnostic criteria in some areas of the world. FOCEM is constituted of neurologists from the six Central American nations, Venezuela, and 26 Caribbean island countries. Most neurological services in these countries have access to MRI, and mostly to 1.5 Tesla equipment; however, practically none of these diagnosticians possess reliable CSF analysis technology to locally perform complimentary analyses. The risk of underdiagnosing in areas of the world where these limitations exist is a realistic concern [40].

It is expected that future availability of economic serological biomarkers will considerably alleviate the diagnostic restrictions existing for MS in some areas of the world.

4. Global MS Care Disparities

MS therapies have flourished in the last three decades whilst becoming more complicated and onerous. The advent of what are recognized as high-efficacy medications applies mostly to DMT for relapsing MS (RMS), with thus far only one MAB approved for primary progressive MS (PPMS). These medications have a greater pharmacological effect than the original first-line, platform, injectable therapies (interferons and glatiramer acetate). International licensing agencies, satisfying an unmet therapeutic need, have approved ocrelizumab, a CD20 cytolytic MAB targeting B lymphocytes, for treatment of PPMS. Several clinical trials are being carried out addressing progressive forms including secondary progressive MS (SPMS). However, making these pharmacological agents accessible to all MS populations is a formidable challenge and realistic socioeconomic preoccupation. Except for the private health enterprise sector of the U.S., most countries of the world rely almost entirely on their official health systems to provide access to MS therapies. For most of the 101 countries that provided data to the MSIF, therapies were partially or fully funded by the government. In the countries affiliated to the MSIF, health services funded by taxation through social security or mandated health insurance covered 76% of the cost of DMT. Global availability of MS medications is notably dissimilar between high-, upper middle-, lower middle- and low-income countries, as described in the Atlas of MS (World Health Organization/MSIF) [41]. The higher the national income, the more availability of medications—not just platform injectable medications, but oral agents and intravenous MAB, as well. Most countries with the lowest national incomes may have access to only one or two first-line DMT. For instance, in Cuba, the only DMT available is the brand Interferon beta 1-a, 44 mcg (Rebif®) [42]; in the Republic of Salvador, the national social security system offers only two medications, both innovators, including a low-dose (Avonex®, 30 mcg) and a high-dose interferon beta 1-a (Rebif®, 44 mcg) [43]. Availability of DMT to MS patients in the world is reviewed in detail at the Atlas of MS 2013, with data provided by the World Bank and the World Health Organization [44]. Availability of medications for all people with MS is not a reality for at least 90 countries of the world. The MSIF document indicates that affordability was ranked as the most common cause of lack of access to therapy in 46% of countries, which rises to 86% in 21 low- and lower-middle-income countries.

The socioeconomic impact of MS in developing countries is a considerable public health concern. These same areas usually display a low prevalence of MS; hence, the disease is not generally appreciated by their health systems. In economically emergent countries in Latin America, for instance, only 9.5% to 42.3% of the MS population have access to a DMT [45]. On the other hand, almost 90% of the economic burden exerted by MS on the country of Colombia is spent just to cover the cost of DMT [46], this cost being dependent on the grade of disability: For a patient with Expanded Disability Score Status (EDSS) 3.0-5.5, the annual cost of MS medications is 25,713 USD, while for a patient with EDSS $\geq$7.0 in Argentina, it is estimated at 50,712 USD. In general, the cost of DMT is less expensive in European countries and elsewhere, in comparison to the United States where, for example, an interferon for Relapsing Remitting MS (RRMS) may cost as much as 5150 USD/month, and oral fingolimod

5372 USD/month. Other tangible and intangible costs, including medical expenses, rehabilitation procedures, other multidisciplinary care required by MS, loss of work productivity, and the emotional and physical impact on the care givers, add exponentially to the price of MS. The cost increases as disability advances [47]. In many countries where access to DMT is limited, escalation to drugs with higher efficacy is not feasible; hence, the ideal goal of obtaining the therapeutic goal of 'no evidence of disease activity' (NEDA) is consequently and fundamentally challenged. Potential strategies to address these concerns would involve increasing public awareness and knowledge, which eventually should also impact health officials' education and attitudes. Transparency in the process of MS medication acquisition by national health systems would be more efficient and cost-containing by involving neurologists with MS knowledge and independently appointed public commissioners with input from patients support groups in this complex undertaking.

5. Impact of Follow-On Therapeutic Molecules and Biosimilar Medications

The appearance of "generic" medications for MS in international public and private health markets, and prescription formularies of social security programs around the world, has been increasing in development. International regulatory agencies, including the U.S. Food and Drug Administration (FDA) and the European Medicines Agency (EMA), have approved follow-on CBND replacing the innovator Copaxone®. This decision was based on bioequivalence shown by molecular and pharmacological similarity, without requiring clinical studies. Neither the FDA nor EMA have determined approval pathways for follow-on biomedicines such interferons and MAB. In both cases, appropriate phase III clinical data, and even "head-to-head" trials performed on the proposed follow-on medication set against the innovator drug as a substitute, should be required by international licensing agencies. The lack of essential clinical and pharmacological data from biosimilar medications is reflected in the fact in that most international MS associations do not include or consider them as yet in their therapeutic guidelines: These include the American Academy of Neurology, the European Academy of Neurology, the Spanish Society of Neurology, the Catalonia Society of Neurology, Consensus from Peru, Central America and Caribbean countries, among others. Some of the follow-on products manufactured in North Korea, India, Iran, Mexico, Argentina, and Uruguay (outside the sphere of the FDA and EMA), lack data on efficacy and safety of their own, in fact utilizing results obtained from the phase III pivotal trials performed by the innovator (original) products. Follow-on medications have been approved by many international licensing agencies outside the U.S. and the European Union, and are basically unchallenged due to lack of local appropriate technology and education on the subject of the responsible health departments, including the ability to evaluate the biological and immunologic behaviors of the proposed product. Substantial molecular differences have been reported [48] between follow-on and innovator interferon drugs. Analytical studies performed on the interferon 1-a innovators Avonex® (30 mcg) and Rebif® (44 mcg), both produced in the U.S., and the follow-on products Juntab® (Mexico) and CinnoVex® (Iran), both 30 mcg preparations, and the 44 mcg presentations Clausen® (Uruguay) and Blastoferon® (Argentina), these latter examples revealing considerable heterogeneity in immunochemical analyses and in "reporter gene assays" among the follow-on products but not in the brand medications. These studies also demonstrated significant pharmacological and biological potency differences between the innovators and the follow-on products [49]. Studies have consistently shown that lack of clinical data, confounded with absence of demonstration of bioequivalence and interchangeability of biosimilars, do not provide at present time evidence for their efficacy and safety. The economic impacts on individual and public health offered by the follow-on products have not been reflected in significant savings for the health systems [50]. Several international initiatives have developed, like the one promoted by the Latin American Committee for Treatment and Research in MS (LACTRIMS) [51], that encourage practitioners, MS study groups, and MS patient associations (most affiliated to the MSIF) from the region (20 countries) to coordinate with local health officials providing information and education on the licensing process, and even participating as independent advisors, striving for the proposed non-innovative follow-on medications to provide adequate clinical efficacy and safety data.

6. Conclusions

Except for rare exceptions, MS has in fact become a global disease affecting virtually every ethnic and racial group. The widespread epidemiologic presence of the disease has carried tremendous socioeconomic challenges due to the limitation of access and barriers to MS management, notably in countries still undergoing economic development. Considering that comorbidities (obesity, hyperlipidemia, migraine, rheumatological conditions) have been reported to increase the risk of relapse in MS [52], emphasis in management of these comorbidities, including a healthy diet and exercise, should be part of the management paradigm across the globe. Ensuring improved diagnosis, access to treatment, information, and available support resources require coordinated efforts from local and regional neurological MS study groups, societal MS organizations, and patient support groups. The 2017 McDonald panel recognizes this need and encourages MS diagnostic validation in non-Western European ethnicity populations (since 2000, the diverse revisions have applied practically to only Caucasian populations), and to geographic areas where the disease has a low prevalence. Revisions to the MS criteria are conducted every 5–7 years, once new or more advanced diagnostic technology and documented clinical data justify updating the diverse criteria of the proposal. It is expected the next revision will include contributions from the international committees for treatment and research in MS from all areas of the world. Tangible and indirect expenses compound the associated costs of necessary but complex multidisciplinary MS care. In this commentary, these aspects are reviewed from an international perspective while providing awareness and potential paths to alleviate these actual concerns, including addressing the concern of insufficient data on follow-on therapeutic molecules.

Author Contributions: V.M.R. designed and wrote the paper.

Funding: There were no funding sponsors for this paper.

Conflicts of Interest: The author declares no conflict of interest.

References

1. Rossi, S.; Studer, V.; Motta, C.; Polidoro, S.; Perugini, J.; Macchiarulo, G.; Giovannetti, A.M.; Pareja-Gutierrez, L.; Calò, A.; Colonna, I.; et al. Neuroinflammation drives anxiety and depression in relapsing-remitting multiple sclerosis. *Neurology* **2017**, *89*, 1338–1347. [CrossRef] [PubMed]
2. Isoupras, A.; Lordan, R.; Zabetakis, I. Inflammation, not Cholesterol, Is a Cause of Chronic Disease. *Nutrients* **2018**, *10*, 604. [CrossRef] [PubMed]
3. Ontaneda, D.; Thompson, A.J.; Cohen, J.A. Progressive multiple sclerosis: Prospects for disease therapy, repair, and restoration of function. *Lancet* **2017**, *389*, 1357–1366. [CrossRef]
4. Corboy, J.R.; Weinshenker, B.G.; Wingerchuk, D.M. Comment on 2018 American Academy of Neurology guidelines on disease-modifying therapies in MS. *Neurology* **2018**, *90*, 1106–1112. [CrossRef] [PubMed]
5. Rivera, V.M. Multiple Sclerosis in Latin America: Reality and challenge. *Neuroepidemiology* **2009**, *32*, 293–295. [CrossRef] [PubMed]
6. Pearson, J.F.; Alla, S.; Clarke, G.; Taylor, B.V.; Miller, D.H.; Richardson, A.; Mason, D.F. Multiple Sclerosis in New Zealand Māori. *Mult. Scler.* **2014**, *20*, 1892–1895. [CrossRef] [PubMed]
7. Heydarpour, P.; Koshkish, S.; Abtahi, S.; Moradi-Lakeh, M.; Sahraian, M.A. Multiple Sclerosis Epidemiology in Middle East and North Africa: A Systematic review and Meta-Analysis. *Neuroepidemiology* **2015**, *44*, 232–244. [CrossRef] [PubMed]
8. Stachowiak, J. Rising Multiple Sclerosis Rates in Middle East. Available online: https://www.msconnection.org/Blog/October-2015-rising-multiple-sclerosis-rates-in-Middle-East (accessed on 6 September 2018).
9. Callegaro, D.; de Lolio, C.A.; Radvany, J.; Tilbery, C.P.; Mendonça, R.A.; Melo, A.C. Prevalence of Multiple Sclerosis in the city of Sao Paulo, Brazil, in 1990. *Neuroepidemiology* **1992**, *11*, 11–14. [CrossRef] [PubMed]

10. Gonzalez, O.; Sotelo, J. Is the Frequency of Multiple Sclerosis Increasing in Mexico? *J. Neurol. Neurosurg. Psychiatry* **1995**, *59*, 528–530. [CrossRef] [PubMed]

11. Charcot, J.M. *Lectures on the Diseases of the Nervous System. Delivered at la Salpêtrière*; New Sydenham Society: London, UK, 1881; Volume II.

12. Wood, H.C., Jr. *Multiple Sclerosis: The History of a Disease*; Demos Medical Publishing: New York, NY, USA, 2005; pp. 224–250.

13. Alter, M.; Olivares, L. Multiple sclerosis in Mexico: An epidemiologic study. *Arch. Neurol.* **1970**, *23*, 451–454. [CrossRef] [PubMed]

14. Cristiano, E.; Rojas, J.; Romano, M.; Frider, N.; Machnicki, G.; Giunta, D.; Calegaro, D.; Corona, T.; Flores, J.; Gracia, F.; et al. The epidemiology of multiple sclerosis in Latin America and the Caribbean: A systematic review. *Mult. Scler.* **2013**, *19*, 844–854. [CrossRef] [PubMed]

15. De la Maza Flores, M.; Arambide Garcia, G. Prevalence of multiple sclerosis in the Municipality of San Pedro Garza García, Nuevo León (Mexico). *Avances* **2006**, *1*, 8–10.

16. Nazr, Z.; Elemadifar, M.; Khalili, B. Epidemiology of Multiple Sclerosis in the Middle East. A systematic review and meta-analysis. *Mult. Scler. Relat. Disord.* **2014**, *3*, 744. [CrossRef]

17. Gracia, F.; Castillo, L.C.; Benzadón, A.; Larreategui, M.; Villareal, F.; Triana, E.; Arango, A.C.; Lee, D.; Pascale, J.M.; Gomez, E.; et al. Prevalence and Incidence of multiple sclerosis in Panama (2000–2005). *Neuroepidemiology* **2009**, *32*, 287–293. [CrossRef] [PubMed]

18. Ordoñez, G.; Romero, S.; Orozco, L.; Pineda, B.; Jiménez-Morales, S.; Nieto, A.; García-Ortiz, H.; Sotelo, J. Genomewide admixture study in Mexican Mestizos with multiple sclerosis. *Clin. Neurol. Neurosurg.* **2015**, *130*, 55–60. [CrossRef] [PubMed]

19. Rivera, V.M. Multiple Sclerosis in Latin Americans: Genetic Aspects. *Curr. Neurol. Neurosci. Rep.* **2017**, *17*, 57–63. [CrossRef] [PubMed]

20. Flores, J.; González, S.; Morales, X.; Yescas, P.; Ochoa, A.; Corona, T. Absence of multiple sclerosis and demyelinating diseases among Lacandonians, a Pure Amerindian Ethnic Group in Mexico. *Mult. Scler. Int.* **2012**. [CrossRef] [PubMed]

21. Liu, X.; Cui, Y.; Han, J. Estimating epidemiological data of Multiple Sclerosis in hospitalized data in Shandong, Province, China. *Orphanet J. Rare Dis.* **2016**, *11*, 73. [CrossRef] [PubMed]

22. Kira, J. Multiple Sclerosis in the Japanese population. *Lancet Neurol.* **2003**, *2*, 117–127. [CrossRef]

23. Kim, N.H.; Kim, H.J.; Cheong, H.K.; Kim, B.J.; Lee, K.H.; Kim, E.-H.; Kim, E.A.; Kim, S.; Park, M.S.; Yoon, W.T.; et al. Prevalnece of multiple sclerosis in Korea. *Neurology* **2018**, *75*, 1432–1438. [CrossRef] [PubMed]

24. Boiko, A.N. Multiple sclerosis prevalence in Russia and other countries of the former USSR. In *Multiple Sclerosis In Europe: An Epidemiological Update*; Firmhaber, W., Lauer, K., Eds.; Leuchtturm: Darmstadt, Germany, 1994; pp. 219–230.

25. Malkova, N.A.; Shperling, L.P.; Riabukhina, O.V.; Merkulova, E.A. Multiple sclerosis in Eastern Siberia: A 20-year prospective study in Novosibirsk city. *Zh. Nevrol. Psikhiatr. Im. S S Korsakova* **2006**, *3*, 11–16.

26. Boyko, A.; Smirnova, N.; Petrov, S.; Gusev, E. Epidemiology of Multiple Sclerosis in Russia, a historical review. *Mult. Scler. Demyelinating Dis.* **2016**, *1*, 13. [CrossRef]

27. Mohammed, E.M.A. Multiple Sclerosis is prominent in the Gulf states: Review. *Pathogenesis* **2016**, *3*, 19–38. [CrossRef]

28. Inshasi, J.; Thakre, M. Prevalence of multiple sclerosis in Dubai, United Arab Emirates. *Int. J. Neurosci.* **2011**, *121*, 393–398. [CrossRef] [PubMed]

29. Eskandarieh, S.; Heydarpour, P.; Elhami, S.-R.; Sahralan, M.A. Prevalence and Incidence of Multiple Sclerosis in Tehran, Iran. *Iran J. Public Health* **2017**, *45*, 699–704.

30. Najim Al-Din, A.S. Multiple Sclerosis in Kuwait: Clinical and epidemiological study. *J. Neurol. Neurosurg. Psychiatry* **1986**, *49*, 928–931. [CrossRef]

31. Deleu, D.; Mir, D.; Al Tabouki, A.; Mesraoua, R.; Mesraoua, B.; Akhtar, N.; Al Hail, H.; D'souza, A.; Melikyan, G.; Imam, Y.Z.; et al. Prevalence, demographics and clinical characteristics of multiple sclerosis in Qatar. *Mult. Scler.* **2013**, *19*, 816–819. [CrossRef] [PubMed]

32. Visser, E.M.; Wilde, K.; Wilson, J.F.; Yong, K.K.; Counsell, C.E. A new prevalence study of Multiple Sclerosis in Orkney, Shetland and Aberdeen City. *J. Neurol. Neurosurg. Psychiatry* **2012**, *83*, 719–724. [CrossRef] [PubMed]

33. Prevalence and Incidence of Multiple Sclerosis in Scotland. Available online: https://www.mstrust.org.uk (accessed on 6 September 2018).

34. Multiple Sclerosis Canada. Available online: https://mssociety.ca (accessed on 6 September 2018).

35. Dilokthornsakul, O.; Valuck, R.J.; Nair, K.V.; Corboy, J.R.; Allen, R.R.; Campbell, J.D. Multiple sclerosis in the United States commercially insured population. *Neurology* **2016**, *86*, 1014–1021. [CrossRef] [PubMed]

36. Thompson, A.J.; Banwell, B.L.; Barkhof, F.; William, M.C.; Timothy, C.; Giancarlo, C.; Jorge, C.; Franz, F.; Massimo, F.; Mark, S.F.; et al. Diagnosis of multiple sclerosis: 2017 revisions of the McDonald criteria. *Lancet Neurol.* **2018**, *17*, 162–173. [CrossRef]

37. Poser, C.M.; Paty, D.W.; Scheinberg, L.; McDonald, W.I.; Davis, F.A.; Ebers, G.C.; Johnson, K.P.; Sibley, W.A.; Silberberg, D.H.; et al. New diagnostic criteria for multiple sclerosis: Guidelines for research protocols. *Ann. Neurol.* **1983**, *13*, 227–231. [CrossRef] [PubMed]

38. Fortini, A.S.; Sanders, E.L.; Weinshenker, B.G.; Katzmann, J.A. Cerebrospinal Fluid Oligoclonal Bands in the Diagnosis of Multiple Sclerosis. *Am. J. Clin. Pathol.* **2003**, *120*, 672–675. [CrossRef] [PubMed]

39. Available online: http://www.focem.org (accessed on 3 October 2018).

40. Gracia, F.; Armién, B.; Rivera, V. Collaborative Multiple Sclerosis Group of Central America and Spanish Caribbean Region. Multiple Sclerosis in Central American and Spanish Caribbean Region: Should it be Recognized as a Public Health Problem? *J. Epid. Prev. Med.* **2017**, *3*, 134.

41. Browne, P.; Chandraratna, D.; Angood, C.; Tremlett, H.; Baker, C.; Taylor, B.V.; Thompson, A.J. Atlas of Multiple Sclerosis 2013: A growing global problem with widespread inequity. *Neurology* **2014**, *83*, 1022–1024. [CrossRef] [PubMed]

42. Diaz de la Fé, A. Treatment of Multiple Sclerosis in Cuba. Centro Internacional de Rehabilitación Neurológica (CIREN): Havana, Cuba. Available online: www.ciren.cu (accessed on 4 May 2017).

43. Rivera, V.M.; Medina, M.T.; Duron, R.M. Multiple Sclerosis Care in Latin America. *Neurology* **2014**, *82*, 1660–1661. [CrossRef] [PubMed]

44. Available online: www.msif.org/wp-content/upload/2014/09/Atlas-of-MS (accessed on 3 October 2018).

45. Rivera, V.M.; Macias, M.A. Access and barriers to MS care in Latin America. *Mult. Scler. J. Exp. Transl. Clin.* **2017**, *3*. [CrossRef] [PubMed]

46. Jimenez-Pérez, C.E.; Zarco-Montero, L.A.; Castañeda-Cardona, C.; Otálora Esteban, M.; Martínez, A.; Rosselli, D. Current state of Multiple Sclerosis in Colombia. *Acta Neurol. Colomb.* **2015**, *31*, 385–390.

47. Rojas, J.L.; Patrucco, L.; Cristiano, E. Current and emerging treatments for relapsing multiple sclerosis in Argentinean patients: A review. *Deg. Neurol. Neuromusc. Dis.* **2014**, *4*, 103–109.

48. Cuevas, C.; Deisenhammer, F.; You, X.; Scolnik, M.; Buffels, R.; Sperling, B.; Flores Ramirez, F.; Macias Islas, M.; Sauri-Suárez, S. Low immunogenicity but reduced bioavailability of an interferon beta-1a biosimilar compared with its biological parent: Results of MATRIX, a cross-sectional multicenter phase 4 study. *Biosimilars* **2015**, *5*, 1–7.

49. Meager, A.; Dolman, C.; Dilger, P.; Bird, C.; Giovannoni, G.; Schellekens, H.; Thorpe, R.; Wadhwa, M. An Assessment of Biological Potency and Molecular Characteristics of Different Innovator and Noninnovator Interferon-Beta Products. *J. Interferon Cytokine Res.* **2011**, *31*, 383–392. [CrossRef] [PubMed]

50. Macias-Islas, M.A.; Soria-Cedillo, I.; Vazquez-Quintana, M.; Rivera, V.M.; Baca-Muro, V.I.; Lemus-Carmona, E.A.; Chiquete, E. Cost of care according to disease-modifying therapies in Mexicans with multiple sclerosis. *Acta Neurol. Belg.* **2013**, *113*, 415–420. [CrossRef] [PubMed]

51. Steinberg, J.; Fragoso, Y.; Garcia Bonitto, J.R.; Guerra, C.; Rodriguez, V.; Correa, P.; Macias, M.; Novarro, N.; Vizcarra, D.; Orozco, G.; et al. Practical aspects and recommendations concerning the approval and use of biosimilar drugs for the treatment of multiple sclerosis in Latin America. In Proceedings of the X Latin American Committee for Treatments and Research in MS, Asuncion, Paraguay, 22–24 November 2018. Abstract 0098.

52. Kowalek, K.; McKay, K.A.; Patten, S.B.; Fisk, J.D.; Evans, C.; Tremlett, H.; Marrie, R.A.; CIHR Team in Epidemiology and Impact of Comorbidity on Multiple Sclerosis (ECoMS). Comorbidity increases the risk of relapse in multiple sclerosis. *Neurology* **2017**, *89*, 2455–2461. [CrossRef] [PubMed]

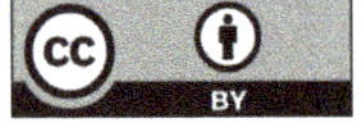

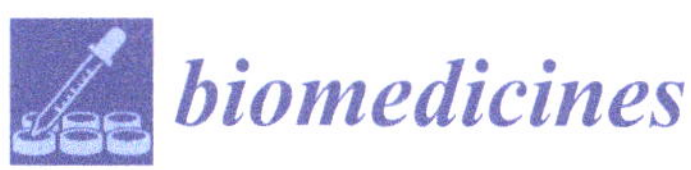 *biomedicines*

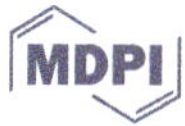

Article

Genetic Association and Altered Gene Expression of *CYBB* in Multiple Sclerosis Patients

Giulia Cardamone [1], Elvezia Maria Paraboschi [1], Giulia Soldà [1,2], Stefano Duga [1,2], Janna Saarela [3] and Rosanna Asselta [1,2,*]

[1] Department of Biomedical Sciences, Humanitas University, Via Rita Levi Montalcini 4, 20090 Pieve Emanuele, Milan, Italy; giulia.cardamone@st.hunimed.eu (G.C.); elvezia_maria.paraboschi@hunimed.eu (E.M.P.); giulia.solda@hunimed.eu (G.S.); stefano.duga@hunimed.eu (S.D.)

[2] Humanitas Clinical and Research Center, Via Manzoni 56, 20089 Rozzano, Milan, Italy

[3] Institute for Molecular Medicine Finland, Helsinki Institute of Life Science (HiLIFE), University of Helsinki, 00290 Helsinki, Finland; janna.saarela@helsinki.fi

* Correspondence: rosanna.asselta@hunimed.eu; Tel.: +39-02-82245215

Received: 21 November 2018; Accepted: 15 December 2018; Published: 18 December 2018

Abstract: Multiple sclerosis (MS) is a chronic neurological disorder characterized by inflammation, demyelination, and axonal damage. Increased levels of reactive oxygen species (ROS), produced by macrophages and leading to oxidative stress, have been implicated as mediators of demyelination and axonal injury in both MS and experimental autoimmune encephalomyelitis, the murine model of the disease. On the other hand, reduced ROS levels can increase susceptibility to autoimmunity. In this work, we screened for association with MS 11 single nucleotide polymorphisms (SNPs) and two microsatellite markers in the five genes (*NCF1*, *NCF2*, *NCF4*, *CYBA*, and *CYBB*) of the nicotinamide adenine dinucleotide phosphate (NADPH) oxidase (NOX2) system, the enzymatic pathway producing ROS in the brain and neural tissues, in 347 Finnish patients with MS and 714 unaffected family members. This analysis showed suggestive association signals for *NCF1* and *CYBB* (lowest $p = 0.038$ and $p = 0.013$, respectively). Functional relevance for disease predisposition was further supported for the *CYBB* gene, by microarray analysis in $CD4^{+/-}$ mononuclear cells of 21 individuals from five Finnish multiplex MS families, as well as by real-time RT-PCRs performed on RNA extracted from peripheral blood mononuclear cells of an Italian replication cohort of 21 MS cases and 21 controls. Our results showed a sex-specific differential expression of *CYBB*, suggesting that this gene, and more in general the NOX2 system, deserve to be further investigated for their possible role in MS.

Keywords: multiple sclerosis; association study; reactive oxygen species; NADPH oxidase; *CYBB*

---

1. Introduction

Multiple sclerosis (MS) (Online Mendelian Inheritance in Men, OMIM #126200) is a chronic disease of the central nervous system (CNS) characterized by multifocal inflammation, plaques of myelin degeneration, axonal damage, and by a high degree of individual variability in the severity and progression of symptoms [1–3]. Among neurological disorders of young adults, MS is the most common: in Europe, where a latitude-correlated distribution of prevalence and incidence rates can be observed, prevalence ranges from 70 to 100 per 100,000, whereas incidence varies between 2 and 4 per 100,000 person/year; the highest prevalence and incidence rates have been reported in Finland [4]. Here, incidence and prevalence reach the exceptional rate of 11.6 and 200 per 100,000 in the Southern Ostrobothnian region (western coast of Finland), reflecting several centuries of genetic drift in a small and isolated population [5].

In agreement with the multigenic character of MS, genome-wide linkage scans, genome-wide association studies (GWAS), as well as meta-analyses performed in large cohorts disclosed more than 200 non-HLA (human leukocyte antigen) single nucleotide polymorphisms (SNPs) associated with MS, each having a small effect size on MS predisposition [6–10]. Typically, the identified association signals point to genes belonging to innate and adaptive pathways [9,10]. The deep involvement of a dysregulated immune system in MS is also supported by the efficacy of drugs targeting T- and B-cell functions in the treatment of the disease, as well as by the numerous studies indicating CD4$^+$ and CD8$^+$ T cells as strong contributors to the pathogenic process [11–14].

Apart from immune-mediated mechanisms, a growing body of evidence indicates that oxidative stress (OS) may play a role in the etiology of MS [15–17]. Increased levels of oxygen-free radicals (collectively called reactive oxygen species, ROS), produced by macrophages and leading to OS, have been implicated as mediators of demyelination and axonal injury in both MS and experimental autoimmune encephalomyelitis, the murine model of the disease [18–20]. Moreover, ROS: (i) activate specific transcription factors, such as the nuclear transcription factor kappa B, which in turn upregulates the expression of genes associated with MS or its progression (e.g., tumor necrosis factor α) [21,22]; (ii) mediate the activity of matrix metalloproteinases, which are involved in T-cell activation and trafficking into the CNS and hence probably involved in some of the early pro-inflammatory events in MS [23–25]; (iii) are produced in increased amount by activated mononuclear cells of patients, resulting in oxygen damage to DNA, lipids, and proteins—these molecules are frequently found in active MS lesions and are associated with apoptotic oligodendrocytes and neurodegeneration in the brains of patients with MS [16,26–28].

Besides reactions involving the electron-transport chain of mitochondria or those related to the metabolism of amino acids and neurotransmitters, in the brain and neural tissue ROS are also produced by enzymatic pathways, such as xanthine oxidase, lipoxygenase, and cyclooxygenase, as well as by the nicotinamide adenine dinucleotide phosphate (NADPH) oxidase (NOX) systems [29,30]. Specifically, the NOX2 system is a complex that, in resting cells, is compartmentalized between cytosol and plasma membrane: the core enzyme is composed of three cytoplasmic polypeptides (p47phox, p67phox, and p40phox, encoded by *NCF1*, *NCF2*, and *NCF4* genes, respectively), and a membrane-bound flavo-hemo-cytochrome, b558, constituted by two components, the p22phox and gp91phox subunits (encoded by *CYBA* and *CYBB*, respectively) [29,30]. When the resting cell is exposed to stimuli (i.e., chemotactic reactants or particulate stimuli, such as bacteria and fungi), p47phox becomes heavily phosphorylated, inducing all cytoplasmic components to translocate to the membrane-bound cytochrome in order to form the active enzyme complex [29,30].

Given the proposed role of OS in MS, its contribution to the pathogenesis of the disease was here investigated by genetic association and expression analyses of the five genes coding for the main components of the NOX2 complex.

2. Results

2.1. NCF1 and CYBB Are Associated with MS in the Finnish Population

For investigating the potential role of OS genes in the pathogenesis of MS, we performed an association analysis on a Finnish cohort of 63 MS families (547 individuals) with two microsatellite markers and 11 SNPs mapping in or located close to the five genes coding for the main components of the NOX2 complex (the soluble factors *NCF1*, *NCF2*, and *NCF4*, and the membrane-bound redox core proteins of the complex, *CYBA* and *CYBB*) (see Table S1 in the Supplementary Materials). No significant deviation from Hardy-Weinberg equilibrium (HWE) and no Mendelian inheritance errors were observed for any of the markers included in this study. The overall average genotype call rate was 96.5%, and the accuracy was >99.5% according to duplicated genotyping (5%) of all samples.

Table 1 shows the results of the allelic association analysis for each of the 11 variants for the whole study cohort. Two polymorphisms, D7S1870 in *NCF1* and rs5963310 in *CYBB*, showed suggestive evidence of association with MS in the transmission/disequilibrium (TDT) test ($p = 0.038$ and $p = 0.027$ for *NCF1* and *CYBB*, respectively; not corrected for multiple testing). By using the more powerful approach based on the TDT statistic implemented with the parental discordance test (see the Materials and Methods section), we confirmed the association signal for the rs5963310 polymorphism in *CYBB* ($p = 0.013$), which confers a protective effect against MS (the minor allele A is untransmitted in MS cases). No significant allelic association between MS and the other NADPH variants could be detected (Table 1).

2.2. CYBB Is Differentially Expressed in MS Cases

To verify the possible functional relevance of NADPH genes for MS predisposition, we performed a genome-wide microarray-based gene expression analysis. We extracted total RNA from CD4$^+$ and CD4$^-$ samples isolated from peripheral blood mononuclear cells (PBMCs) of 21 individuals from five Finnish multiplex MS families. An adequate amount of high-quality total RNA was obtained from nine MS cases (four males, five females) and ten controls (four males, six females) for the CD4$^-$ cells, and from nine cases (five males, four females) and 11 controls (six males, five females) for the CD4$^+$ cells. All patients had a relapsing-remitting (RR) subtype, i.e., the most common form of MS (~80% of cases), which is characterized by periods of acute intensification of symptoms followed by phases of almost complete remission [31].

To screen for differential expression of the genes of interest in MS, we specifically searched for probe sets corresponding to *NCF1*, *NCF2*, *NCF4*, *CYBA*, and *CYBB* in the NetAffx annotation site (http://www.affymetrix.com/analysis/index.affx). The 11 identified probes were individually searched in the University of California Santa Cruz (UCSC) Genome Browser (hg19; Blat search) to identify the correct target gene (http://genome.ucsc.edu/cgi-bin/hgGateway). Probe sets recognizing only intronic sequences or mapping to several loci were excluded: in this way expression data were available for seven probes mapping in the five genes.

As for the *NCF1* gene, none of the probes were mapping correctly/specifically. As for *NCF2*, it did not show appreciable expression signals in any of the CD4$^+$/CD4$^-$ samples. We hence monitored for potential differential expression of these two genes by using the more sensitive semi-quantitative real-time reverse transcription-PCR (RT-PCR) approach. Figure 1 shows the results of RT-PCR assays: no significant difference between cases and controls in the expression levels of either genes was evidenced (no significant difference between cases and controls was seen even stratifying individuals on the basis of the D7S1870 genotype in *NCF1*; data not shown).

Table 1. NADPH polymorphisms: Results of family-based association TDT and haplotype relative risk (HRR) tests.

Gene	Marker	ANALYZE Analyses [1]				PLINK Analyses				
		HRR *p* Value	TDT *p* Value	Minor Allele [2]	MAF	Transmitted/Untransmitted [3]	TDT *p* Value	OR [95% CI]	*p* Par [4]	*p* Comb [4]
NCF1	D7S1870	**0.0491**	**0.0383**	20 repeats	0.4533	Untransmitted	0.330	0.727 [0.38–1.385]	0.157	0.206
	D7S2518	0.376	0.431	7 repeats	0.3986	/	1	1 [0.351–2.851]	0.414	0.655
NCF2	rs796860	0.895	0.500	C	0.06548	/	1	1 [0.250–3.998]	1	1
	rs2296164	0.568	0.399	T	0.4861	Untransmitted	0.297	0.643 [0.278–1.485]	0.564	0.239
	rs3818364	0.604	0.500	T	0.4688	Transmitted	0.847	1.0770 [0.506–2.291]	0.564	0.715
	rs789192	0.183	0.253	G	0.4268	Transmitted	0.144	1.727 [0.822–3.630]	0.317	0.423
	rs2274065	0.293	0.500	C	0.0974	Transmitted	0.180	4 [0.447–35.790]	0.317	0.414
NCF4	rs1883112	0.991	0.500	A	0.3861	Transmitted	0.353	1.417 [0.677–2.966]	0.257	0.182
	rs741999	0.680	0.444	A	0.4444	Transmitted	0.336	1.455 [0.675–3.134]	0.479	0.237
CYBA	rs4673	0.319	0.199	T	0.1795	Untransmitted	0.317	0.600 [0.218–1.651]	0.564	0.251
	rs2306422	0.661	0.500	T	0.494	Transmitted	0.739	1.118 [0.581–2.150]	0.655	0.876
CYBB	rs5963310	0.239	**0.0274**	A	0.09848	Untransmitted	0.0578	0.250 [0.0531–1.177]	0.0833	**0.0126**
	rs9330580	0.663	0.206	A	0.1203	Untransmitted	0.366	0.571 [0.167–1.952]	0.0833	0.109

Suggestive *p* values (*p* < 0.05) are indicated in bold. Results are presented not corrected for multiple testing (total number of performed analyses for each test: 11; Bonferroni threshold for significance: *p* < 0.0045). [1] Analyses were run both considering MS frequency of 0.01 and penetrance of 0.05, as well as considering MS frequency of 0.0006 and penetrance of 0.76 (identical results). [2] In the case of multiallelic markers (D7S1870, D7S2518), the minor allele corresponds to the most frequent repeat, which was analyzed against all the others clumped together. [3] Indication referred to the minor allele. [4] *p* par (*p* values for parents) and *p* comb (combined *p* value, deriving from the asymptotic TDT *p* value and the *p* par value). NADPH, nicotinamide adenine dinucleotide phosphate; CI, confidence interval; HRR, haplotype relative risk; MAF, minor allele frequency; OR, odds ratio; TDT, transmission disequilibrium test.

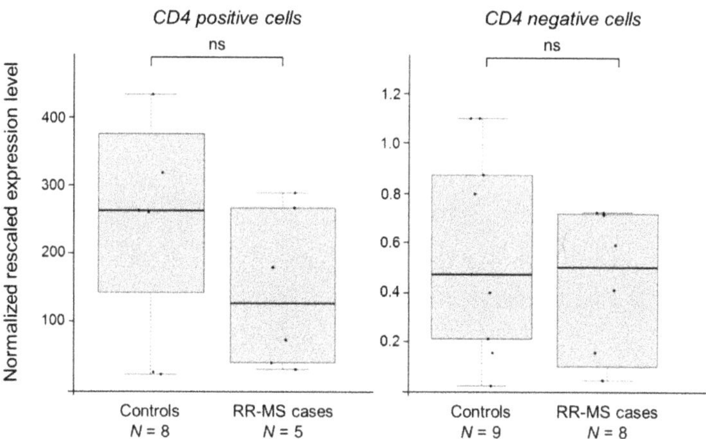

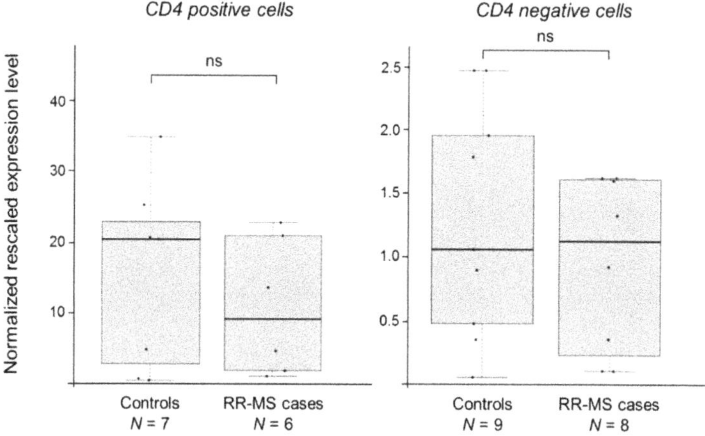

Figure 1. *NCF1* and *NCF2* do not show any significant difference between MS cases and controls. Boxplots show the expression levels of the *NCF1* and *NCF2* genes measured by semi-quantitative real-time RT-PCR in CD4$^+$ and CD4$^-$ cells (prepared from peripheral blood mononuclear cells, PBMCs). MS cases and controls belong to five multiplex Finnish families (comprising both male and female individuals). Boxes define the interquartile range; the thick line refers to the median. Results were normalized to expression levels of the *HMBS* and *ACTB* housekeeping genes and are presented as rescaled values. The number of subjects belonging to each group is indicated (*N*). The significance level of *t*-tests was in all cases not significant (ns).

Concerning *NCF4*, *CYBA*, and *CYBB*, probes were correctly mapping on the corresponding transcripts and gave appreciable signals. In Figure 2a, differential expression analysis for MS cases and controls is shown for both CD4$^-$ and CD4$^+$ cells, again indicating no differences between the two groups. However, considering that the *CYBB* gene is located on chromosome X, we stratified patients according to gender. Interestingly, this analysis allowed us to highlight an opposite molecular signature not only between males and females, but also between CD4$^-$ and CD4$^+$ cells (Figure 2b). In particular, we found a 1.76-fold significant up-regulation ($p = 0.021$) of *CYBB* in RR-MS male patients in CD4$^-$ cells (with females showing an opposite, though not significant, trend; 0.80-fold decrease). Conversely, in CD4$^+$ cells, we noticed the opposite situation, with a 1.75-fold significant *CYBB* increased expression in RR-MS females patients ($p = 0.014$) and a 0.74-fold decrease (not significant) in MS male cases compared to healthy controls.

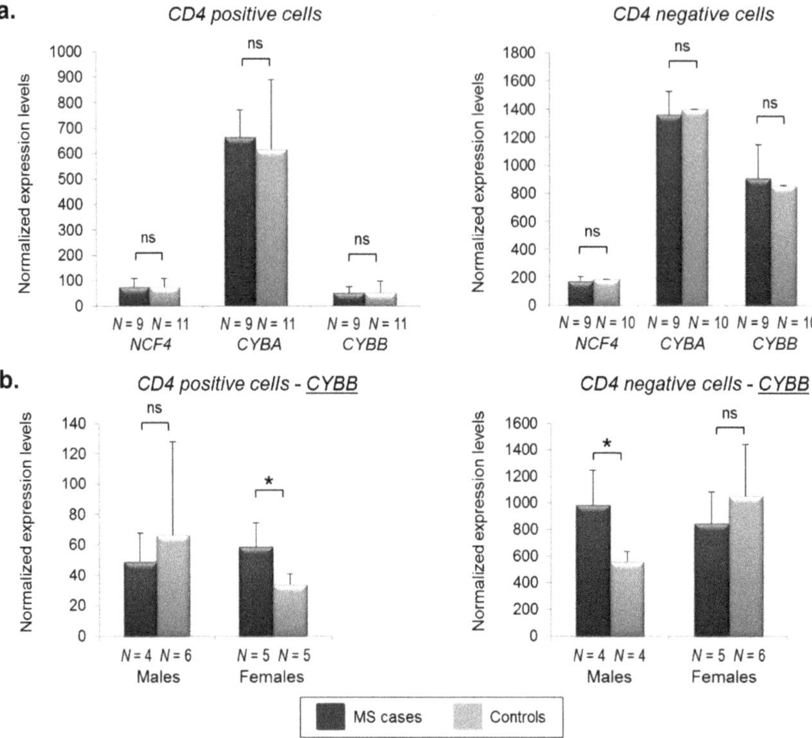

Figure 2. *CYBB* shows sex-related and cell-specific differential expression in MS cases and controls. *NCF4*, *CYBA*, and *CYBB* expression levels (shown by histograms) were measured by means of microarray-based experiments (see the "Materials and Methods" section). The number of subjects belonging to each group is indicated (*N*). Error bars represent means + SD (standard deviation). Significance levels of *t*-tests are shown. *: $p < 0.05$.

To validate the most interesting result obtained from the microarray profiling, expression of *CYBB* was quantitated by real-time RT-PCR assays, performed on RNA extracted from PBMCs of an independent cohort of 21 RR-MS Italian cases and an equal number of age-matched controls. Only females were included in this analysis. We found a 1.43-fold significant up-regulation ($p = 0.032$) of *CYBB* in RR-MS patients (Figure 3), which is consistent with the high abundance of CD4$^+$ cells in the heterogeneous pool of PBMCs (25–60% of PBMC is composed of CD4$^+$ cells) [32].

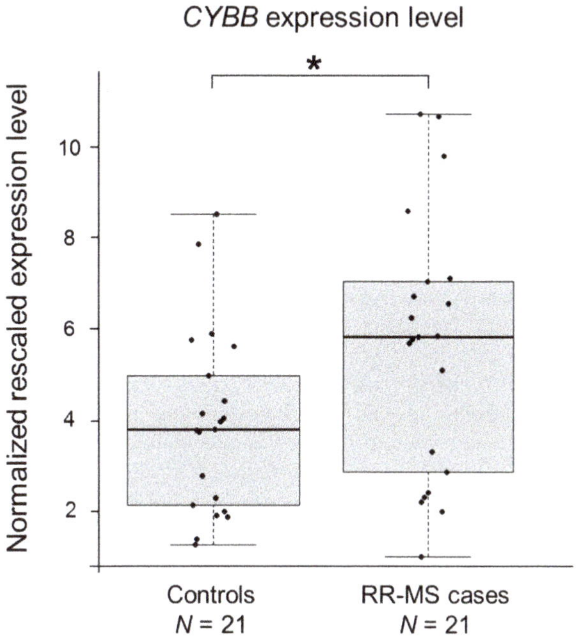

Figure 3. *CYBB* is upregulated in MS patients. Boxplots show the expression levels of the *CYBB* gene measured by semi-quantitative real-time RT-PCR in PBMCs of an Italian case-control cohort (only female individuals). Boxes define the interquartile range; the thick line refers to the median. Results were normalized to expression levels of the *HMBS* and *ACTB* housekeeping genes and are presented as rescaled values. The number of subjects belonging to each group is indicated (*N*). Significance levels of *t*-tests are shown. * $p < 0.05$.

3. Discussion

Apart from the well-known implication of mutations affecting the NOX2 complex in the pathogenesis of chronic granulomatous disease (CGD) [33], some information is currently available in the literature on the possible predisposing role of polymorphisms in *NCF1*, *NCF2*, *NCF4*, *CYBA*, and *CYBB* genes in other immune disorders. Among others, missense variants in the *NCF1* gene have been associated with systemic lupus erythematosus (SLE), Sjögren's syndrome, and rheumatoid arthritis (RA) [34]; two missense polymorphisms in *NCF2* were described as predisposing to SLE [35]; and common polymorphisms in *NCF4* were associated both with RA and Crohn's disease [36,37]. In our exploratory study, we aimed at investigating the possible genetic association between MS and all of the five genes coding for the NADPH oxidase complex. We found suggestive association signals for the *NCF1* and *CYBB* genes (lowest $p = 0.038$ and $p = 0.013$, respectively), which were paralleled, in the case of *CYBB*, by a gender-specific differential gene expression between MS cases and controls.

However, we acknowledge the limited size of our study material, and a lack of a replication step confirming the association of *CYBB* with MS. No significant association between the *CYBB* locus and MS was reported in the previous GWAS analyses, which, however, excluded the X chromosome harboring the *CYBB* gene from the genome-wide analysis. The role of the X chromosome in MS—a pathology characterized by higher susceptibility in females than males—remains still largely unknown. For instance, in the largest MS-related meta-analysis so far published, genome-wide, a total of 233 loci were found to be significantly associated with the disease, and only one maps to chromosome X [10]. The case-control analysis did not take gender into account, while the study presented here was utilizing family-based transmission analysis. Overall, the lack of association signals on chromosome X is indeed a common feature of complex traits: the X chromosome accounts for 5% of the nuclear genome and underlies almost 10% of Mendelian disorders [38]. Nonetheless, only 114 associations (0.8%) at $p \leq 5 \times 10^{-8}$ have been reported on the X chromosome, on a total of more than 14,700 signals identified by GWAS for ~300 traits [39]. These data could potentially be explained by the fact that the vast majority of GWAS have not included chromosome X in their analyses and have not considered gender. There is also a lack of specific bioinformatics pipelines to adopt in the analytic steps [40].

To overcome the limitation of the lack of a replication cohort in the association study, we focused on the investigation of an "intermediate phenotype", i.e., the gene expression profile of NOX2 components in CD4$^+$ and CD4$^-$ cells. We used a two-tiered approach, based on both microarray and real-time RT-PCR experiments. The most striking result was the differential gene expression for the *CYBB* gene in MS cases, with opposite molecular signatures not only between males and females, but also between CD4$^-$ and CD4$^+$ cells. Indeed, sex-differential expression has recently emerged as a common feature of many genes. For instance, by comprehensively analyzing the Genotype-Tissue Expression (GTEx) data across 53 tissues (publicly available at https://www.gtexportal.org/home/), Gershoni and Pietrokovski were able to demonstrate that more than 6500 protein-coding genes showed significant sex-differential expression in one or more tissues [41]. In most of the cases, these genes are differentially expressed according to gender in just one or a few tissues. The *CYBB* gene seems to conform to this rule, showing a certain degree of sex-differential expression in kidney cortex, bladder, and thyroid (see Figure S1 in the Supplementary Materials); similar observations can be made for *NCF1*, *NCF2*, *NCF4*, and *CYBA*. Of note, data relative to blood cell sub-populations are missing in the GTEx portal.

The differential gene expression evidenced by stratifying patients and controls on the basis of the gender and, above all, according to the cell type, could contribute to explaining—if confirmed in other immune disorders—some of the puzzling observations that have accumulated over the years on CGD, SLE, or RA. For instance, RA patients show in blood a marked increase in ROS formation, protein oxidation, as well as lipid peroxidation [42]. In addition, they also present a synovial tissue that is invaded by inflammatory cells, a large proportion of which are activated CD4$^+$ T cells [43]. Both these phenomena can collectively account for tissue damage and for the chronicity of the disease. However, the development of RA has been associated with a lower copy number of the *NCF1* gene [44], and this association was supported by *ncf1* mutant rodents [45,46]. In this regard, it could be speculated that lower expression levels of the NOX2 complex could be protective against the chronic inflammation in RA relevant tissues; on the other hand, a lower oxidative burst response in antigen-presenting cells, especially in the thymus during priming, could change the antigen-presentation capacity of the cells, thus inducing autoimmunity [46]. Besides RA and SLE, previously shown examples of immune pathology characterized by inappropriate over-activation or down-regulation of ROS also include psoriasis, Hashimoto thyroiditis, vitiligo, and inflammatory bowel disease [47,48].

Concerning specifically MS, our results well fit with the observations of Fischer and colleagues [16], who described a global NOX2 over-expression in microglia and infiltrating macrophages of MS patients' autopsy brain tissues. These data also suggest that an inflammation-associated oxidative burst could play a fundamental role in the demyelination process typical of MS.

In conclusion, our work adds another piece of information on the possible involvement of NOX2 in the pathogenesis of MS, suggesting that this particular topic deserves to be further investigated, especially in the light of potential therapies based on decreasing/enhancing the oxidative burst.

4. Materials and Methods

4.1. Materials

All oligonucleotides for SNP genotyping and quantitative real-time RT-PCRs were purchased from Proligo (Paris, France). Primer couples for microsatellite analysis were from Applied Biosystems (Foster City, CA, USA). All sequences can be provided on request. The AmpliTaq Gold, DynaZyme, and HotStar Taq DNA polymerases were from Applied Biosystems, Finnzymes (Espoo, Finland), and Qiagen (Hilden, Germany), respectively.

4.2. MS Pedigrees

The study was approved by the ethical committee of the Helsinki and Uusimaa hospital district (Decision 46/2002, #192/E9/02), and all individuals included in the study gave their informed consent. The study material consisted of a total of 63 families: 22 of them were multiplex MS families, having two to six affected cases per pedigree, whereas the remaining 41 families were composed of MS patients with their parents and unaffected siblings. These families were previously described [49] and they all originate from the high-risk region for MS in Southern Ostrobothnia, Finland. In total, the cohort consisted of 547 individuals, 116 being MS cases. Patient selection was hospital-based; only definite cases were included (clinically or laboratory-supported definite). Diagnosis of MS in affected individuals strictly followed Poser's diagnostic criteria [50].

4.3. Genotyping

Genomic DNA was extracted from peripheral blood cells following standard procedures.

Two non-chimeric microsatellite markers (D7S1870 and D7S2518) were selected from databases for the association analysis of the *NCF1* gene, avoiding the highly duplicated regions characterizing this chromosomal locus (7q11.23). Microsatellite markers were PCR amplified in two-plex format in 10-µL reaction mixtures under standard conditions, using VIC (D7S1870) or PET (D7S2518) labeled primers, the AmpliTaq Gold DNA polymerase, a MJ Tetrad thermal cycler (MJ Research INC, Waltham, MA, USA), and a touch-down thermal profile. PCR products were run on an ABI-3730 Genetic Analyzer (Applied Biosystems) and analyzed using the Genotyper software (Applied Biosystems).

For the association analysis of the other genes, we selected 21 SNPs, having heterozygosity >10%. Primers flanking the putative SNPs were designed for multiplex PCR amplification using the web-based program MPprimer (https://omictools.com/mpprimer-tool?t=tab-tool-variant-0). SNPs were first tested for polymorphic content by direct sequencing the relevant PCR-amplified fragment in 32 healthy Finnish individuals. Nine SNPs were monomorphic in the Finnish population, whereas one was tri-allelic; those ten SNPs were not further investigated. The remaining 11 SNPs were typed in MS samples using an in-house developed microarray, based on allele-specific primer extension [51]. In particular, two allele-specific detection oligonucleotides were designed for each SNP: these primers were characterized by the presence of a 5′ aminolinker and a stretch of 9T (poly-T), followed by the SNP-specific sequence. The 5′ aminolinker and the poly-T served to spot and anchor detection oligonucleotides onto silane/isothiocyanate-coated chrome mirror microscope slides (Evaporated Coatings, Willow Grove, PA, USA). Spotting was performed in duplicate using an OmniGrid 100 arrayer (Discovery Scientific, Vancouver, BC, Canada). Regions containing the SNPs were PCR amplified with a touch-down protocol from genomic DNA in two multiplex reactions, using SNP-specific primers with a T3 (forward) or a T7 (reverse) tail. Multiplex reactions were in-vitro transcribed using the AmpliScribe T7 or T3 High Yield Transcription Kit (Epicentre Technologies, Madison, WI, USA). The DNAseI-treated T3 or T7 RNA pools were hybridized to the arrays in a hybridization buffer (1.67 M NaCl) at 42 °C for 20 min. Arrays were washed twice in a washing buffer (0.3 M NaCl, 0.5× TE, 0.1% TritonX-100) and subsequently rinsed in ice-cold water. The allele-specific extension was performed using the MMLV Reverse Transcriptase (Epicentre Technologies) in a 20-µL reaction containing 50 mM Tris-HCl (pH 8.3), 10 mM $MgCl_2$, 75 mM KCl, 10 mM DTT, 0.5 µM dATP, 0.5 µM dGTP, 0.5 µM ddATP, 0.5 µM ddGTP, 1 µM Cy5-labeled dCTP, 1 µM Cy5-labeled dUTP (Cy5-labeled nucleotides were from Amersham Pharmacia Biotech, Uppsala, Sweden), 15% glycerol, and 0.24 M trehalose. Reverse transcription was carried out at 52 °C for 20 min. Finally, arrays were put in washing buffer under mild agitation for 15 min, dipped quickly in 50 mM NaOH, washed again in washing buffer, rinsed in ice-cold water, air dried, and scanned using a ScanArray 4000 instrument (Packard Biochip Technologies, Perkin Elmer Life Sciences, Boston, MA, USA). The image was analyzed using the ScanArray software (Packard Biochip Technologies, Perkin Elmer Life Sciences). Genotypes were called using an in-house developed software (W. Wong and C. Li, unpublished data).

The list of selected polymorphisms is presented in the Supplementary Materials (Table S1).

Important note: the entire analysis was performed a while ago, i.e., before the genomic databases became available with all the associated information on allele frequencies in different ethnicities.

4.4. Statistical Analyses

All genotypes were checked for Mendelian errors using PedCheck [52]. The check for the HWE was performed using the Genepop program (option 1), which also admits multiallelic markers [53]; only genotypes of women were considered for X-linked SNPs.

TDT [54] and HRR (a modified TDT test that uses siblings as "pseudo-controls") [55] analyses, both implemented in the ANALYZE package [55], were used in the association study. Since the inheritance pattern of MS is unknown, analyses were performed using two different modes of inheritance, i.e., dominant with reduced penetrance of $f = 0.05$ (with disease allele-frequency estimate of 0.01) or $f = 0.76$ (with disease allele-frequency estimate of 0.0006) [56].

Analyses were repeated using the PLINK software v.1.07 [57] by applying a more powerful method based on the TDT statistic implemented with the parental discordance test. This test is based on counting the number of alleles in affected versus unaffected parents (using each nuclear-family parental pair as a matched pair). These counts are then combined with the transmitted and untransmitted counts of the basic TDT to give a combined test statistic [58]. In this analysis, multiallelic markers were analyzed as biallelic, considering from one hand the most common allele, and from the other all the remaining ones clumped together as they were a unique alternative allele. In the text, p values, ORs, and 95% CIs always referred to the minor allele.

Considering the exploratory hypothesis-generating nature of the present study and the limited sample size as compared to the number of investigated genetic variants, we did not adjust for multiple testing, and p values < 0.05 were considered to be statistically significant. However, the total number of performed tests as well as the threshold of significance based on the over-conservative Bonferroni correction has been indicated in the footnote of the relevant table.

4.5. RNA Samples

Fresh blood samples from 25 members (both male and female subjects) belonging to five of the above-mentioned multiplex MS families were collected. PBMCs were separated using a Ficoll-Paque (Amersham Pharmacia Biotech) density gradient centrifugation, and hence stratified to CD4$^+$ and CD4$^-$ cell populations by negative selection using the CD4$^+$ T-cell isolation kit (Miltenyi Biotec, Auburn, CA, USA) and an autoMACS instrument (Miltenyi Biotec). Total RNA was extracted from CD4$^+$ and CD4$^-$ samples using the Trizol reagent (Ambion, Austin, TX, USA), treated with DNAse-I, and further purified with RNeasy Mini Kit columns (Qiagen, Valencia, CA, USA) according to the manufacturers' instruction. RNA quality was assessed using the RNA 6000 Nano assay in a Bioanalyzer (Agilent Technologies, Foster City, CA, USA).

As for the replication cohort, we collected PBMCs from 21 unrelated RR-MS patients and 21 healthy subjects, all females and Caucasians (coming from Northern Italy). Controls were age-matched with cases. To avoid possible confounding effects, we focused only on RR-MS cases in remitting phase, who had not received any immune-modulatory therapy within the month prior to blood withdrawal. PBMCs were isolated from heparinized blood immediately after phlebotomy by centrifugation on a Lympholyte Cell separation media (Cederlane Laboratories Limited, Hornby, ON, Canada) gradient. Total RNA was isolated using the Eurozol kit (Euroclone, Wetherby, UK).

4.6. Sample Preparation, Microarray Processing, and Data Analysis

RNA samples were prepared for hybridization on the Affymetrix GeneChip Human Genome U133 Plus 2.0 Array (Affymetrix, Santa Clara, CA, USA) according to the manufacturer's recommendations.

In brief, 1 µg of total RNA was converted to biotin-labelled cRNA using the Affymetrix HT One-Cycle cDNA Synthesis Kit and the HT IVT Labelling Kit. Fifteen µg of cRNA were then fragmented and hybridized for 16 hours at 45 °C, washed in Affymetrix Fluidics Station 450, and then scanned with Affymetrix GeneChip Scanner 3000. Hybridization, washing, staining, and scanning were conducted using the same instruments for all samples.

Raw intensity data files were imported to GeneSpring 7.3 (Agilent Technologies) and GC Robust Multi-array Average (GC-RMA) normalized. We then excluded probe sets with low signal intensity (GC-RMA normalized signal < 50). Probe sets with a $p \leq 0.05$ were considered to be differentially expressed.

4.7. Semi-Quantitative Real-Time RT-PCRs

Random hexamers and the TaqMan Gold RT-PCR kit (Applied Biosystems) were used to perform first-strand cDNA synthesis starting from 1 µg of total RNA from $CD4^{+/-}$ cells, according to the manufacturer's instructions. From a total of 20 µL of the RT reaction, 4 µL were used as template for semi-quantitative real-time RT-PCRs for the quantitation of the *NCF1* and *NCF2* mRNAs. Assays were carried out using the SYBR-Green Kit (Applied Biosystems) and a standard PCR thermal protocol on the ABI Prism 7900 HT Sequence Detection System. Data were analyzed with the Sequence Detector version 2.0 software (Applied Biosystems).

As for *CYBB* evaluation, random hexamers and the Superscript-III Reverse Transcriptase (Invitrogen, Carlsbad, CA, USA) were used in the RT step starting from 1 µg of RNA extracted from PBMCs of MS patients and controls. From a total of 20 µL of the RT reaction, 1 µL was used as a template for amplifications, using the FastStart SYBR Green Master Mix (Roche, Basel, Switzerland) on a LightCycler 480 (Roche), following a touch-down thermal protocol. Data were analyzed by the GeNorm software [59].

In all cases, RT-PCRs were performed at least in triplicate. Expression levels were normalized using *HMBS* (hydroxymethylbilane synthase gene) and *ACTB* (β-actin) as housekeeping genes. Primer sequences can be provided on request.

Supplementary Materials: Supplementary materials can be found at http://www.mdpi.com/2227-9059/6/4/117/s1.

Author Contributions: R.A. and J.S. conceived and designed the experiments; R.A., G.C., and E.M.P. performed the experiments; R.A., G.S., S.D., and J.S. analyzed the data; R.A. wrote the paper; J.S. and R.A. supervised the entire study.

Funding: This research received no external funding.

Acknowledgments: The European Science foundation is acknowledged for the support to R.A. (Grant program GENOMICS/2003/19).

Conflicts of Interest: The authors declare no conflict of interest.

Abbreviations

ACTB	β-actin
$CD4^+$	Cluster of differentiation 4 positive
$CD4^-$	Cluster of differentiation 4 negative
CGD	Chronic granulomatous disease
CI	Confidence interval
CNS	Central nervous system
CYBA	Cytochrome B-245 alpha chain, coding for the p22phox subunit of the NOX2 system
CYBB	Cytochrome B-245 beta chain, coding for the gp91phox subunit of the NOX2 system
GC-RMA	GC Robust Multi-array Average
GWAS	Genome-wide association study
HLA	Human leukocyte antigen
HMBS	Hydroxymethylbilane synthase gene

HRR	Haplotype relative risk
HWE	Hardy-Weinberg equilibrium
MMLV	Moloney Murine Leukemia Virus
MS	Multiple sclerosis
NADPH	nicotinamide adenine dinucleotide phosphate
NCF1	Neutrophil cytosolic factor 1, coding for the p47phox subunit of the NOX2 system
NCF2	Neutrophil cytosolic factor 2, coding for the p67phox subunit of the NOX2 system
NCF4	Neutrophil cytosolic factor 4, coding for the p40phox subunit of the NOX2 system
NOX	NADPH oxidase system
NOX2	NADPH oxidase system 2 (isoform 2 of the complex)
OMIM	Online Mendelian Inheritance in Men
OR	Odds ratio
OS	Oxidative stress
PBMCs	Peripheral blood mononuclear cells
RA	Rheumatoid arthritis
ROS	Reactive oxygen species
RR	Relapsing-remitting
RT-PCR	Reverse-transcription polymerase chain reactions
SD	Standard deviation
SLE	Systemic lupus erythematosus
SNP	Single nucleotide polymorphism
TDT	Transmission/disequilibrium test

References

1. Trapp, B.D.; Peterson, J.; Ransohoff, R.M.; Rudick, R.; Mörk, S.; Bö, L. Axonal transection in the lesions of multiple sclerosis. *N. Engl. J. Med.* **1998**, *338*, 278–285. [CrossRef] [PubMed]
2. Hauser, S.L.; Oksenberg, J.R. The neurobiology of multiple sclerosis: Genes, inflammation, and neurodegeneration. *Neuron* **2006**, *52*, 61–76. [CrossRef] [PubMed]
3. Thompson, A.J. Multiple sclerosis—A global disorder and still poorly managed. *Lancet Neurol.* **2008**, *7*, 1078–1079. [CrossRef]
4. Kingwell, E.; Marriott, J.J.; Jetté, N.; Pringsheim, T.; Makhani, N.; Morrow, S.A.; Fisk, J.D.; Evans, C.; Béland, S.G.; Kulaga, S.; et al. Incidence and prevalence of multiple sclerosis in Europe: A systematic review. *BMC Neurol.* **2013**, *13*, 128. [CrossRef] [PubMed]
5. Sumelahti, M.L.; Tienari, P.J.; Wikström, J.; Palo, J.; Hakama, M. Regional and temporal variation in the incidence of multiple sclerosis in Finland 1979–1993. *Neuroepidemiology* **2000**, *19*, 67–75. [CrossRef] [PubMed]
6. International Multiple Sclerosis Genetics Consortium; Hafler, D.A.; Compston, A.; Sawcer, S.; Lander, E.S.; Daly, M.J.; De Jager, P.L.; de Bakker, P.I.; Gabriel, S.B.; Mirel, D.B.; et al. Risk alleles for multiple sclerosis identified by a genomewide study. *N. Engl. J. Med.* **2007**, *357*, 851–862. [CrossRef] [PubMed]
7. Sawcer, S.; Hellenthal, G.; Pirinen, M.; Spencer, C.C.; Patsopoulos, N.A.; Moutsianas, L.; Dilthey, A.; Su, Z.; Freeman, C.; Hunt, S.E.; et al. Genetic risk and a primary role for cell-mediated immune mechanisms in multiple sclerosis. *Nature* **2011**, *476*, 214–219. [CrossRef] [PubMed]
8. International Multiple Sclerosis Genetics Consortium (IMSGC); Beecham, A.H.; Patsopoulos, N.A.; Xifara, D.K.; Davis, M.F.; Kemppinen, A.; Cotsapas, C.; Shah, T.S.; Spencer, C.; Booth, D.; et al. Analysis of immune-related loci identifies 48 new susceptibility variants for multiple sclerosis. *Nat. Genet.* **2013**, *45*, 1353–1360. [CrossRef] [PubMed]
9. Bos, S.D.; Berge, T.; Celius, E.G.; Harbo, H.F. From genetic associations to functional studies in multiple sclerosis. *Eur. J. Neurol.* **2016**, *23*, 847–853. [CrossRef] [PubMed]
10. Patsopoulos, N.; Baranzini, S.E.; Santaniello, A.; Shoostari, P.; Cotsapas, C.; Wong, G.; Beecham, A.H.; James, T.; Replogle, J.; Vlachos, I.; et al. The Multiple Sclerosis Genomic Map: Role of peripheral immune cells and resident microglia in susceptibility. *bioRxiv* **2017**. [CrossRef]
11. Linker, R.A.; Kieseier, B.C.; Gold, R. Identification and development of new therapeutics for multiple sclerosis. *Trends Pharm. Sci.* **2008**, *29*, 558–565. [CrossRef] [PubMed]

12. Broux, B.; Stinissen, P.; Hellings, N. Which immune cells matter? The immunopathogenesis of multiple sclerosis. *Crit. Rev. Immunol.* **2013**, *33*, 283–306. [CrossRef] [PubMed]
13. Salou, M.; Nicol, B.; Garcia, A.; Laplaud, D.A. Involvement of CD8(+) T Cells in Multiple Sclerosis. *Front. Immunol.* **2015**, *6*, 604. [CrossRef] [PubMed]
14. Jones, A.P.; Kermode, A.G.; Lucas, R.M.; Carroll, W.M.; Nolan, D.; Hart, P.H. Circulating immune cells in multiple sclerosis. *Clin. Exp. Immunol.* **2017**, *187*, 193–203. [CrossRef] [PubMed]
15. Gilgun-Sherki, Y.; Melamed, E.; Offen, D. The role of oxidative stress in the pathogenesis of multiple sclerosis: The need for effective antioxidant therapy. *J. Neurol.* **2004**, *251*, 261–268. [CrossRef] [PubMed]
16. Fischer, M.T.; Sharma, R.; Lim, J.L.; Haider, L.; Frischer, J.M.; Drexhage, J.; Mahad, D.; Bradl, M.; van Horssen, J.; Lassmann, H. NADPH oxidase expression in active multiple sclerosis lesions in relation to oxidative tissue damage and mitochondrial injury. *Brain* **2012**, *135*, 886–899. [CrossRef] [PubMed]
17. Adamczyk, B.; Adamczyk-Sowa, M. New Insights into the Role of Oxidative Stress Mechanisms in the Pathophysiology and Treatment of Multiple Sclerosis. *Oxidative Med. Cell. Longev.* **2016**, *2016*, 1973834. [CrossRef] [PubMed]
18. Van der Goes, A.; Brouwer, J.; Hoekstra, K.; Roos, D.; van den Berg, T.K.; Dijkstra, C.D. Reactive oxygen species are required for the phagocytosis of myelin by macrophages. *J. Neuroimmunol.* **1998**, *92*, 67–75. [CrossRef]
19. Nikić, I.; Merkler, D.; Sorbara, C.; Brinkoetter, M.; Kreutzfeldt, M.; Bareyre, F.M.; Brück, W.; Bishop, D.; Misgeld, T.; Kerschensteiner, M. A reversible form of axon damage in experimental autoimmune encephalomyelitis and multiple sclerosis. *Nat. Med.* **2011**, *17*, 495–499. [CrossRef] [PubMed]
20. Friese, M.A.; Schattling, B.; Fugger, L. Mechanisms of neurodegeneration and axonal dysfunction in multiple sclerosis. *Nat. Rev. Neurol.* **2014**, *10*, 225–238. [CrossRef] [PubMed]
21. Barnes, P.J.; Karin, M. Nuclear factor-kappaB: A pivotal transcription factor in chronic inflammatory diseases. *N. Engl. J. Med.* **1997**, *336*, 1066–1071. [CrossRef] [PubMed]
22. Srinivasan, M.; Lahiri, D.K. Significance of NF-κB as a pivotal therapeutic target in the neurodegenerative pathologies of Alzheimer's disease and multiple sclerosis. *Expert Opin. Ther. Targets* **2015**, *19*, 471–487. [CrossRef] [PubMed]
23. Romanic, A.M.; Madri, J.A. Extracellular matrix-degrading proteinases in the nervous system. *Brain Pathol.* **1994**, *4*, 145–156. [CrossRef] [PubMed]
24. Merrill, J.E.; Murphy, S.P. Inflammatory events at the blood brain barrier: Regulation of adhesion molecules, cytokines, and chemokines by reactive nitrogen and oxygen species. *Brain Behav. Immun.* **1997**, *11*, 245–263. [CrossRef] [PubMed]
25. Chiurchiù, V.; Orlacchio, A.; Maccarrone, M. Is Modulation of Oxidative Stress an Answer? The State of the Art of Redox Therapeutic Actions in Neurodegenerative Diseases. *Oxidative Med. Cell. Longev.* **2016**, *2016*, 7909380. [CrossRef] [PubMed]
26. Vladimirova, O.; Lu, F.M.; Shawver, L.; Kalman, B. The activation of protein kinase C induces higher production of reactive oxygen species by mononuclear cells in patients with multiple sclerosis than in controls. *Inflamm. Res.* **1999**, *48*, 412–416. [CrossRef] [PubMed]
27. Lu, F.; Selak, M.; O'Connor, J.; Croul, S.; Lorenzana, C.; Butunoi, C.; Kalman, B. Oxidative damage to mitochondrial DNA and activity of mitochondrial enzymes in chronic active lesions of multiple sclerosis. *J. Neurol. Sci.* **2000**, *177*, 95–103. [CrossRef]
28. Van Horssen, J.; Witte, M.E.; Schreibelt, G.; de Vries, H.E. Radical changes in multiple sclerosis pathogenesis. *Biochim. Biophys. Acta* **2011**, *1812*, 141–150. [CrossRef] [PubMed]
29. Babior, B.M. NADPH Oxidase: An update. *Blood* **1999**, *93*, 1464–1476. [PubMed]
30. Vignais, P.V. The superoxide-generating NADPH oxidase: Structural aspects and activation mechanism. *Cell. Mol. Life Sci.* **2002**, *59*, 1428–1459. [CrossRef] [PubMed]
31. Trapp, B.D.; Nave, K.A. Multiple sclerosis: An immune or neurodegenerative disorder? *Annu. Rev. Neurosci.* **2008**, *31*, 247–269. [CrossRef] [PubMed]
32. Kleiveland, C.R. Peripheral Blood Mononuclear Cells. In *The Impact of Food Bioactives on Health*; Verhoeckx, K., Cotter, P., López-Expósito, I., Kleiveland, C., Lea, T., Mackie, A., Requena, T., Swiateck, D., Wicher, H., Eds.; Springer: Cham, Switzerland, 2015. [CrossRef]

33. Wu, J.; Wang, W.F.; Zhang, Y.D.; Chen, T.X. Clinical Features and Genetic Analysis of 48 Patients with Chronic Granulomatous Disease in a Single Center Study from Shanghai, China (2005–2015): New Studies and a Literature Review. *J. Immunol. Res.* **2017**, *2017*, 8745254. [CrossRef] [PubMed]

34. Zhao, J.; Ma, J.; Deng, Y.; Kelly, J.A.; Kim, K.; Bang, S.Y.; Lee, H.S.; Li, Q.Z.; Wakeland, E.K.; Qiu, R.; et al. A missense variant in NCF1 is associated with susceptibility to multiple autoimmune diseases. *Nat. Genet.* **2017**, *49*, 433–437. [CrossRef] [PubMed]

35. Armstrong, D.L.; Eisenstein, M.; Zidovetzki, R.; Jacob, C.O. Systemic lupus erythematosus-associated neutrophil cytosolic factor 2 mutation affects the structure of NADPH oxidase complex. *J. Biol. Chem.* **2015**, *290*, 12595–12602. [CrossRef] [PubMed]

36. Olsson, L.M.; Lindqvist, A.K.; Källberg, H.; Padyukov, L.; Burkhardt, H.; Alfredsson, L.; Klareskog, L.; Holmdahl, R. A case-control study of rheumatoid arthritis identifies an associated single nucleotide polymorphism in the NCF4 gene, supporting a role for the NADPH-oxidase complex in autoimmunity. *Arthritis Res. Ther.* **2007**, *9*, R98. [CrossRef] [PubMed]

37. Rioux, J.D.; Xavier, R.J.; Taylor, K.D.; Silverberg, M.S.; Goyette, P.; Huett, A.; Green, T.; Kuballa, P.; Barmada, M.M.; Datta, L.W.; et al. Genome-wide association study identifies new susceptibility loci for Crohn disease and implicates autophagy in disease pathogenesis. *Nat. Genet.* **2007**, *39*, 596–604. [CrossRef] [PubMed]

38. Amberger, J.; Bocchini, C.A.; Scott, A.F.; Hamosh, A. McKusick's Online Mendelian Inheritance in Man (OMIM). *Nucleic Acids Res.* **2009**, *37*, D793–D796. [CrossRef] [PubMed]

39. MacArthur, J.; Bowler, E.; Cerezo, M.; Gil, L.; Hall, P.; Hastings, E.; Junkins, H.; McMahon, A.; Milano, A.; Morales, J.; et al. The new NHGRI-EBI Catalog of published genome-wide association studies (GWAS Catalog). *Nucleic Acids Res.* **2017**, *45*, D896–D901. [CrossRef] [PubMed]

40. Wise, A.L.; Gyi, L.; Manolio, T.A. eXclusion: Toward integrating the X chromosome in genome-wide association analyses. *Am. J. Hum. Genet.* **2013**, *92*, 643–647. [CrossRef] [PubMed]

41. Gershoni, M.; Pietrokovski, S. The landscape of sex-differential transcriptome and its consequent selection in human adults. *BMC Biol.* **2017**, *15*, 7. [CrossRef] [PubMed]

42. Mateen, S.; Moin, S.; Khan, A.Q.; Zafar, A.; Fatima, N. Increased Reactive Oxygen Species Formation and Oxidative Stress in Rheumatoid Arthritis. *PLoS ONE* **2016**, *11*, e0152925. [CrossRef] [PubMed]

43. Kondo, Y.; Yokosawa, M.; Kaneko, S.; Furuyama, K.; Segawa, S.; Tsuboi, H.; Matsumoto, I.; Sumida, T. Review: Transcriptional Regulation of CD4+ T Cell Differentiation in Experimentally Induced Arthritis and Rheumatoid Arthritis. *Arthritis Rheumatol.* **2018**, *70*, 653–661. [CrossRef] [PubMed]

44. Olsson, L.M.; Nerstedt, A.; Lindqvist, A.K.; Johansson, S.C.; Medstrand, P.; Olofsson, P.; Holmdahl, R. Copy number variation of the gene NCF1 is associated with rheumatoid arthritis. *Antioxid Redox Signal* **2012**, *16*, 71–78. [CrossRef] [PubMed]

45. Olofsson, P.; Holmberg, J.; Tordsson, J.; Lu, S.; Akerström, B.; Holmdahl, R. Positional identification of Ncf1 as a gene that regulates arthritis severity in rats. *Nat. Genet.* **2003**, *33*, 25–32. [CrossRef] [PubMed]

46. Hultqvist, M.; Olofsson, P.; Holmberg, J.; Bäckström, B.T.; Tordsson, J.; Holmdahl, R. Enhanced autoimmunity, arthritis, and encephalomyelitis in mice with a reduced oxidative burst due to a mutation in the Ncf1 gene. *Proc. Natl. Acad. Sci. USA* **2004**, *101*, 12646–12651. [CrossRef] [PubMed]

47. Kienhöfer, D.; Boeltz, S.; Hoffmann, M.H. Reactive oxygen homeostasis—The balance for preventing autoimmunity. *Lupus* **2016**, *25*, 943–954. [CrossRef] [PubMed]

48. Di Dalmazi, G.; Hirshberg, J.; Lyle, D.; Freij, J.B.; Caturegli, P. Reactive oxygen species in organ-specific autoimmunity. *Autoimmun. Highlights* **2016**, *7*, 11. [CrossRef] [PubMed]

49. Saarela, J.; Kallio, S.P.; Chen, D.; Montpetit, A.; Jokiaho, A.; Choi, E.; Asselta, R.; Bronnikov, D.; Lincoln, M.R.; Sadovnick, A.D.; et al. PRKCA and multiple sclerosis: Association in two independent populations. *PLoS Genet.* **2006**, *2*, e42. [CrossRef] [PubMed]

50. Poser, C.M.; Paty, D.W.; Scheinberg, L.; McDonald, W.I.; Davis, F.A.; Ebers, G.C.; Johnson, K.P.; Sibley, W.A.; Silberberg, D.H.; Tourtellotte, W.W. New diagnostic criteria for multiple sclerosis: Guidelines for research protocols. *Ann. Neurol.* **1983**, *13*, 227–231. [CrossRef] [PubMed]

51. Pastinen, T.; Raitio, M.; Lindroos, K.; Tainola, P.; Peltonen, L.; Syvänen, A.C. A system for specific, high-throughput genotyping by allele-specific primer extension on microarrays. *Genome Res.* **2000**, *10*, 1031–1042. [CrossRef] [PubMed]

52. O'Connell, J.R.; Weeks, D.E. PedCheck: A program for identification of genotype incompatibilities in linkage analysis. *Am. J. Hum. Genet.* **1998**, *63*, 259–266. [CrossRef] [PubMed]

53. Raymond, M.; Rousset, F. GENEPOP (version 1.2): Population genetics software for exact tests and ecumenicism. *J. Hered.* **1995**, *86*, 248–249. [CrossRef]

54. Spielman, R.S.; McGinnis, R.E.; Ewens, W.J. Transmission test for linkage disequilibrium: The insulin gene region and insulin-dependent diabetes mellitus (IDDM). *Am. J. Hum. Genet.* **1993**, *52*, 506–516. [PubMed]

55. Terwilliger, J.D.; Ott, J. A haplotype-based 'haplotype relative risk' approach to detecting allelic associations. *Hum. Hered.* **1992**, *42*, 337–346. [CrossRef] [PubMed]

56. Kuokkanen, S.; Sundvall, M.; Terwilliger, J.D.; Tienari, P.J.; Wikström, J.; Holmdahl, R.; Pettersson, U.; Peltonen, L. A putative vulnerability locus to multiple sclerosis maps to 5p14-p12 in a region syntenic to the murine locus Eae2. *Nat. Genet.* **1996**, *13*, 477–480. [CrossRef] [PubMed]

57. Purcell, S.; Neale, B.; Todd-Brown, K.; Thomas, L.; Ferreira, M.A.; Bender, D.; Maller, J.; Sklar, P.; de Bakker, P.I.; Daly, M.J.; et al. PLINK: A tool set for whole-genome association and population-based linkage analyses. *Am. J. Hum. Genet.* **2007**, *8*, 559–575. [CrossRef] [PubMed]

58. Purcell, S.; Sham, P.; Daly, M.J. Parental phenotypes in family-based association analysis. *Am. J. Hum. Genet.* **2005**, *76*, 249–259. [CrossRef] [PubMed]

59. Vandesompele, J.; De Preter, K.; Pattyn, F.; Poppe, B.; Van Roy, N.; De Paepe, A.; Speleman, F. Accurate normalization of real-time quantitative RT-PCR data by geometric averaging of multiple internal control genes. *Genome Biol.* **2002**, *3*, RESEARCH0034. [CrossRef] [PubMed]

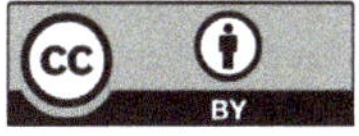

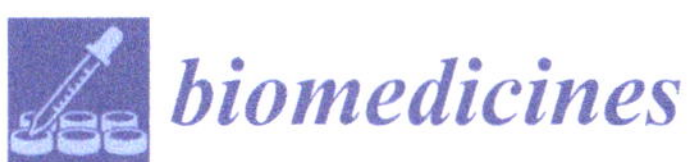 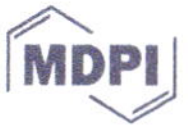

Review

Mechanisms of Neurodegeneration and Axonal Dysfunction in Progressive Multiple Sclerosis

Jorge Correale *, Mariano Marrodan and María Célica Ysrraelit

Department of Neurology, FLENI, Buenos Aires 1428, Argentina; mmarrodan@fleni.org.ar (M.M.); mcysrraelit@fleni.org.ar (M.C.Y.)

* Correspondence: jcorreale@fleni.org.ar or jorge.correale@gmail.com; Tel.: +54-11-5777-3200-2704/2456; Fax: +54-11-5777-3209

Received: 29 January 2019; Accepted: 18 February 2019; Published: 20 February 2019

Abstract: Multiple Sclerosis (MS) is a major cause of neurological disability, which increases predominantly during disease progression as a result of cortical and grey matter structures involvement. The gradual accumulation of disability characteristic of the disease seems to also result from a different set of mechanisms, including in particular immune reactions confined to the Central Nervous System such as: (a) B-cell dysregulation, (b) CD8$^+$ T cells causing demyelination or axonal/neuronal damage, and (c) microglial cell activation associated with neuritic transection found in cortical demyelinating lesions. Other potential drivers of neurodegeneration are generation of oxygen and nitrogen reactive species, and mitochondrial damage, inducing impaired energy production, and intra-axonal accumulation of Ca^{2+}, which in turn activates a variety of catabolic enzymes ultimately leading to progressive proteolytic degradation of cytoskeleton proteins. Loss of axon energy provided by oligodendrocytes determines further axonal degeneration and neuronal loss. Clearly, these different mechanisms are not mutually exclusive and could act in combination. Given the multifactorial pathophysiology of progressive MS, many potential therapeutic targets could be investigated in the future. This remains however, an objective that has yet to be undertaken.

Keywords: autoimmunity; axon; cortex; demyelination; mitochondria; multiple sclerosis; myelin; neurodegeneration; oligodendrocyte; progressive multiple sclerosis

---

1. Introduction

Multiple Sclerosis (MS) is a chronic inflammatory disease of the Central Nervous System (CNS) leading to demyelination and diffuse neurodegeneration in both brain and spinal cord grey and white matter of the brain and spinal cord [1,2]. Although its etiology remains elusive results from immunological, genetic, and histopathology studies of patients with MS support the concept that autoimmunity plays a major role in disease pathogenesis [1,3]. Disease course can be highly variable, however most patients present recurring clinical symptoms from onset followed by total or partial recovery, the classic relapsing–remitting form of the disease (RRMS). After 10–15 years the pattern becomes progressive in up to 50% of untreated patients, and symptoms slowly progress over a period of many years. This stage is defined as secondary progressive MS (SPMS). Fifteen percent of MS patients can present a progressive from onset, and is named primary progressive MS (PPMS) [4]. Actually, it is not known to whether PPMS is a different form of MS or is simply SPMS, without identifiable clinical relapses.

The most characteristic brain tissue injury in MS is primary demyelination with partial preservation of axons [2]. In general, actively demyelinating plaques in RRMS involves the movement of immune cells from the periphery into the CNS, which is associated with disruption of the blood-brain-barrier (BBB). In contrast, progressive disease involves the development of compartmentalized pathological processes within the brain mediated mainly by resident CNS cells. Evidence of this comes from MRI showing decreased gadolinium (Gd) enhancement in CNS lesions found in progressive MS patients, indicating reduced BBB breakdown and less movement of immune cells into the CNS. Several tissue pathology findings are associated with progressive MS. The most prominent is brain atrophy, caused chiefly by degeneration and chronic demyelination of axons, ultimately leading to neuronal loss [5]. Representing a major cause of irreversible neurological disability [6]. Although imaging and neuropathological studies have shown that both axonal degeneration and neuronal death are present in acute or active MS lesions [7], progression likely occurs once axonal loss exceeds CNS compensatory capacity. Whether inflammation and neurodegeneration are primary or secondary processes, and how they interact during the course of disease remains unclear. Another major pathological substrate of progressive MS is cortical demyelination. Grey matter demyelination is also observed in cerebellar cortex, the hippocampus, and in deep grey matter nuclei [8–11]. In addition to demyelination and oligodendrocyte loss, demyelinating cortical lesions show neuritic transection, neuronal death and reduced presynaptic terminal numbers [8,12]. In progressive MS lesions diffuse pathology is also present in normal appearing white and grey matter, reflected by diffuse axonal injury with profound microglia activation within a background of a global inflammation of the entire brain and the meninges [13]. Interestingly, MRI studies suggest that cortical atrophy may be more closely related to diffuse neurodegeneration in the normal appearing white matter than to the extent of focal white-matter demyelination [14].

In recent decades, better understanding of mechanisms underlying RRMS has led to the development of different disease-modifying therapies, reducing both severity and frequency of new relapses through immune system modulation [15,16]. In contrast, therapeutic options available for progressive MS are comparatively disappointing, and remain a challenge. One possible reason may be lack of knowledge regarding the pathogenic mechanisms driving progressive MS. At present, abnormal tissue findings seen in progressive MS remain poorly represented in experimental animal models.

This review discusses present knowledge on grey matter involvement in progressive MS, as well as the putative mechanisms that can determine the processes of neurodegeneration and neuronal death.

2. Grey Matter Changes Observed in MS

2.1. Cortical Compromise in MS

Even though MS was considered early on to be a demyelinating disease of CNS white matter mediated by inflammation, the possibility has been raised in recent years that cortical and deep grey matter demyelination may exceed that of white-matter demyelination, with both postmortem and in vivo studies revealing presence of extensive lesions in grey matter (GM) structures [8,17,18]. Initially articles explained GM compromise as a phenomenon associated exclusively with prolonged disease duration and progressive forms. Recently, however, cortical and deep grey matter lesions in the thalamus, caudate, putamen and cerebellum cortex have been detected during early stages of disease independent of white-matter pathology [19–22]. Indeed, evidence establishing that grey matter involvement related to disease activity and more aggressive forms is growing [23]. In contrast to other neurodegenerative diseases, it is not known whether cortical atrophy in MS is a more diffuse process or develops instead following distinct anatomical patterns. Cortical regions of the frontal lobe, posterior cingulate, insula and temporal lobes (especially hippocampus) as well as of the cerebellum are by far the most frequent areas affected early on, causing disability progression and cognitive impairment [24]. Recently different patterns of cortical atrophy with or without concomitant white-matter lesions have been described in patients with long-lasting MS. Most of these show a non-random and symmetric distribution, as well as, stronger associations with clinical dysfunction than global cortical atrophy [25]. In CNS tissue samples obtained at autopsy, different cortical lesions have been detected [8,17] in around 60% of the cases, while more recent 7T MRI protocols estimate a frequency above 90% [8,17,26]. Three types of cortical lesions have been reported in MS brain tissue: leukocortical, intracortical and subpial [27]. Leukocortical lesions or type 1 lesions seems to start in the subcortical white matter and extend into the cortex to layers V and VI (Figure 1A,B). Cortical sectors of these lesions showed increased numbers of lymphocytes and microglia/monocytes compared to normal appearing cortex from the same brain or from aged-matched control brains, although numbers of these cells are substantially less abundant than those seen in subcortical white matter [8]. Leukocortical lesions have been detected in patients even during the earliest stages of MS. Intracortical lesions or type 2 lesions are located entirely within the cerebral cortex, are not in direct contact with subcortical white matter or pia mater, and are in general small and perivascular. Finally, subpial lesions or type 3 lesions represent the most abundant type of cortical lesions, and are most prominent during progressive stages. These lesions often show myelin loss in cortical layers I through IV spanning several gyri. On occasion, they can involve all six cortical layers, but rarely invade subcortical white matter, and are mostly associated with meningeal inflammation [17,28,29]. With the exception of loss of myelin, subpial lesions lack most of the other pathological signature findings described in white-matter lesions such as blood-brain-barrier breakdown, as well as immune cells infiltration, perivascular cuffs, astrogliosis, loss of oligodendrocyte progenitor cells, and complement activation. Active tissue damage is also associated with microglial activation [22,30]. However, no correlation has been observed between subpial and white-matter lesion loads [31,32], suggesting subpial demyelination occurs independently of white-matter demyelination. General consensus from autopsy studies would indicate subpial lesions are abundant in progressive stages of MS (both PPMS and SPMS) and rare in MS patients with acute disease or during early stages of RRMS.

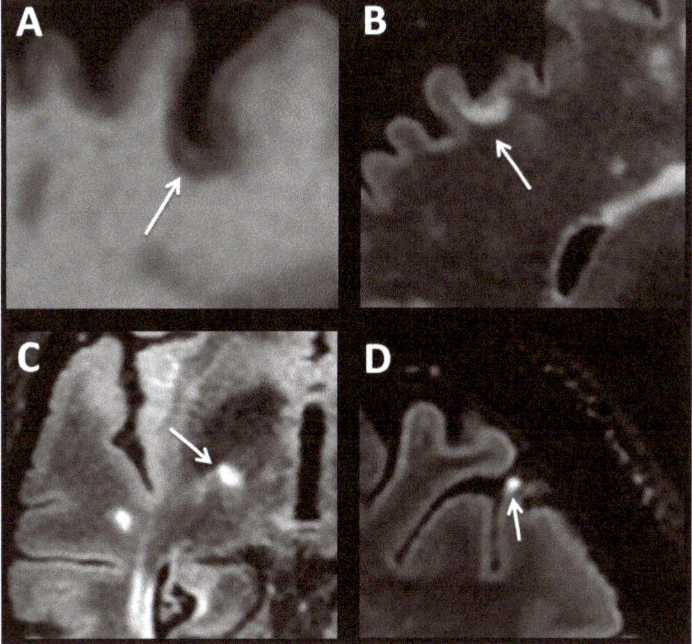

Figure 1. (**A**) Three-dimension sagittal T1-weighted. Hypointense cortical lesion (white arrow). (**B**) Three-dimension sagittal T2-Fluid Attenuated Inversion Recovery (FLAIR). Hyperintense leukocortical lesion (white arrow). (**C**) Axial FLAIR. Subcortical temporal demyelinating plaque and perithalamic internal capsule lesion (white arrow). (**D**) Post-contrast 3D sagittal FLAIR. Focal area of leptomeningeal enhancement (white arrow).

2.2. Deep Grey Matter (DGM) Structures Changes in MS

Although less well studied, DGM structures involvement is often present together with cortical atrophy, particularly of the thalamus. To date estimation of whole-brain volume has been used most often as a surrogate marker of atrophy in MS, because it is relatively easy to measure. However, there is growing evidence that grey matter volume loss may be more pronounced than that of white matter and be more strongly linked to long-term disability [33,34]. The thalamus may be particularly susceptible to neurodegeneration through different mechanisms, of which two are particularly prominent. First, demyelinating lesions can occur in the thalamus and in perithalamic regions (Figure 1C). Indeed, DGM demyelination can be frequently observed in postmortem MS brain, particularly in the caudate, and in the medial and anterior thalamic nuclei [11]. Histopathologic characterization of the thalamic lesions recapitulates the spectrum of active, chronically demyelinated, lesions observed in the white matter. Similar to changes found in cortical grey matter at autopsy, parenchymal infiltration by T and B cells is limited when compared to levels observed in classic active white-matter lesions. Second, recent work has shown clear patterns of grey matter atrophy in patients with MS that are focused in regions that are strongly connected with diverse neuronal networks [25]. Because DGM structures are extensively connected to cortical grey matter regions, atrophy could also be due to a retrograde event resulting from axonal transection in white-matter tracts projecting from the thalamus, or secondary to trans-synaptic deafferentation of thalamic neurons [11,35]. Interestingly, recent studies have shown that volume loss in DGM over time is faster than in other brain regions across all clinical phenotypes, and drives disability [21,36,37]. Together these studies provide strong evidence that thalamic volume and DGM volume more broadly, are dramatically affected in MS.

3. Mechanisms of Neurodegeneration

Different theories have been put forward to explain how progressive MS is triggered. One suggestion is that although brain damage is driven by inflammatory processes similar to those observed during RRMS, during progressive disease stages, a microenvironment is created within the CNS favoring homing and retention of inflammatory cells, ultimately making disease-modifying therapies ineffective [38]. A second possibility is that MS starts out as an inflammatory disease, but after several years a neurodegenerative process independent of inflammatory responses becomes the key mechanism behind disease progression [39]. Finally, MS could be a neurodegenerative disease, with inflammation occurring as a secondary response, amplifying progressive states [40,41]. Clearly, these different mechanisms are not mutually exclusive and could occur in combination. Therefore, in MS neurodegeneration and ultimately progression of disease and chronic disability develop as a result of many different molecular mechanisms. These have been summarized in Table 1.

Table 1. Mechanisms proposed to explain Multiple Sclerosis progression.

Immunological Mechanisms and Effectors	Mechanisms of Neurodegeneration and Axonal Dysfunction
B Cells	**Mitochondrial Injury**
Antibody production, Ag presentation, ectopic formation of follicle-like structures	Impaired activity of respiratory chain complexes (I, III and IV)
Induction of compartmentalized population driving CNS injury, independent of peripheral immune activity.	Alterations in mitochondrial molecular motors mtDNA deletions
Secretion of IL-6, TNF-α, IL-10, and IL-35: Complement activation and T cell functions	Energy deficiency: failure of Na$^+$/K$^+$ ATPase, reverse activity of NCX, and excess of intra-axonal Ca^{2+}.
EBV-infected B-cell Induce CD8-mediated immune responses against brain tissue	Amplify oxidative stress. Mediates histotoxic hypoxia, which magnifies energy deficiency
CD8$^+$ cytotoxic T lymphocytes	**Release of Fe^{3+}**
Release of TNF-α: neuronal cell death via p55 receptor; IFN-γ: increased Glutamate neurotoxicity and Ca^{2+} influx; secretion of perforin and granzyme: cellular membrane damage, associated to Na$^+$ and Ca^{2+} influx	Iron accumulates with aging. The release of Fe^{3+} from damaged OGD amplifies oxidative injury

Table 1. *Cont.*

Immunological Mechanisms and Effectors	Mechanisms of Neurodegeneration and Axonal Dysfunction
Astrocytes *	**Anomalous Distribution of Ion Channels**
Secretion of pro-inflammatory cytokines (IL-1, IL-6, TNF-α), chemokines (CCL-2, CCL-5, IP-10, CXCL-12, IL-8) and BAFF. Blood-brain-barrier breakthrough: action on endothelial cells and tight junctions Activation of microglia: secretion of CXCL-10/CXR3, GM-CSF, M-CSF and TGF-β. Production of Lactosylceramide: induces secretion of CCL2 and GM-CSF Production of ROS, RNS, NO and ONOO-limited Glutamate transporters, increasing Glutamate excitotoxicity Reactive astrogliosis: inhibition of remyelination and axonal regeneration by over-secretion of FGF-2, CSPGs and EPH. Upregulation of purinergic receptors: increased responsiveness to ATP, formation of membrane pores and increased of Ca^{2+} influx Cellular senescence: low level of chronic inflammation, altered Ca^{2+} homeostasis	Redistribution of Na^{+} channels (Na_V, 1.2, 1.6 and 1.8) along the denuded axon: increased energy demand. Activation of VGCC, ASIC1 and TRPM4 contributes to excess of intra-axonal Ca^{2+} Glutamate excitotoxicity mediates massive influx of Ca^{2+} into neurons Excess of intra-axonal Ca^{2+} stimulates catabolic enzyme systems: leading to proteolytic degradation of cytoskeletal proteins
Microglia *	**Loss of Myelin-Derived Trophic Support and Deficit in Axonal Transport**
Decreased expression of immunosuppressive factors: fractalkine-CX3CR1, and CD200-CD200R. Secretion of pro-inflammatory cytokines: IL-1, IL-6, TNF-α, IFN-γ. Ag presentation of CD4^{+} T cells via Major Histocompatibility Complex (MHC) Class II Oxidative burst: production of ROS and RNS Acquisition of aging phenotype: expression of AGE and RAGE	Alteration of a single myelin protein synthesis (PLP, MGA, or CNP) can cause axonal dysfunction Deficit in axonal transport can reduced expression of kinesins (anterograde transport) and dyneins (retrograde transport)

* Only deleterious mechanisms are presented. Ag: antigen; AGE: Advanced glycation end products; ASIC1: acid-sensing ion channel; BAFF: B-cell-activating factor; CNP: 2′3′ cyclic-nucleotide 3′ phosphodiesterase; CNS: Central Nervous System; CSPGs: chondroitin sulphate proteoglycans; EBV: Epstein–Barr virus; EPH: ephrins; FGF-2: fibroblast growth factor 2; GM-CSF: granulocyte-macrophage-colony stimulating factor; MAG: myelin-associated glycoprotein; M-CSF: macrophage-colony stimulating factor; mtDNA: mitochondrial DNA; NCX: sodium calcium exchanger; NO: nitric oxide; OGD: oligodendrocytes; ONOO^{-}: peroxynitrite; PLP: proteolipid-protein; RAGE: AGE receptor; RNS: reactive nitrogen species; ROS: reactive oxygen species; TRPM4: transient potential receptor melastatin 4; VGCC: Voltage-gated Ca^{2+} channel.

4. Inflammatory Events

Evidence from animal models and immunological studies in MS patients suggests that peripheral immune response targeting the CNS drives the disease process during early phases, whereas immune reactions confined to the CNS dominate later phases of progression [42,43]. The composition of the inflammatory infiltrate within the CNS results from the combination of peripheral immune cells influx, and resident cell activation, particularly of microglial cells, which can change their intrinsic "resting" state in response to prolonged inflammation. Among potential candidates driving inflammation during progressive MS, the role of B cells appears to be prominent. B-cell functions that could be of relevance in progressive MS include: antibody production, increased secretion of pro-inflammatory cytokines, deficient production of regulatory cytokines which impact complement activation and T cell function, as well as antigen presentation and ectopic formation of follicle-like structures [44,45]. Ectopic follicle-like structures are pathological tissue formations resembling tertiary lymph nodes, found in the subarachnoid space of leptomeninges close to inflamed blood vessels (Figure 1D), and also present in other chronic inflammatory diseases [46,47]. They can be induced by follicular T- helper cells cytokine networks acting as positive (i.e., IL-21, and IL-22) and negative (i.e., IL-27) regulators, as well by changes in the stromal networks in connective tissue [48,49]. Composition of these pathologic structures is characterized by aggregates of T and B cells often showing T/B segregation, and development of high endothelial venules, and follicular dendritic cell networks [19,46]. They are capable of sustaining in situ antibody diversification, isotype switching, B-cell differentiation and oligoclonal expansion similar to ectopic germinal centers, which can also support the production of autoreactive plasma cells at the site of local inflammation [48]. These structures co-localize with grey matter lesions and parenchymal infiltrates [50], and are present during different stages of development, ranging from simple T and B-cell clusters to highly organized follicles encapsulated by reticulin lining [51]. Once follicle-like develop, lymphoid chemokines CCL19, CCL21, CXCL12, and CXCL13 are critical for their perpetuation and function, controlling homing recruitment, maturation and antigenic selection of B cells [52], which in turn sustain a high level of humoral response within the CNS independent of peripheral inflammation. This is of particular relevance during progressive MS, when the BBB is intact and contribution to disease activity from entry of peripheral immune cells into the brain is negligible. Antibodies against both myelin antigens and to non-myelin antigens such as neurofascin, neurofilaments and the glial potassium channel KIR 4. 1 has been shown to play an important role in axonal and neuronal damage through complement cascade activation [53–55]. In progressive MS cortical demyelination, neurodegeneration and atrophy show positive correlation with diffuse inflammatory infiltrates and lymphoid-follicle structures in leptomeninges, indicating activation of these structures contribute to cortical pathology [2,19,23]. As in other chronic inflammatory diseases follicle-like structures occur in around 40% of SPMS cases [45,56], but are uncommon in PPMS cases. However, it is not known whether follicle-like structures are a typical feature of different disease subtypes from the beginning, or develop as a result of persistent tissue damage and antigen release [20,49]. Notably, meningeal inflammation in SPMS is associated with damage of glial limitans, and a gradient of neuronal loss, which is greater in superficial cortical layers (I-III) nearer the pial surface than in inner cortical layers [23]. These findings suggest cytotoxic factors diffusing from the infiltrated meninges may play a major role in subpial cortical lesions development. Indeed, presence of follicle-like structures in patients with SPMS has been associated with a more severe clinical course, shorter disease duration and earlier death [28,57,58]. Despite this evidence, some studies have reported no substantial perivascular infiltration in pure intracortical lesions found postmortem in patients with longstanding progressive MS [8,17]. These contradictory findings could be due to a reduced sample size, or to insufficient inflammatory activity in the tissue analyzed. Of note, questions remaining regarding neurodegenerative and immunological mechanisms underlying PPMS and SPMS pathology are different. In both cases diffuse meningeal inflammation and cortical neuronal pathology may be significant contributors to clinical progression, suggesting similar pathogenic mechanisms, irrespective of a prior relapsing–remitting course, or the presence of follicle-like structures [59]. Differences observed between both forms of the disease are more quantitative than qualitative in nature [60]. Because serological and epidemiological studies have found an association between B-lymphotropic Epstein–Barr virus (EBV) infection and MS [61], it has been hypothesized that EBV infection of CNS- infiltrating B cells may drive MS pathology [62]. Analysis of postmortem brain tissue from MS patients with different forms of disease, have shown that accumulation of EBV-infected B cells/plasma cells in the meninges and perivascular compartment of white-matter lesions is common and that numbers of EBV-harboring cells correlates with the degree of brain inflammation. Absence of EBV in brain-infiltrating B cells in other inflammatory neurological diseases indicates that homing of EBV-infected B cells to the CNS is specific to MS and not a general phenomenon driven by inflammation [63]. Colonization of cortical lesions has been associated with EBV-encoded small nuclear mRNA (EBER) transcripts in B cells and plasma cells, predominantly expressed during the latent phase of viral infection. Expression of the latency proteins EBNA2 and LMP1, which provide proliferative and prosurvival signals to B cells, in active white-matter lesions and in the meninges in most MS cases, as well as the presence of foci of B-cell proliferation in the MS brain tissue, support a mechanism of EBV-driven B-cell expansion. Ectopic follicle-like structures contained numerous LMP1$^+$, but no EBNA2$^+$ cells. Meanwhile lytic proteins BZLF1 and BERF1 were found restricted to plasma cells located in active cortical lesions, indicating these structures represent main sites of viral reactivation [63]. Because cells expressing EBNA2 and LMP1 are usually not found in blood, their presence in brain suggests complete disruption of EBV regulation [64]. However, other authors report absence of CNS EBV infection in MS [65]. Interestingly, early lytic EBV antigens elicited CD8-mediated immune responses, triggering strong cytotoxic effects in brain tissue [66]. Indeed, the most active cortical MS lesions are often crowded with CD8$^+$ T cells, and contain few B cells o plasma cells, suggesting cortical inflammation correlate with reduction in both B and plasma cell numbers [67]. These observations suggest that EBV reactivation combined with a strong cytotoxic antiviral response mediated by CD8$^+$ T cells may drive acute inflammation in both white and grey matter, as well as within the meningeal compartment. CD8$^+$ T cells can also recognize specific antigens present on oligodendrocytes, neurons or axons. Once activated, they may be partly responsible for demyelination or axonal/neuronal damage in MS [68–70]. Most CD8$^+$ T lymphocytes recovered from MS lesions belonged to a few clones [71]. Samples obtained from patients studied longitudinally have shown that certain CD8$^+$ T cell clones found in MS patients may persisted over many years in CSF and/or CNS tissue [5,72]. In sharp contrast, the repertoire of CD4$^+$ T cells recovered from the CNS in MS patients is heterogeneous [5,71,72]. Overall, these findings reinforce the concept that CD8$^+$ T lymphocytes present in the CNS of MS patients are not just bystander cells but are engaged in active immune responses [73]. Axonal damage in white-matter lesions correlates with the number of both CD8$^+$ T cells [74] and of activated microglia/macrophages [75] and resident CNS cells which show intense MHC I expression in all types of inflammatory lesions [76]. These observations collectively suggest that in white-matter lesions, CD8$^+$ T cells contribute as effector cells causing oligodendrocyte as well as axonal damage. However, there is still controversy over the underlying mechanisms, through which cytotoxic CD8$^+$ T lymphocytes harm axons and neurons in MS. Cytotoxic CD8$^+$ T lymphocytes release cytokines, such as IFN-γ, and TNF-α, as well as perforin, and granzymes A and B [70,77,78]. IFN-γ for instance, can increase glutamate neurotoxicity and Ca^{2+} influx into neurons through modulation of the IFN-γ/AMPA Glutamate receptor complex [78]. TNF-α on the other hand triggers cell death via the p55 receptor present on neurons [79]. Perforin and granzymes directly damage the cell membrane, causing Na$^+$ and Ca^{2+} influx, ultimately leading to energy breakdown and consequent activation of lytic cell enzymes (see below). Granzymes disrupted calcium homeostasis by increasing resting levels, and enhancing IP3-mediated endoplasmic reticulum calcium release. Elevated concentrations of Ca^{2+} are sufficient to activate calcium-dependent death effectors, including caspases [80]. Although perforin did enhance GrB-mediated neurotoxicity, recombinant GrB can itself induce neurotoxicity, independently of perforin [80]. Likewise, interactions between Fas antigen on CD8$^+$ cytotoxic T lymphocytes and Fas ligand on neurons triggers Ca $^{2+}$ release from intracellular storage sites resulting in additional activation of the intracellular caspase cascade causing further axonal/neuronal damage [81].

The role of cytotoxic CD4$^+$ T cells in progressive MS has not always been highlighted. However, recent studies demonstrated an increase of this T cell population in late/chronic Experimental Autoimmune Encephalomyelits (EAE) lesions as compared with acute lesions. Moreover, proportions of cytotoxic CD4$^+$ T cells were further enriched in the CSF from SPMS patients as compared with corresponding blood samples [82]. These cells arise from repeated antigenic stimulation, after which they lose the co-stimulatory molecule CD28, presenting a cytotoxic phenotype, comparable with NK and CD8$^+$ T cells [83]. In addition, CD4$^+$CD28$^-$ T cells lose their sensitivity to apoptosis induction [84], and are resistant to the suppressive actions of regulatory T cells [85]. Expansion of CD4$^+$CD28$^-$ T cells is associated with several autoimmune and chronic inflammatory conditions, including MS [86,87], whereas in healthy individuals they are almost undetectable [88]. They have been identified not just in the circulation of patients with chronic inflammatory diseases, but also in target tissues. In MS CD4$^+$CD28$^-$ T cells are capable of migrating to the CNS mainly through the fractalkine (CX$_3$CL1-CX$_3$CR1) system. It comes as no surprise that patients who have high numbers of these cells have more severe disease and poor prognosis. Indeed, recently baseline percentage of CD4$^+$CD28$^-$ T cells was associated with multimodal evoked potential (EP), indicating a link between these cells and disease severity. In addition, the baseline CD4 $^+$CD28$^-$ T cells percentage had a prognostic value since it was associated with EP after 3 years and with EP and Expanded Disability Status Scale (EDSS) after 5 years [89]. Notably, in patients with chronic inflammatory disorders it has been shown that CD4$^+$CD28$^-$ T cells have oligoclonal antigen receptors [90], produce high levels of inflammatory cytokines such as IFN-γ, and GM-CSF, and express cytotoxic molecules (e.g., NKG2D, perforin and Granzyme B), features similar to innate-like T cells, which together could lead to neuronal and axonal loss similar as described by CD8$^+$ T cell [68,83]. It remains unclear to date which are the antigens or cues that trigger and/or drive the expansion of CD4$^+$CD28$^-$ T cells and what stage they acquire cytotoxic activity that contributes to tissue damage and consequent disease progression in MS.

Active demyelination and neurodegeneration have also been linked to microglial activation in early lesions [91]. While in the surveillance state, microglia monitor brain parenchyma detecting danger signals. This state seems to be maintained through a number of interactions with neurons. For example, interactions have been described between CD200-CD200R, CD47-CD172a, and fractalkine-CX3CR1 interactions. As a consequence of brain injury or disease these interactions are lost and resident microglia change their phenotype developing an "activated" state. This change can be induced through several mechanisms including: production of pro-inflammatory cytokines released by Th1 or Th17 T cells, presence of microbial pathogens (PAMPs) recognized by Toll-like receptors (TLRs) or leucine-rich repeat containing receptors (NLRs), release of intracellular components from necrotic or apoptotic cells, as well as presence of heat shock proteins, misfolded proteins (DAMPs) or components of the complement cascade [92]. Microglial activation is not restricted to lesions, but is also diffusely present in normal appearing white and grey matter [13]. In normal appearing white matter (NAWM) for example clustering of activated microglia, so-called microglial nodules, are abundant in areas adjacent to plaques, particularly in patients with progressive MS [93]. Notably, microglia nodules have been associated with damaged axons expressing amyloid precursor protein (APP) accumulation, and changes in neurofilament phosphorylation in the periplaque white matter. Furthermore, direct spatial association has been observed between microglial nodules and axons undergoing Wallerian degeneration [94]. These findings indicate microglial activation is associated with signs of neuronal damage and tissue atrophy strongly suggesting microglial cells contribute to CNS damage in progressive MS.

Damage induced by microglial cells in MS is mediated through different mechanisms (Figure 2A), including secretion of pro-inflammatory cytokines such as IL-1, IL-6, TNF-α, and IFN-γ, phagocytic activity and presentation of antigens to CD4$^+$ T cells via MHC Class II molecules [95,96]. Pro-inflammatory cytokines can also induce mitochondrial injury both in neurons and glial cells. In addition, reactive oxygen and nitrogen species (ROS/RNS), produced by microglial cells, cause direct damage to neuron through loss of cytochrome C oxidase (COX1), as well as mitochondrial respiratory chain complex IV activity, leading to mitochondrial dysfunction (see below) [97]. Importantly, release of Fe^{2+} into the extracellular space from injured oligodendrocytes may amplify oxidative damage by generating highly toxic hydroxyl (OH) radicals, from H$_2$O$_2$. Fe^{2+} uptake by activated microglia determines their fragmentation and degeneration, leading to a second wave of Fe^{2+} release, which can increase susceptibility of surrounding tissues to free radicals-driven axonal and neuronal destruction [98].

Interestingly, cortical demyelinated lesions lack inflammatory lymphocyte or macrophage infiltrates in progressive MS and does not show complement deposition. The majority of phagocytic cells are ramified microglia in close apposition to neurites and neuronal cell bodies [8]. Activated microglia also possesses a puzzling array of neuroprotective functions, including debris phagocytosis and clearance, growth factors production and neuronal-circuit shaping [95]. Distinguish neuroprotective from pro-inflammatory phenotypes remains a challenge when interpreting microglial function.

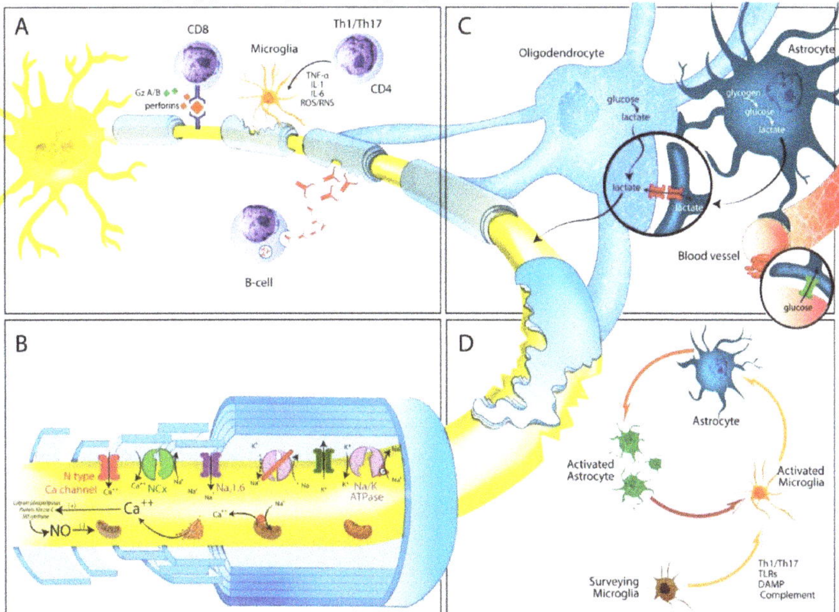

Figure 2. Possible mechanisms involved in MS progression. (**A**) In progressive MS the inflammatory phenomena eventually leading to axonal degeneration and loss are compartmentalized within the CNS. Cellular components are represented by cells that come from the periphery (T and B lymphocytes), as well as by resident CNS cells (microglia cells and astrocytes). B cells can form ectopic follicle-like structures resembling tertiary lymph nodes, producing antibodies against myelin and non-myelin antigens, shown to play an important role in axonal and neuronal damage through complement cascade activation. In turn, CD8$^+$ lymphocytes can recognize specific axonal antigens and produce tissue damage through secretion of perforin or granzymes A and B. Autoreactive CD4$^+$ Th1 and Th17 lymphocytes can activate microglial cells, which in turn produce pro-inflammatory cytokines (IL-1, IL-6, TNF-α) or oxygen or nitrogen free radicals (ROS/RNS) causing axonal damage and neuronal loss through a bystander mechanism. (**B**) Following demyelination, energy requirements increase due to disruption of paranodal myelin loops. Reduction in neuronal ATP production may lead to failure of the Na$^+$/K$^+$ pump failure, generating a sustained sodium current, which drives reverse sodium/calcium exchange and accumulation of intra-axonal calcium. This, in turn activates degradative enzymes, including proteases, phospholipases, and calpains, resulting in further neuronal and/or axonal damage as well as impaired ATP production. (**C**) Axonal damage could be cause by poor trophic support. Oligodendrocytes capture glucose from circulation, breaking it down glucose to form pyruvate or lactate, which can enter axons, and be imported by mitochondria for ATP synthesis. An alternative source of energy for axons comes from glycogen stored in astrocytes, which can be transformed into glucose and later into pyruvate or lactate, depending on oxygen availability. (**D**) Several mechanisms cause surveillance microglia activation including Th1 or Th17 T cells; presence of microbial pathogens (PAMPs) recognized by Toll-like receptors (TLRs) or leucin-rich repeat containing receptors (NLRs); release of intracellular components from necrotic or apoptotic cells; presence of heat shock proteins, misfolded proteins (DAMPs), or components of the complement cascade. Once activated they in induce activation and proliferation of astrocytes, leading to astrogliosis.

As previously mentioned, postmortem tissue studies have shown increased microglial numbers and increased activation are associated with variable degrees of axonal/neuritic injury, demyelination, and neuronal loss in cortical grey matter during progressive stages of MS. However, it is as yet unclear how early during the course of MS these degenerative events begin. Future longitudinal in vivo studies linking microglial activation to local cortical atrophy or dysfunction levels as well as to progression of disability in individual subjects should help to improve our understanding of the consequences of cortical pathology at different disease stages. In this context, in vivo positron emission tomography (PET) images of microglia, could clarify the role of activated microglia in MS-related neurodegeneration. Use of a selective translocator protein (TSPO) radioligand 11C-PK11195 allows detection of activated microglia on PET. TSPO is a protein, expressed on the outer mitochondrial membrane of microglial cells, at low levels in the healthy CNS, but up-regulated upon microglial activation [99] making TSPO a sensitive "real-time" marker of activation [100,101]. In non-neoplastic injury to CNS without BBB damage, microglial are the main cell population expressing TSPO. However, blood-derived macrophages, reactive astrocytes, and endothelial cells in the vasculature express TSPO [100,102]. Imaging studies in MS patients using the TSPO radioligand 11C-PK11195 have shown microglial cells activation occurs early on and appears to be linked to disability and brain atrophy [103]. In the NAWM of SPMS patients TSPO binding is significantly increased compared to age-matched healthy controls [102,104]. PET imaging can also be used to differentiate active from inactive chronic lesions. Slowly expanding chronic active lesions are thought to contribute to MS progression. Detection of plaque kinetics in vivo will likely provide new information on underlying pathology driving progression [105].

As in other neurodegenerative disorders, expansion and activation of microglia is the primary mechanism behind astrocytosis (Figure 2D). Although astrocytes survive oxidative stress induced by inflammation and ROS/RNS, they still shown signs of injury, mainly reflected by changes in cell morphology and molecular expression [106]. Scar tissue is composed primarily of astrocytes, however in severe lesions, interaction with other cell types including oligodendrocyte progenitor cells, and fibromeningeal cells also occurs [107]. Several specific molecular and morphologic features have been observed in astrocytes during reactive astrogliosis both in human pathology and animal models [108], of which upregulation of Glial fibrillary acidic protein (GFAP), vimentin, nestin, and the less investigated synemin are hallmarks. Glial scars are evident in tissue from MS patients and mice with EAE and surround areas of demyelination [109]. The purpose of scar formation would appear to be isolation of damaged CNS areas, to prevent spread of tissue destruction. However, glial scar rigidity results in inhibition of both remyelination and axonal regeneration, both negative effects mediated through different mechanisms. Over-secretion of FGF-2 by astrocytes may be detrimental for remyelination, which in turn promotes oliogodendrocytes precursor cells (OPC) proliferation and survival, but prevents maturation [110]. Another molecule that appears to play an important role in preventing OPC maturation is the glycosaminoglycan hyaluronan, which is found throughout the extracellular matrix and CNS white matter [111]. Oligodendrocytes that co-localize with hyaluronan express an immature phenotype, and in vitro treatment of oligodendrocytes precursor cells with hyaluronan in vitro prevents maturation [112]. In addition, astrocytes in injured areas release inhibitory extracellular matrix molecules known as chondroitin sulphate proteoglycans (CSPGs) which can severely in injured areas, affect both cytoskeleton and membrane components of growth cone architecture [113]. CSPGs are a family of molecules characterized by a protein core to which highly sulphated glycosaminoglycan (GAG) chains are attached. Neurocan (secreted) and brevican (cell bound) are the major proteoglycans produced by astrocytes in vitro and both have been shown to inhibit axon growth, following CNS damage [114]. There is clear evidence that CSPGs are produced in excess by astrocytes when they become reactive and that CSPGs inhibitory activity depends on GAG content, as removal of GAG chains from the protein core suppresses CSPG- mediated inhibition [114]. Aside from CSPGs, other less studied inhibitory molecules expressed by astrocytes can suppress axonal growth. Ephrins (EPH) and their receptors for example are secreted by normal astrocytes and increased in MS lesions, inducing axonal growth cone collapse through activation of axon-bound EPH tyrosine-receptor kinase [115].

Likewise, astrocytes as part of the immune system could contribute to disease progression through several mechanisms. First, they can directly affect cell entry to the CNS, via de the BBB, by regulating expression of adhesion molecules, particularly vascular adhesion-molecule-1 (VCAM-1), and intercellular adhesion-molecule-1 (ICAM-1), that bind to lymphocyte receptors very late antigen-4 (VLA4), and lymphocyte function-associated antigen-1 (LFA-1), respectively [116,117]. Second, astrocytes secrete different chemokines such as CCL-2 (MCP-1), CCL5 (RANTES), IP-10 (CXCL10), CXCL12 (SDF-1) and IL-8 (CXCL8), which attract both peripheral immune cells (e.g., T cells, monocytes, and DCs), as well as resident CNS cells (microglia) to lesion sites [118]. In addition, astrocytes can secrete GM-CSF, M-CSF or TGF-β, which can regulate MHC Class II molecule expression by microglia and even their phagocytosis [119]. This could represent the primary mechanism through which astrocytes perpetuate immune-mediated demyelination and neurodegeneration. Recent investigations have demonstrated that in chronic phases of EAE, astrocyte depletion ameliorates disease severity. This deleterious effect of astrocytes on EAE is mediated by preferential expression of 4-galactosyltransferase 5 and 6 (B4GALT5 and B4GALT6) [120]. Notably, B4GALT6 is also expressed by reactive astrocytes in human MS lesions. These enzymes synthesize the signaling molecule lactosylceramide (LacCer), the CNS expression of which is significantly increased during progressive phases of EAE. LacCer promotes astrocyte activation in an autocrine manner [120,121], inducing GM-CSF and CCL2 genes, activating microglia and causing infiltration of monocytes from blood, respectively. Remarkably, inhibition or knockout of B4GALT6 in mice suppresses disease progression, local CNS innate immunity and neurodegeneration in EAE, and interferes with human astrocyte activation in vitro [120].

Third, B-cell-activating factor (BAFF), critical for both B-cell development and survival, as well as for immunoglobulin production, is constitutively expressed by astrocytes in normal CNS. BAFF expression in astrocytes is up-regulated in MS lesions and in EAE affected mice, suggesting astrocytes may contribute to drive B-cell-dependent autoimmunity [122], an important mechanism in disease progression as described above. Finally, an important function of innate immune cells is to act as antigen-presenting cells. However, although astrocytes express MHC Class I and Class II molecules in vitro capable of presenting myelin antigens, their ability to also express co-stimulatory molecules including CD40, CD80, and CD86 challenges this function, making their final effect unclear [123]. Nor is it clear to what degree astrocytes can perform phagocytosis, or process and present antigens, particularly under physiological conditions in vivo [124].

In addition to being part of the immune system, astrocytes contribute to MS progression through production of cytotoxic factors. In rodents, astrocytes stimulated with IL-17 or IFN-γ induce nitric oxide synthase (iNOS) [125]. Likewise, IL-1 as well as combined treatment with TGF-β plus IFN-γ increases the percentage of astrocyte secreted nitric oxide (NO), which is one of the most prominent damage-inducing molecules in neurodegeneration [126,127]. Simultaneously, NO stimulates glutamate release from astrocytes which further increase excitotoxicity [128]. Remarkably, the predominant contribution of NO to excitotoxicity depends on increased superoxide ion O_2^- production, which reacts with NO forming peroxynitrite (ONOO$^-$) resulting in neuronal necrosis or apoptosis, depending on its concentration [129]. Furthermore, ONOO$^-$ inactivates glutamate transporters in astrocytes, directly damaging myelin, oligodendrocytes, and axons [130]. Decreased uptake of glutamate by astrocyte transporters could also contribute to abnormal levels of extracellular glutamate, which are directly toxic to oligodendrocytes, axons and neurons [131]. Excitotoxicity is caused mainly by sustained activation of glutamate receptors and massive subsequent influx of Ca^{2+} into viable neurons, which in turn results in changes in microtubules and neurofilament phosphorylation, ultimately leading to axon cytoskeleton breakdown (see below) [132].

It is important to note astrocytes have a dual role, not only aiding axonal degeneration, but also creating a permissive environment promoting remyelination [133]. The actual impact of astrocytes on pathogenesis and repair of inflammation therefore, will be dependent on a number of factors, including timing after injury, type of lesion and surrounding microenvironment, as well as interaction with other cell types and factors influencing their activation [134].

5. Redistribution of Ion Channels and Axonal Damage

Because pathology findings and number of transected axons correlate with degree of inflammation in MS [7,135], great interest has been focused on neurotoxic products release by the innate immune system, in particular, ROS, RNS, and NO produced by macrophages, microglia, and astrocytes both in MS and EAE [136]. Mitochondria and mitochondrial DNA (mtDNA) are highly susceptible to oxidative injury. ROS and RNS generate mitochondrial enzymes deficit which can be either reversible or irreversible. In MS highly active lesions show diffuse mitochondrial damage, making energy failure the main mechanisms behind functional and structural loss [137]. During progressive MS mitochondrial injury emerges in grey matter, and neuronal cell bodies in deeper layers of the cortex show both impaired mitochondrial activity in the respiratory chain complexes as well as alterations in motor proteins responsible for mitochondria movement from the cell body to axons [96,138]. Axonal transport is essential for neuronal health, and has been implicated in different neurodegenerative conditions. Mitochondria, like other membranous organelles are transported along the axon by two major families of microtubule-based molecular motors, the kinesin family which mediates anterograde transport away from the cell body toward the axon terminal, and cytoplasmic dynein which drives retrograde transport from the distal axon toward the cell body [139]. Notably, in non-demyelinated cortex in progressive MS patients mitochondrial transport deficits, associated with kinesin decrease, preceded structural axons alterations, and morphological changes in mitochondria [140,141]. Additionally, progressive MS neurons in deeper cortical layers present mitochondrias with mtDNA deletions, indicative of an accelerated aging phenotype [138]. Consequences of mitochondrial abnormalities in neuronal cell bodies and axons are two-fold. First, mitochondrial dysfunction results in energy deficiency, which in mild forms will induce functional disturbances, in the absence of structural damage. However, when injury surpasses a certain threshold, energy deficiency will lead to axonal degeneration and cell death [142]. Once a neuronal system has lost it reserves capacity, it is less capable of spontaneous recovery and hence less prone to functional improvement. Second, mitochondrial injury may amplify oxidative stress through release of oxygen radicals, generated as a result of impaired respiratory chain function, establishing a vicious cycle of tissue destruction [143]. Following demyelination, redistribution of certain isoforms of Na^+ channels (Na_v 1.1 and Na_v 1.6) along the unmyelinated segment ensues, resulting in increased sodium influx. Early redistribution of Na^+ channels along denuded axons in white matter of MS plaques and EAE may allow continuation of action potentials in the context of MS recovery of clinical function [144,145]. Interestingly, Na_v 1.6, which generates persistent electrical current much larger than those of Na_v 1. 2 [146], is co-localized with Na^+/Ca^{2+} exchanger and with APP, a marker of axonal injury. Conversely, Na_v 1. 2 channels may serve an adaptive function with limited ability to sustain high-frequency conduction of action potentials and may contribute to slow depolarization, promoting ectopic firing patterns after demyelination [137]. Slow axonal transport of mitochondria as well as, mitochondrial damage may lead to failure of the Na^+/K^+ ATPase pump, generating a persistent sodium current. Na^+ accumulated in the axoplasm is replaced by Ca^{2+} through a reverse action of the Na^+/Ca^{2+} exchanger. Increased intra-axonal Ca^{2+} activate a variety of catabolic enzymes including proteases, phospholipases and calpains, ultimately leading to progressive proteolytic degradation of cytoskeletal proteins [147]; (Figure 2B). Moreover, intracellular Ca^{2+} increase results in changes in microtubules and neurofilaments (NF) phosphorylation, ultimately causing cytoskeleton breakdown [132]. Additional deleterious accumulation of Ca^{2+} in axons results from influx via L- and N-type Ca^{2+} channels [148], as well as release from intracellular stores in the axoplasmic reticulum. Abnormal axonal accumulation of Ca^{2+} may also result from glutamate neurotoxicity, which alters intracellular Ca^{2+} homeostasis through a mechanism mediated by axonal AMPA/kainate and metabotropic glutamate receptors, located in the intermodal region of the axons [149]. In addition to Na^+ channels, others ion channels show parallel adaptive changes to inflammatory stimuli by altering their distribution in neurons as an initial compensatory mechanism, to preserve conductance and axonal integrity. Redistribution of voltage-gated Ca^{2+} channels transient potential receptors melastatin 4 (TRPM4), and acid-sensing ion channels 1 (ASIC1) induce additional overload of Ca^{2+}, eliciting further deleterious effects on axons [142].

Abnormal accumulations of NF are a pathological hallmark of many human neurodegenerative disorders. Therefore, neurofilament light chain protein (NfL) together with the neurofilament medium (NfM) and heavy (NfH) subunits, are gaining increasing attention as candidate biomarkers of neuroaxonal injury because they are abundant structural scaffolding proteins of the cytoskeleton, with important roles in axon radial growth and stability, enabling effective nerve conduction velocity, as well as dendritic branching and growth [150]. They are exclusively expressed in neurons and reach abnormal levels as a result of axonal damage and eventual neuronal death. Under normal conditions NF are highly stable within axons and their turnover is low. Pathological processes that cause axonal damage release NF proteins into the CSF and peripheral blood, depending on the extent of damage. Initial studies in MS revealed that CSF levels of NfL were associated with the degree of disease activity and disability [151,152]. Furthermore, CSF levels of NfL, fall as a consequence of disease modifying therapies (DMT), suggesting that NfL can be used to monitor therapeutic efficacy [153–155]. However, despite these promising results in MS, a major barrier to widespread adoption of NfL assessment in MS research and clinical practice has been the need for CSF sampling, a problem overcome by use fourth-generation immunoassays, which allow evaluation of serum NfL levels [155]. High serum NfL levels have been associated with disability worsening and relapse status [155,156]. Patients under DMT have lower levels of serum NfL than untreated patients, indicating they are a marker of response to treatment [155]. Notably, a longitudinal study demonstrated patients with increased serum levels of NfL at baseline, independent of MRI variables, experience significantly more brain and spinal cord atrophy over 2 and 5 years of follow-up [156]. Collectively, these observations indicate serum NfL levels can be a useful marker of axonal damage, when applying adequate detection technique.

6. Loss of Myelin Trophism Induces Axonal Degeneration

Although myelin is traditionally viewed as a passive insulating structure, recent reports indicate it may exert a more dynamic role. It has become clear that myelin is metabolically active, allowing movement of macromolecules into the periaxonal space with important contributions to axonal health and neuronal survival. Indeed, once myelination is completed, a major task of oligodendrocytes is the provision of energy-rich substrates to axons required for fast axonal transport and propagation of action potentials. Furthermore, bi-directional signaling exists for efficient recruitment of resources, whereby the axons inform their myelinating cells of their metabolic needs proportionally to their activity. The myelin sheath and its subjacent axon should therefore be regarded as a functional unit coupled not only at the morphologic, but also at the metabolic level [157].

Animal studies have shown that oligodendrocytes exert a critical role in maintenance and long-term survival of axons and neurons. Mice mutant of the oligodendrocyte-specific *Plp1* gene, encoding PLP/DM20 a structural component of the myelin sheath, develop progressive axonal CNS degeneration at an older age. However, in this model PLP/DM20 absence has minimal impact on myelination [158]. Likewise, 2'3' cyclic-nucleotide 3' phosphodiesterase (CNP) knockout mice develop progressive axonopathy and die prematurely. Interestingly, these mice do not show demyelination at ages when axon degeneration is prominent [159,160]. This is surprising because there is strong evidence that CNP is expressed exclusively by oligodendrocytes. Although the pathology in both mutants is similar, mice deficient in both CNP and PLP develop a more severe axonal phenotype than either single mutant, indicating that each oligodendroglial protein serves a distinct role in supporting myelinated axon function [160]. Axonal pathology preceding axonal degeneration includes altered axonal transport and axonal ovoid formation. These findings are more prominent in paranodal regions, where myelin-axonal communication is most likely to occur, and are highly reminiscent of changes found in CNS tissue from MS patients [158,159]. Studies have also investigated the impact of acute death of oligodendroglia on neuron function and survival. Selective ablation of mature oligodendrocytes induced by diphtheria toxin produces axonal injury characterized by accumulation of non-phosphorylated neurofilaments and APP, without spread of myelin degradation Although some mice exhibited abnormalities in myelin composition, overall myelination was not affected, suggesting axonal injury is not due to demyelination [161]. Taken together, these observations from animal models suggest that the myelin-producing function of oligodendrocytes is not coupled to their role in axon preservation, and that oligodendrocytes themselves are critical for axonal function maintenance and survival in adult life.

During development oligodendrocytes import glucose and lactate to allow rapid myelination synthesize large amounts of lipids. When myelination is complete, oligodendrocytes-derived lactate and piruvate can be taken up by energy-deprived axons for mitochondrial ATP production supporting their energy needs [162]. Several experiments indicate monocarboxylic acid transporters (MCTs) are critical to maintain axonal integrity. Based on sequence homology, 16 MCTs members have been identified, of which only MCT1, 2 and 4 are found in the CNS [163]. As oligodendrocytes accumulate intracellular lactate, this substrate can flow through MCT1 into the periaxonal space, where neurons capture it through MCT2 and metabolize it to supplement energy requirements [162,164]. (Figure 2C). Notably, both genetic and pharmacologic down-regulation of MCT1, which is present almost exclusively in oligodendrocytes, results in axon degeneration and neuronal loss both in vivo and in vitro, without obvious oligodendrocyte damage [165]. Although the observations mentioned above provide strong evidence for a role of oligodendrocytes in directly supplying energy support to axons, other cells including astrocytes may also participate [166]. Astrocytes are essentially the only cells containing glycogen in the adult CNS, and glycogen metabolism followed by glyscolisis provides a source of lactate for other cells [167]. Studies show astrocytes transfer energy metabolites directly to oligodendrocytes, which in turn support neurons and axons metabolism as previously discussed (Figure 2C). Connections between astrcytes and myelinating cells occur via gap junctions formed by connexins (Cx). These gap junctions comprise Cx32 and Cx47 expressed on oligodendrocytes which form heteromeric channels with astrocytes through Cx30 and Cx43 respectively. Double mutant CX32- and Cx43-deficient mice exhibit profound CNS demyelination and axonal injury [168]. Likewise, CX47 and Cx30 double null mice, in which connections between astrocytes and oligodendrcoytes are altered, also developed myelin pathology and severe axonal degeneration [169]. Similarly, loss of Cx43 inhibits glucose delivery to progenitor oligodendrocytes cells and their proliferation, which can in turn influence oligodendrogenesis, and oligodendrocyte metabolic support [170]. Overall these findings provide new insights into the role of oligodendrocytes and astrocytes biology. Identification of bi-directional signaling pathways by which oligodendrocytes influence the axonal metabolism, is highly relevant to understanding MS progression.

7. Conclusions and Future Perspectives

Identification of effective therapies for progressive MS remains a priority and a challenge for the MS community. In order to develop new and effective treatment strategies it is necessary to better understand the pathological mechanisms driving disease. Unfortunately, absence of adequate animal models makes identification of potential therapeutic targets even more difficult. In this article we have recapitulated some of the main mechanisms involved in MS progression. Undoubtedly more research will lead to a better understanding of the processes of demyelination/remyelination, as well as of the importance of glial cells in neuronal homeostasis and neuronal degeneration. Clearly, identifying effective therapies for progressive MS would largely be contingent upon a comprehensive understanding of its pathogenesis, animal models incorporating these pathogenic characteristics, novel trial designs including more sensitive outcome measures, and new models of collaboration between physicians and basic science researchers.

Author Contributions: J.C. contributed to the conception and design of the manuscript, drafted the original, designed the figures, revised the draft and provided important intellectual contributions. M.M. contributed to drafting of the original manuscript, design of the figures, and providing important intellectual contributions.

M.C.Y. contributed to drafting the original manuscript, designing the figures, and providing important intellectual contributions.

Funding: This study was supported by an internal grant from FLENI (J.C.).

Acknowledgments: We thank the collaboration of María Inés Gaitán, and Ismael Calandri for the preparation of the figures.

Conflicts of Interest: J.C. is a board member of Merck-Serono Argentina, Biogen-Idec LATAM, Merck-Serono LATAM, and Genzyme global. Jorge Correale has received reimbursement for developing educational presentations for Merck-Serono Argentina, Merck-Serono LATAM, Biogen-Idec Argentina, Genzyme Argentina, and TEVA Argentina as well as professional travel/accommodations stipends. M.M. has nothing to disclose. M.C.Y. has received reimbursement for developing educational presentations and for travel/accommodations stipends from Merck-Serono Argentina, Biogen-Idec Argentina, Genzyme Argentina, Bayer Inc, Novartis Argentina and TEVA-Tuteur Argentina.

References

1. Thomson, A.J.; Baranzini, S.E.; Geurts, J.; Hemmer, B.; Ciccarelli, O. Multiple Sclerosis. *Lancet* **2018**, *391*, 1622–1636. [CrossRef]
2. Lassmann, H.; Brück, W.; Lucchinetti, C.F. The immunopathology of multiple sclerosis: An overview. *Brain Pathol.* **2007**, *17*, 210–218. [CrossRef] [PubMed]
3. Baecher-Allan, C.; Kaskow, B.J.; Weiner, H.L. Multiple sclerosis: Mechanisms and immunotherapy. *Neuron* **2018**, *97*, 742–768. [CrossRef] [PubMed]
4. Lublin, F.D.; Reingold, S.C. Defining the clinical course of multiple sclerosis: Results of an international survey. *Neurology* **1996**, *46*, 907–911. [CrossRef] [PubMed]
5. Skulina, C.; Schmidt, S.; Dornmair, K.; Babbe, H.; Roers, A.; Rajewsky, K.; Wekerle, H.; Hohlfeld, R.; Goebels, N. Multiple sclerosis: Brain-infiltrating CD8$^+$ T cells persist as clonal expansions in the cerebrospinal fluid and blood. *Proc. Natl. Acad. Sci. USA* **2004**, *101*, 2428–2433. [CrossRef] [PubMed]
6. Ghione, E.; Bergsland, N.; Ghione, E.; Bergsland, N.; Dwyer, M.G.; Hagemeier, J.; Jakimovski, D.; Paunkoski, I.; Ramasamy, D.P.; Silva, D.; et al. Brain Atrophy Is Associated with Disability Progression in Patients with MS followed in a Clinical Routine. *Am. J. Neuroradiol.* **2018**, *39*, 2237–2242. [CrossRef] [PubMed]
7. Trapp, B.D.; Peterson, J.; Ransohoff, R.M.; Rudick, R.; Mörk, S.; Bö, L. Axonal transection in lesions of Multiple Sclerosis. *N. Engl. J. Med.* **1998**, *338*, 278–285. [CrossRef] [PubMed]
8. Peterson, J.W.; Bö, L.; Mörk, S.; Chang, A.; Trapp, B.D. Transected neurites, apoptotic neurons, and reduced inflammation in cortical multiple sclerosis lesions. *Ann. Neurol.* **2001**, *50*, 389–400. [CrossRef]
9. Kutzelnigg, A.; Faber-Rod, J.C.; Bauer, J.; Lucchinetti, C.F.; Sorensen, P.S.; Laursen, H.; Stadelmann, C.; Brück, W.; Rauschka, H.; Schmidbauer, M.; et al. Widespread demyelination in the cerebellar cortex in multiple sclerosis. *Brain Pathol.* **2007**, *17*, 38–44. [CrossRef]
10. Geurts, J.J.; Bö, L.; Roosendaal, S.D.; Hazes, T.; Daniëls, R.; Barkhof, F.; Witter, M.P.; Huitinga, I.; van der Valk, P. Extensive hippocampal demyelination in multiple sclerosis. *J. Neuropathol. Exp. Neurol.* **2007**, *66*, 819–827. [CrossRef]
11. Vercellino, M.; Masera, S.; Lorenzatti, M.; Condello, C.; Merola, A.; Mattioda, A.; Tribolo, A.; Capello, E.; Mancardi, G.L.; Mutani, R.; et al. Demyelination, inflammation, and neurodegeneration in multiple sclerosis deep gray matter. *J. Neuropathol. Exp. Neurol.* **2009**, *68*, 489–502. [CrossRef] [PubMed]
12. Wegner, C.; Esiri, M.M.; Chance, S.A.; Palace, J.; Matthews, P.M. Neocortical neuronal, synaptic, and glial loss in multiple sclerosis. *Neurology* **2006**, *67*, 960–967. [CrossRef] [PubMed]
13. Kutzelnigg, A.; Lucchinetti, C.F.; Stadelmann, C.; Brück, W.; Rauschka, H.; Bergmann, M.; Schmidbauer, M.; Parisi, J.E.; Lassmann, H. Cortical demyelination and diffuse white matter injury in multiple sclerosis. *Brain* **2005**, *128*, 2705–2712. [CrossRef] [PubMed]
14. De Stefano, N.; Matthews, P.M. Evidence of early cortical atrophy in MS Relevance to white matter changes and disability. *Neurology* **2003**, *60*, 1157–1162. [CrossRef] [PubMed]
15. Montalban, X.; Gold, R.; Thompson, A.J.; Otero-Romero, S.; Amato, M.P.; Chandraratna, D.; Clanet, M.; Comi, G.; Derfuss, T.; Fazekas, F.; et al. ECTRIMS/EAN guideline on the pharmacological treatment of people with multiple sclerosis. *Eur. J. Neurol.* **2018**, *25*, 215–237. [CrossRef] [PubMed]

16. Rae-Grant, A.; Day, G.S.; Marrie, R.A.; Rabinstein, A.; Cree, B.A.C.; Gronseth, G.S.; Haboubi, M.; Halper, J.; Hosey, J.P.; Jones, D.E.; et al. Comprehensive systematic review summary: Disease-modifying therapies for adults with multiple sclerosis: Report of the Guideline Development, Dissemination, and Implementation Subcommittee of the American Academy of Neurology. *Neurology* **2018**, *90*, 789–800. [CrossRef] [PubMed]

17. Bø, L.; Vedeler, C.A.; Nyland, H.I.; Trapp, B.D.; Mørk, S.J. Subpial demyelination in the cerebral cortex of multiple sclerosis patients. *J. Neuropathol. Exp. Neurol.* **2003**, *62*, 723–732. [CrossRef] [PubMed]

18. Bø, L.; Geurts, J.J.G.; Nyland, H.I.; Trapp, B.D.; Mørk, S.J. Grey matter pathology in multiple sclerosis. *Acta Neurol. Scand.* **2006**, *113*, 48–50. [CrossRef]

19. Magliozzi, R.; Howell, O.; Vora, A.; Serafini, B.; Nicholas, R.; Puopolo, M.; Reynolds, R.; Aloisi, F. Meningeal B-cell follicles in secondary progressive multiple sclerosis associate with early onset of disease and severe cortical pathology. *Brain* **2007**, *130*, 1089–1104. [CrossRef]

20. Bevan, R.J.; Evans, R.; Griffiths, L.; Watkins, L.M.; Rees, M.I.; Magliozzi, R.; Allen, I.; McDonnell, G.; Kee, R.; Naughton, M.; et al. Meningeal inflammation and cortical demyelination in acute multiple sclerosis. *Ann. Neurol.* **2018**, *84*, 829–842. [CrossRef]

21. Eshaghi, A.; Prados, F.; Brownlee, W.J.; Altmann, D.R.; Tur, C.; Cardoso, M.J.; De Angelis, F.; van de Pavert, S.H.; Cawley, N.; De Stefano, N.; et al. Deep gray matter volume loss drives disability worsening in multiple sclerosis. *Ann. Neurol.* **2018**, *83*, 210–222. [CrossRef] [PubMed]

22. Lucchinetti, C.F.; Popescu, B.F.; Bunyan, R.F.; Moll, N.M.; Roemer, S.F.; Lassmann, H.; Brück, W.; Parisi, J.E.; Scheithauer, B.W.; Giannini, C.; et al. Inflammatory cortical demyelination in early multiple sclerosis. *N. Engl. J. Med.* **2011**, *365*, 2188–2197. [CrossRef] [PubMed]

23. Magliozzi, R.; Howell, O.W.; Reeves, C.; Roncaroli, F.; Nicholas, R.; Serafini, B.; Aloisi, F.; Reynolds, R. A gradient of neuronal loss and meningeal inflammation in multiple sclerosis. *Ann. Neurol.* **2010**, *68*, 477–493. [CrossRef] [PubMed]

24. Popescu, B.F.; Lucchinetti, C.F. Meningeal and cortical grey matter pathology in multiple sclerosis. *BMC Neurol.* **2012**, *12*, 11. [CrossRef] [PubMed]

25. Steenwijk, M.D.; Geurts, J.J.G.; Daams, M.; Tijms, B.M.; Wink, A.M.; Balk, L.J.; Tewarie, P.K.; Uitdehaag, B.M.; Barkhof, F.; Vrenken, H.; et al. Cortical atrophy patterns in multiple sclerosis are non-random and clinically relevant. *Brain* **2016**, *139*, 115–126. [CrossRef]

26. Granberg, T.; Fan, Q.; Treaba, C.A.; Ouellette, R.; Herranz, E.; Mangeat, G.; Louapre, C.; Cohen-Adad, J.; Klawiter, E.C.; Sloane, J.A.; et al. In vivo characterization of cortical and white matter neuroaxonal pathology in early multiple sclerosis. *Brain* **2017**, *140*, 2912–2926. [CrossRef] [PubMed]

27. Geurts, J.J.; Barkhof, F. Grey matter pathology in multiple sclerosis. *Lancet* **2008**, *7*, 841–851. [CrossRef]

28. Popescu, B.F.; Pirko, I.; Lucchinetti, C.F. Pathology of multiple sclerosis: Where do we stand? *Continuum* **2013**, *19*, 901–921. [CrossRef]

29. Lagumersindez-Denis, N.; Wrzos, C.; Mack, M.; Winkler, A.; van der Meer, F.; Reinert, M..; Hollasch, H.; Flach, A.; Brühl, H.; Cullen, E.; et al. Differential contribution of immune effector mechanisms to cortical demyelination in multiple scleosis. *Acta Neuropathol.* **2017**, *134*, 15–34. [CrossRef]

30. Chang, A.; Staugaitis, S.M.; Dutta, R.; Batt, C.E.; Easley, K.E.; Chomyk, A.M.; Yong, V.W.; Fox, R.J.; Kidd, G.J.; Trapp, B.D. Cortical remyelination: A new target for repair therapies in multiple sclerosis. *Ann. Neurol.* **2012**, *72*, 918–926. [CrossRef]

31. Bø, L.; Vedeler, C.A.; Nyland, H.; Trapp, B.D.; Mørk, S.J. Intracortical multiple sclerosis lesions are not associated with increased lymphocyte infiltration. *Mult. Scler.* **2003**, *9*, 323–331. [CrossRef] [PubMed]

32. Bö, L.; Geurts, J.J.; van der Valk, P.; Polman, C.; Barkhof, F. Lack of correlation between cortical demyelination and white matter pathologic changes in multiple sclerosis. *Arch. Neurol.* **2007**, *64*, 76–80. [CrossRef] [PubMed]

33. Fisniku, L.K.; Chard, D.T.; Jackson, J.S.; Anderson, V.M.; Altmann, D.R.; Miszkiel, K.A.; Thompson, A.J.; Miller, D.H. Gray matter atrophy is related to long-term disability in multiple sclerosis. *Ann. Neurol.* **2008**, *64*, 247–254. [CrossRef] [PubMed]

34. Fisher, E.; Lee, J.C.; Nakamura, K.; Rudick, R.A. Gray matter atrophy in multiple sclerosis: A longitudinal study. *Ann. Neurol.* **2008**, *64*, 255–265. [CrossRef] [PubMed]

35. Evangelou, N.; Konz, D.; Esiri, M.M.; Smith, S.; Palace, J.; Matthews, P.M. Size-selective neuronal changes in the anterior optic pathways suggest a differential susceptibility to injury in multiple sclerosis. *Brain* **2001**, *124*, 1813–1820. [CrossRef] [PubMed]

36. Azevedo, C.J.; Cen, S.Y.; Khadka, S.; Liu, S.; Kornak, J.; Shi, Y.; Zheng, L.; Hauser, S.L.; Pelletier, D. Thalamic atrophy in multiple sclerosis: A magnetic resonance imaging marker of neurodegeneration throughout disease. *Ann. Neurol.* **2018**, *83*, 223–234. [CrossRef] [PubMed]

37. Gaetano, L.; Häring, D.A.; Radue, E.W.; Mueller-Lenke, N.; Thakur, A.; Tomic, D.; Kappos, L.; Sprenger, T. Fingolimod effect on gray matter, thalamus, and white matter in patients with multiple sclerosis. *Neurology* **2018**, *90*, e1324–e1332. [CrossRef] [PubMed]

38. Fischer, M.T.; Wimmer, I.; Höftberger, R.; Gerlach, S.; Haider, L.; Zrzavy, T.; Hametner, S.; Mahad, D.; Binder, C.J.; Krumbholz, M.; et al. Disease-specific molecular events in cortical multiple sclerosis lesions. *Brain* **2013**, *136*, 1799–1815. [CrossRef]

39. Meuth, S.G.; Simon, O.J.; Grimm, A.; Melzer, N.; Herrmann, A.M.; Spitzer, P.; Landgraf, P.; Wiendl, H. CNS inflammation and neuronal degeneration is aggravated by impaired CD200–CD200R-mediated macrophage silencing. *J. Neuroimmunol.* **2008**, *194*, 62–69. [CrossRef]

40. Barnett, M.H.; Prineas, J.W. Relapsing and remitting multiple sclerosis: Pathology of the newly forming lesion. *Ann. Neurol.* **2004**, *55*, 458–468. [CrossRef]

41. Kassmann, C.M.; Lappe-Siefke, C.; Baes, M.; Brügger, B.; Mildner, A.; Werner, H.B.; Natt, O.; Michaelis, T.; Prinz, M.; Frahm, J.; Nave, K.A. Axonal loss and neuroinflammation caused by peroxisome-deficient oligodendrocytes. *Nat. Genet.* **2007**, *39*, 969. [CrossRef] [PubMed]

42. Hemmer, B.; Kerschensteiner, M.; Korn, T. Role of the innate and adaptive immune responses in the course of multiple sclerosis. *Lancet Neurol.* **2015**, *14*, 406–419. [CrossRef]

43. Magliozzi, R.; Howell, O.W.; Nicholas, R.; Cruciani, C.; Castellaro, M.; Romualdi, C.; Rossi, S.; Pitteri, M.; Benedetti, M.D.; Gajofatto, A.; et al. Inflammatory intrathecal profiles and cortical damage in multiple sclerosis. *Ann. Neurol.* **2018**, *83*, 739–755. [CrossRef] [PubMed]

44. Bar-Or, A.; Fawaz, L.; Fan, B.; Darlington, P.J.; Rieger, A.; Ghorayeb, C.; Calabresi, P.A.; Waubant, E.; Hauser, S.L.; Zhang, J.; et al. Abnormal B-cell cytokine responses a trigger of T-cell–mediated disease in MS? *Ann. Neurol.* **2010**, *67*, 452–461. [CrossRef] [PubMed]

45. Aloisi, F.; Pujol-Borrell, R. Lymphoid neogenesis in chronic inflammatory diseases. *Nat. Rev. Immunol.* **2006**, *6*, 205–217. [CrossRef] [PubMed]

46. Serafini, B.; Rosicarelli, B.; Magliozzi, R.; Stigliano, E.; Aloisi, F. Detection of ectopic B-cell follicles with germinal centers in the meninges of patients with secondary progressive multiple sclerosis. *Brain Pathol.* **2004**, *14*, 164–174. [CrossRef] [PubMed]

47. Pitzalis, C.; Jones, G.W.; Bombardieri, M.; Jones, S.A. Ectopic lymphoid-like structures in infection, cancer and autoimmunity. *Nat. Rev. Immunol.* **2014**, *14*, 447. [CrossRef] [PubMed]

48. Corsiero, E.; Nerviani, A.; Bombardieri, M.; Pitzalis, C. Ectopic lymphoid structures: Powerhouse of autoimmunity. *Front. Immunol.* **2016**, *7*, 430. [CrossRef] [PubMed]

49. Jones, G.W.; Jones, S.A. Ectopic lymphoid follicles: Inducible centers for generating antigen-specific immune responses within tissues. *Immunology* **2016**, *147*, 141–151. [CrossRef] [PubMed]

50. Lovato, L.; Willis, S.N.; Rodig, S.J.; Caron, T.; Almendinger, S.E.; Howell, O.W.; Reynolds, R.; O'Connor, K.C.; Hafler, D.A. Related B cell clones populate the meninges and parenchyma of patients with multiple sclerosis. *Brain* **2011**, *134*, 534–541. [CrossRef] [PubMed]

51. Howell, O.W.; Reeves, C.A.; Nicholas, R.; Carassiti, D.; Radotra, B.; Gentleman, S.M.; Serafini, B.; Aloisi, F.; Roncaroli, F.; Magliozzi, R.; et al. Meningeal inflammation is widespread and linked to cortical pathology in multiple sclerosis. *Brain* **2011**, *134*, 2755–2771. [CrossRef] [PubMed]

52. Corsiero, E.; Bombardieri, M.; Manzo, A.; Bugatti, S.; Uguccioni, M.; Pitzalis, C. Role of lymphoid chemokines in the development of functional ectopic lymphoid structures in rheumatic autoimmune diseases. *Immunol. Lett.* **2012**, *145*, 62–67. [CrossRef] [PubMed]

53. Vanguri, P.; Shin, M.L. Activation of complement by myelin: Identification of C1-binding proteins of human myelin from central nervous tissue. *J. Neurochem.* **1986**, *46*, 1535–1541. [CrossRef] [PubMed]

54. Huizinga, R.; Heijmans, N.; Schubert, P.; Gschmeissner, S.; 't Hart, B.A.; Herrmann, H.; Amor, S. Immunization with neurofilament light protein induces spastic paresis and axonal degeneration in Biozzi ABH mice. *J. Neuropathol. Exp. Neurol.* **2007**, *66*, 295–304. [CrossRef] [PubMed]

55. Mathey, E.K.; Derfuss, T.; Storch, M.K.; Williams, K.R.; Hales, K.; Woolley, D.R.; Al-Hayani, A.; Davies, S.N.; Rasband, M.N.; Olsson, T.; et al. Neurofascin as a novel target for autoantibody-mediated axonal injury. *J. Exp. Med.* **2007**, *204*, 2363–2372. [CrossRef] [PubMed]

56. Manzo, A.; Bombardieri, M.; Humby, F.; Pitzalis, C. Secondary and ectopic lymphoid tissue responses in rheumatoid arthritis: From inflammation to autoimmunity and tissue damage/remodeling. *Immunol. Rev.* **2010**, *233*, 267–285. [CrossRef] [PubMed]

57. Makshakov, G.; Magonov, E.; Totolyan, N.; Nazarov, V.; Lapin, S.; Mazing, A.; Verbitskaya, E.; Trofimova, T.; Krasnov, V.; Shumilina, M.; et al. Leptomeningeal contrast enhancement is associated with disability progression and grey matter atrophy in multiple sclerosis. *Neurol. Res. Int.* **2017**. [CrossRef] [PubMed]

58. Zivadinov, R.; Ramasamy, D.P.; Vaneckova, M.; Gandhi, S.; Chandra, A.; Hagemeier, J.; Bergsland, N.; Polak, P.; Benedict, R.H.; Hojnacki, D.; et al. Leptomeningeal contrast enhancement is associated with progression of cortical atrophy in MS: A retrospective, pilot, observational longitudinal study. *Mult. Scler.* **2016**, *23*, 1336–1345. [CrossRef] [PubMed]

59. Choi, S.R.; Howell, O.W.; Carassiti, D.; Magliozzi, R.; Gveric, D.; Muraro, P.A.; Nicholas, R.; Roncaroli, F.; Reynolds, R. Meningeal inflammation plays a role in the pathology of primary progressive multiple sclerosis. *Brain* **2012**, *135*, 2925–2937. [CrossRef] [PubMed]

60. Antel, J.; Antel, S.; Caramanos, Z.; Arnold, D.L.; Kuhlmann, T. Primary progressive multiple sclerosis: Part of the MS disease spectrum or separate disease entity? *Acta Neuropathol.* **2012**, *123*, 627–638. [CrossRef] [PubMed]

61. Ascherio, A.; Munger, K.L.; Lennette, E.T.; Spiegelman, D.; Hernán, M.A.; Olek, M.J.; Hankinson, S.E.; Hunter, D.J. Epstein-Barr virus antibodies and risk of multiple sclerosis: A prospective study. *JAMA* **2001**, *286*, 3083–3088. [CrossRef] [PubMed]

62. Warner, H.B.; Carp, R.I. Multiple Sclerosis and Epstein-Barr virus. *Lancet* **1981**, *2*, 1290. [CrossRef]

63. Serafini, B.; Rosicarelli, B.; Franciotta, D.; Magliozzi, R.; Reynolds, R.; Cinque, P.; Andreoni, L.; Trivedi., P.; Salvetti, M.; Faggioni, A.; et al. Dysregulated Epstein-Barr virus infection in the multiple sclerosis brain. *J. Exp. Med.* **2007**, *204*, 2899–2912. [CrossRef] [PubMed]

64. Küppers, R. B cells under influence: Transformation of B cells by Epstein–Barr virus. *Nat. Rev. Immunol.* **2003**, *3*, 801. [CrossRef] [PubMed]

65. Willis, S.N.; Stadelmann, C.; Rodig, S.J.; Caron, T.; Gattenloehner, S.; Mallozzi, S.S.; Roughan, J.E.; Almendinger, S.E.; Blewett, M.M.; Brück, W.; et al. Epstein–Barr virus infection is not a characteristic feature of multiple sclerosis brain. *Brain* **2009**, *132*, 3318–3328. [CrossRef] [PubMed]

66. Hislop, A.D.; Taylor, G.S.; Sauce, D.; Rickinson, A.B. Cellular responses to viral infection in humans: Lessons from Epstein-Barr virus. *Annu. Rev. Immunol.* **2007**, *25*, 587–617. [CrossRef] [PubMed]

67. Magliozzi, R.; Serafini, B.; Rosicarel, B.; Chiappetta, G.; Veroni, C.; Reynolds, R.; Aloisi, F. B-cell enrichment and Epstein-Barr virus infection in inflammatory cortical lesions in secondary progressive multiple sclerosis. *J. Neuropathol. Exp. Neurol.* **2013**, *72*, 29–41. [CrossRef] [PubMed]

68. Bitsch, A.; Schuchardt, J.; Bunkowski, S.; Kuhlmann, T.; Brück, W. Acute axonal injury in multiple sclerosis: Correlation with demyelination and inflammation. *Brain* **2000**, *123*, 1174–1183. [CrossRef] [PubMed]

69. Medana, I.M.; Gallimore, A.; Oxenius, A.; Martinic, M.M.; Wekerle, H.; Neumann, H. MHC class I-restricted killing of neurons by virus-specific CD8$^+$ T lymphocytes is effected through the Fas/FasL, but not the perforin pathway. *Eur. J. Immunol.* **2000**, *30*, 3623–3633. [CrossRef]

70. Meuth, S.G.; Herrmann, A.M.; Simon, O.J.; Siffrin, V.; Melzer, N.; Bittner, S.; Meuth, P.; Langer, H.F.; Hallermann, S.; Boldakowa, N.; et al. Cytotoxic CD8$^+$ T cell–neuron interactions: Perforin-dependent electrical silencing precedes but is not causally linked to neuronal cell death. *J. Neurosci.* **2009**, *29*, 15397–15409. [CrossRef] [PubMed]

71. Junker, A.; Ivanidze, J.; Malotka, J.; Eiglmeier, I.; Lassmann, H.; Wekerle, H.; Meinl, E.; Hohlfeld, R.; Dornmair, K. Multiple sclerosis: T-cell receptor expression in distinct brain regions. *Brain* **2007**, *130*, 2789–2799. [CrossRef] [PubMed]

72. Jacobsen, M.; Cepok, S.; Quak, E.; Happel, M.; Gaber, R.; Ziegler, A.; Schock, S.; Oertel, W.H.; Sommer, N.; Hemmer, B. Oligoclonal expansion of memory CD8$^+$ T cells in cerebrospinal fluid from multiple sclerosis patients. *Brain* **2002**, *125*, 538–550. [CrossRef] [PubMed]

73. Mars, L.T.; Saikali, P.; Liblau, R.S.; Arbour, N. Contribution of CD8 T lymphocytes to the immuno-pathogenesis of multiple sclerosis and its animal models. *Biochim. Biophys. Acta* **2011**, *1812*, 151–161. [CrossRef] [PubMed]

74. Kuhlmann, T.; Lingfeld, G.; Bitsch, A.; Schuchardt, J.; Brück, W. Acute axonal damage in multiple sclerosis is most extensive in early disease stages and decreases over time. *Brain* **2002**, *125*, 2202–2212. [CrossRef] [PubMed]

75. Ferguson, B.; Matyszak, M.K.; Esiri, M.M.; Perry, V.H. Axonal damage in acute multiple sclerosis lesions. *Brain* **1997**, *120*, 393–399. [CrossRef] [PubMed]

76. Höftberger, R.; Aboul-Enein, F.; Brueck, W.; Lucchinetti, C.; Rodriguez, M.; Schmidbauer, M.; Jellinger, K.; Lassmann, H. Expression of major histocompatibility complex class I molecules on the different cell types in multiple sclerosis lesions. *Brain Pathol.* **2004**, *14*, 43–50. [CrossRef] [PubMed]

77. Huse, M.; Quann, E.J.; Davis, M.M. Shouts, whispers and the kiss of death: Directional secretion in T cells. *Nat. Immunol.* **2008**, *9*, 1105. [CrossRef] [PubMed]

78. Mizuno, T.; Zhang, G.; Takeuchi, H.; Kawanokuchi, J.; Wang, J.; Sonobe, Y.; Jin, S.; Takada, N.; Komatsu, Y.; Suzumura, A. Interferon-γ directly induces neurotoxicity through a neuron specific, calcium-permeable complex of IFN-γ receptor and AMPA GluR1 receptor. *FASEB J.* **2008**, *22*, 1797–1806. [CrossRef] [PubMed]

79. Venters, H.D.; Dantzer, R.; Kelley, K.W. A new concept in neurodegeneration: TNFα is a silencer of survival signals. *Trend Neurosci.* **2000**, *23*, 175–180. [CrossRef]

80. Wang, T.; Allie, R.; Conant, K.; Haughey, N.; Turchan-Chelowo, J.; Hahn, K.; Rosen, A.; Steiner, J.; Keswani, S.; Jones, M.; et al. Granzyme B mediates neurotoxicity through a G-protein-coupled receptor. *FASEB J.* **2006**, *20*, 1209–1211. [CrossRef] [PubMed]

81. Giuliani, F.; Goodyer, C.G.; Antel, J.P.; Yong, V.W. Vulnerability of human neurons to T cell-mediated cytotoxicity. *J. Immunol.* **2003**, *171*, 368–379. [CrossRef] [PubMed]

82. Raveney, B.J.E.; Oki, O.; Hohjoh, H.; Nakamura, M.; Sato, W.; Murata, M.; Yamamura, T. Eomesodermin-expressing T-helper cells are essential for chronic neuroinflammation. *Nat. Commun.* **2015**, *6*, 8437. [CrossRef] [PubMed]

83. Broux, B.; Markovic-Plese, S.; Stinissen, P.; Hellings, N. Pathogenic features of CD4$^+$CD28$^-$ T cells in immune disorders. *Trends Mol. Med.* **2012**, *18*, 446–453. [CrossRef] [PubMed]

84. Kovalcsik, E.; Antunes, R.F.; Baruah, P.; Kaski, J.C.; Dumitriu, J.E. Proteasome-mediated reduction in proapoptotic molecule Bim renders CD4$^+$CD28^{null} T cell resistant to apoptosis in acute coronary syndrome. *Circulation* **2015**, *131*, 709–720. [CrossRef] [PubMed]

85. Thewissen, M.; Somers, V.; Hellings, N.; Fraussen, J.; Damoiseaux, J.; Stinissen, P. CD4$^+$CD28^{null} T cells in autoimmune disease: Pathogenic features and decreased susceptibility to immunoregualtion. *J. Immunol.* **2007**, *179*, 6514–6523. [CrossRef] [PubMed]

86. Markovic-Plese, S.; Cortese, I.; Wandinger, K.P.; McFarland, H.F.; Martin, R. CD4$^+$CD28$^-$ costimualtion-independent T cells in multiple sclerosis. *J. Clin. Investig.* **2001**, *108*, 1185–1194. [CrossRef] [PubMed]

87. Scholz, C.; Patton, K.T.; Anderson, D.E.; Freeman, G.J.; Hafler, D.A. Expansion of autoreactive T cells in multiple sclerosis is independent of exogenous B7 costimulation. *J. Immunol.* **1998**, *160*, 1532–1538. [PubMed]

88. Dumitriu, I.E.; Araguás, E.T.; Baboorian, C.; Kaski, J.C. CD4$^+$CD28^{null} T cells in coronary artery disease: When helpers become killers. *Cardiovasc. Res.* **2009**, *81*, 11–19. [CrossRef]

89. Peeters, L.M.; Vanheusden, M.; Somers, V.; Van Wijmeersch, B.; Stinissen, P.; Broux, B.; Hellings, N. Cytotoxic CD4$^+$ T cells drive multiple sclerosis progression. *Front. Immunol.* **2017**, *8*, 1160. [CrossRef]

90. Schmidt, D.; Goronzy, J.J.; Weyand, C.M. CD4$^+$ CD7$^-$ CD28$^-$ T cells are expanded in rheumatoid arthritis and are characterized by autoreactivity. *J. Clin. Investig.* **1996**, *97*, 2027–2037. [CrossRef]

91. Lassmann, H. Multiple sclerosis: Lessons from molecular neuropathology. *Exp. Neurol.* **2014**, *262*, 2–7. [CrossRef] [PubMed]

92. Kigerl, K.A.; de Rivero Vaccari, J.P.; Dietrich, W.D.; Popovich, P.G.; Keane, R.W. Pattern recognition recpetors and central nervous system repair. *Exp. Neurol.* **2014**, *258*, 5–16. [CrossRef] [PubMed]

93. De Groot, C.J.A.; Bergers, E.; Kamphorst, W.; Ravid, R.; Polman, C.H.; Barkhof, F.; van der Valk, P. Post-mortem MRI-guided sampling of multiple sclerosis brain lesions: Increased yield of active demyelinating and (p) reactive lesions. *Brain* **2001**, *124*, 1635–1645. [CrossRef] [PubMed]

94. Singh, S.; Metz, I.; Amor, S.; van der Valk, P.; Stadelmann, C.; Brück, W. Microglial nodules in early multiple sclerosis white matter are associated with degenerating axons. *Acta Neuropathol.* **2013**, *125*, 595–608. [CrossRef] [PubMed]

95. Correale, J. The role of microglial activation in disease progression. *Mult. Scler.* **2014**, *20*, 1288–1295. [CrossRef] [PubMed]

96. Campbell, G.R.; Ziabreva, I.; Ziabreva, I.; Reeve, A.K.; Krishnan, K.J.; Reynolds, R.; Howell, O.; Lassmann, H.; Turnbull, D.M.; Mahad, D.J. Mitochondrial DNA deletions and neurodegeneration in multiple sclerosis. *Ann. Neurol.* **2011**, *69*, 481–492. [CrossRef]

97. Nikić, I.; Merkler, D.; Sorbara, C.; Brinkoetter, M.; Kreutzfeldt, M.; Bareyre, F.M.; Brück, W.; Bishop, D.; Misgeld, T.; Kerschensteiner, M. A reversible form of axon damage in experimental autoimmune encephalomyelitis and multiple sclerosis. *Nat. Med.* **2011**, *17*, 495. [CrossRef]

98. Hametner, S.; Wimmer, I.; Haider, L.; Pfeifenbring, S.; Brück, W.; Lassmann, H. Iron and neurodegeneration in the multiple sclerosis brain. *Ann. Neurol.* **2013**, *74*, 848–861. [CrossRef]

99. Politis, M.; Su, P.; Piccini, P. Imaging of microglia in patients with neurodegenerative disorders. *Front. Pharmacol.* **2012**, *3*, 96. [CrossRef]

100. Cosenza-Nashat, M.; Zhao, M.L.; Suh, H.S.; Morgan, J.; Natividad., R.; Morgello, S.; Lee, S.C. Expression of the translocator protein of 18 kDa by microglia, macrophages and astrocytes based on immunohistochemical localization in abnormal human brain. *Neuropathol. Appl. Neurobiol.* **2009**, *35*, 306–328. [CrossRef]

101. Maeda, J.; Higuchi, M.; Inaji, M.; Ji, B.; Haneda, E.; Okauchi, T.; Zhang, M.R.; Suzuki, K.; Suhara, T. Phase-dependent roles of reactive microglia and astrocytes in nervous system injury as delineated by imaging of peripheral benzodiazepine receptor. *Brain Res.* **2007**, *1157*, 100–111. [CrossRef] [PubMed]

102. Banati, R.B.; Newcombe, J.; Gunn, R.N.; Cagnin, A.; Turkheimer, F.; Heppner, F.; Price, G.; Wegner, F.; Giovannoni, G.; Miller, D.H.; et al. The peripheral benzodiazepine binding site in the brain in multiple sclerosis: Quantitative in vivo imaging of microglia as a measure of disease activity. *Brain* **2000**, *123*, 2321–2337. [CrossRef] [PubMed]

103. Versijpt, J.; Debruyne, J.C.; Van Laere, K.J.; De Vos, F.; Keppens, J.; Strijckmans, K.; Achten, E.; Slegers, G.; Dierckx, R.A.; Korf, J.; et al. Microglial imaging with positron emission tomography and atrophy measurements with magnetic resonance imaging in multiple sclerosis: A correlative study. *Mult. Scler.* **2005**, *11*, 127–134. [CrossRef] [PubMed]

104. Politis, M.; Giannetti, P.; Su, P.; Turkheimer, F.; Keihaninejad, S.; Wu, K.; Waldman, A.; Malik, O.; Matthews, P.M.; Reynolds, R.; et al. Increased PK11195 PET binding in the cortex of patients with MS correlates with disability. *Neurology* **2012**, *79*, 523–530. [CrossRef] [PubMed]

105. Airas, L.; Nylund, M.; Rissanen, E. Evaluation of Microglial Activation in Multiple Sclerosis Patients Using Positron Emission Tomography. *Front. Neurol.* **2018**, *9*, 181. [CrossRef] [PubMed]

106. Sharma, R.; Fischer, M.T.; Bauer, J.; Felts, P.A.; Smith, K.J.; Misu, T.; Fujihara, K.; Bradl, M.; Lassmann, H. Inflammation induced by innate immunity in the central nervous system leads to primary astrocyte dysfunction followed by demyelination. *Acta Neuropathol.* **2010**, *120*, 223–236. [CrossRef] [PubMed]

107. Grinnell, A.D.; Chen, B.M.; Kashani, A.; Lin, J.; Suzuki, K.; Kidokoro, Y. The role of integrins in the modulation of neurotransmitter release from motor nerve terminals by stretch and hypertonicity. *J. Neurocytol.* **2003**, *32*, 489–503. [CrossRef] [PubMed]

108. Cuddapah, V.A.; Robel, S.; Watkins, S.; Sontheimer, H. A neurocentric perspective on glioma invasion. *Nat. Rev. Neurosci.* **2014**, *15*, 455. [CrossRef] [PubMed]

109. Goddard, D.R.; Berry, M.; Butt, A.M. In vivo actions of fibroblast growth factor-2 and insulin-like growth factor-I on oligodendrocyte development and myelination in the central nervous system. *J. Neurosci. Res.* **1999**, *57*, 74–85. [CrossRef]

110. Sherman, L.S.; Struve, J.N.; Rangwala, R.; Wallingford, N.M.; Tuohy, T.M.; Kuntz, C., 4th. Hyaluronate-based extracellular matrix: Keeping glia in their place. *Glia* **2002**, *38*, 93–102. [CrossRef]

111. Soilu-Hänninen, M.; Laaksonen, M.; Hänninen, A.; Erälinna, J.P.; Panelius, M. Downregulation of VLA-4 on T cells as a marker of long term treatment response to interferon beta-1a in MS. *J. Neuroimmunol.* **2005**, *167*, 175–182. [CrossRef] [PubMed]

112. Johnson-Green, P.C.; Dow, K.E.; Riopelle, R.J. Characterization of glycosaminoglycans produced by primary astrocytes in vitro. *Glia* **1991**, *4*, 314–321. [CrossRef]

113. Bradbury, E.J.; Moon, L.D.; Popat, R.J.; King, V.R.; Bennett, G.S.; Patel, P.N.; Fawcett, J.W.; McMahon, S.B. Chondroitinase ABC promotes functional recovery after spinal cord injury. *Nature* **2002**, *416*, 636. [CrossRef] [PubMed]

114. Yiu, G.; He, Z. Glial inhibition of CNS axon regeneration. *Nat. Rev. Neurosci.* **2006**, *7*, 617. [CrossRef] [PubMed]

115. Fujita, Y.; Takashima, R.; Endo, S.; Takai, T.; Yamashita, T. The p75 receptor mediates axon growth inhibition through an association with PIR-B. *Cell Death Dis.* **2011**, *2*, e198. [CrossRef] [PubMed]

116. Gimenez, M.A.T.; Sim, J.E.; Russell, J.H. TNFR1-dependent VCAM-1 expression by astrocytes exposes the CNS to destructive inflammation. *J. Neuroimmunol.* **2004**, *151*, 116–125. [CrossRef] [PubMed]

117. Sobel, R.A.; Mitchell, M.E.; Fondren, G. Intercellular adhesion molecule-1 (ICAM-1) in cellular immune reactions in the human central nervous system. *Am. J. Pathol.* **1990**, *136*, 1309.

118. Dong, Y.; Benveniste, E.N. Immune function of astrocytes. *Glia* **2001**, *36*, 180–190. [CrossRef]

119. DeWitt, D.A.; Perry, G.; Cohen, M.; Doller, C.; Silver, J. Astrocytes regulate microglial phagocytosis of senile plaque cores of Alzheimer's disease. *Exp. Neurol.* **1998**, *149*, 329–340. [CrossRef]

120. Mayo, L.; Trauger, S.A.; Blain, M.; Nadeau, M.; Patel, B.; Alvarez, J.I.; Mascanfroni, I.D.; Yeste, A.; Kivisäkk, P.; Kallas, K.; et al. Regulation of astrocyte activation by glycolipids drives chronic CNS inflammation. *Nat. Med.* **2014**, *20*, 1147. [CrossRef]

121. Pannu, R.; Won, J.S.; Khan, M.; Singh, A.K.; Singh, I. A novel role of lactosylceramide in the regulation of lipopolysaccharide/interferon-γ-mediated inducible nitric oxide synthase gene expression: Implications for neuroinflammatory diseases. *J. Neurosci.* **2004**, *24*, 5942–5954. [CrossRef] [PubMed]

122. Krumbholz, M.; Theil, D.; Cepok, S.; Hemmer, B.; Kivisäkk, P.; Ransohoff, R.M.; Hofbauer, M.; Farina, C.; Derfuss, T.; Hartle, C.; et al. Chemokines in multiple sclerosis: CXCL12 and CXCL13 up-regulation is differentially linked to CNS immune cell recruitment. *Brain* **2005**, *129*, 200–211. [CrossRef] [PubMed]

123. Chastain, E.M.; D'Anne, S.D.; Rodgers, J.M.; Miller, S.D. The role of antigen presenting cells in multiple sclerosis. *Biochim. Biophys. Acta* **2011**, *1812*, 265–274. [CrossRef] [PubMed]

124. Kort, J.J.; Kawamura, K.; Fugger, L.; Weissert, R.; Forsthuber, T.G. Efficient presentation of myelin oligodendrocyte glycoprotein peptides but not protein by astrocytes from HLA-DR2 and HLA-DR4 transgenic mice. *J. Neuroimmunol.* **2006**, *173*, 23–34. [CrossRef] [PubMed]

125. Bal-Price, A.; Brown, G.C. Inflammatory neurodegeneration mediated by nitric oxide from activated glia-inhibiting neuronal respiration, causing glutamate release and excitotoxicity. *J. Neurosci.* **2001**, *21*, 6480–6491. [CrossRef] [PubMed]

126. Hamby, M.E.; Hewett, J.A.; Hewett, S.J. TGF-β1 potentiates astrocytic nitric oxide production by expanding the population of astrocytes that express NOS-2. *Glia* **2006**, *54*, 566–577. [CrossRef] [PubMed]

127. Lee, S.J.; Benveniste, E.N. Adhesion molecule expression and regulation on cells of the central nervous system. *J. Neuroimmunol.* **1999**, *98*, 77–88. [CrossRef]

128. Stojanovic, I.R.; Kostic, M.; Ljubisavljevic, S. The role of glutamate and its receptors in multiple sclerosis. *J. Neural Transm.* **2014**, *121*, 945–955. [CrossRef]

129. Kumar, P.; Kalonia, H.; Kumar, A. Possible GABAergic mechanism in the neuroprotective effect of gabapentin and lamotrigine against 3-nitropropionic acid induced neurotoxicity. *Eur. J. Pharmacol.* **2012**, *674*, 265–274. [CrossRef]

130. Rossi, S.; Motta, C.; Studer, V.; Barbieri, F.; Buttari, F.; Bergami, A.; Sancesario, G.; Bernardini, S.; De Angelis, G.; Martino, G.; et al. Tumor necrosis factor is elevated in progressive multiple sclerosis and causes excitotoxic neurodegeneration. *Mult. Scler.* **2014**, *20*, 304–312. [CrossRef]

131. Matute, C. Excitotoxicity in glial cells. *Proc. Natl. Acad. Sci. USA* **1997**, *94*, 8830–8835. [CrossRef] [PubMed]

132. Nicholls, D.G. Mitochondrial dysfunction and glutamate excitotoxicity studied in primary neuronal cultures. *Curr. Mol. Med.* **2004**, *4*, 149–177. [CrossRef] [PubMed]

133. Correale, J.; Farez, M.F. The role of astrocytes in multiple sclerosis progression. *Front. Neurol.* **2015**, *6*, 180. [CrossRef] [PubMed]

134. Williams, A.; Piaton, G.; Lubetzki, C. Astrocytes—friends or foes in multiple sclerosis? *Glia* **2007**, *55*, 1300–1312. [CrossRef] [PubMed]

135. Frischer, J.M.; Bramow, S.; Dal-Bianco, A.; Lucchinetti, C.F.; Rauschka, H.; Schmidbauer, M.; Laursen, H.; Sorensen, P.S.; Lassmann, H. The relation between inflammation and neurodegeneration in multiple sclerosis brains. *Brain* **2009**, *132*, 1175–1182. [CrossRef] [PubMed]

136. Haider, L.; Fischer, M.T.; Frischer, J.M.; Bauer, J.; Höftberger, R.; Botond, G.; Esterbauer, H.; Binder, C.J.; Witztum, J.L.; Lassmann, H. Oxidative damage in multiple sclerosis lesions. *Brain* **2011**, *134*, 1914–1924. [CrossRef]

137. Mahad, D.J.; Ziabreva, I.; Campbell, G.; Lax, N.; White, K.; Hanson, P.S.; Lassmann, H.; Turnbull, D.M. Mitochondrial changes within axons in multiple Sclerosis. *Brain* **2009**, *132*, 1161–1174. [CrossRef]

138. Campbell, G.R.; Worrall, J.T.; Mahad, D.J. The central role of mitochondria in axonal degeneration in multiple sclerosis. *Mult. Scler.* **2014**, *20*, 1806–1813. [CrossRef]
139. Hirokawa, N.; Niwa, S.; Tanaka, Y. Molecular motors in neurons: Transport mechanisms and roles in brain function, development and disease. *Neuron* **2010**, *68*, 610–638. [CrossRef]
140. Campbell, G.; Mahad, D. Neurodegeneration in progressive multiple sclerosis. *Cold Spring Harb. Perspect. Med.* **2018**, *8*. [CrossRef]
141. Hares, K.; Kemp, K.; Rice, C.; Gray, E.; Scolding, N.; Wilkins, A. Reduced axonal motor protein expression in non-lesional grey matter in multiple sclerosis. *Mult. Scler.* **2014**, *20*, 812–821. [CrossRef] [PubMed]
142. Friese, M.A.; Schattling, B.; Fugger, L. Mechanisms of neurodegeneration and axonal dysfunction in multiple sclerosis. *Nat. Rev. Neurol.* **2014**, *10*, 225–238. [CrossRef] [PubMed]
143. Murphy, M.P. How mitochondria produce reactive oxygen species. *Biochem. J.* **2009**, *417*, 1–13. [CrossRef] [PubMed]
144. Craner, M.J.; Hains, B.C.; Lo, A.C.; Black, J.A.; Waxman, S.G. Co-localization of sodium channel $Na_v1. 6$ and the sodium-calcium exchanger at sites of axonal injury in the spinal cord in EAE. *Brain* **2004**, *127*, 294–303. [CrossRef] [PubMed]
145. Craner, M.J.; Newcombe, J.; Black, J.A.; Hartle, C.; Cuzner, M.L.; Waxman, S.G. Molecualr changes in neurons in multiple sclerosis: Altered axonal expression of $Na_v1.2$ and $Na_v1.6$ sodium channels and Na^+/Ca^{2+} exchanger. *Proc. Natl. Acad. Sci. USA* **2004**, *101*, 8168–8173. [CrossRef] [PubMed]
146. Rush, A.M.; Dib-Hajj, S.D.; Waxman, S.G. Electrophysiological properties of two axonal sodium channels, $Na_v1. 2$ and $Na_v1. 6$, expressed in mouse spinal sensory neurons. *J. Physiol.* **2005**, *564*, 803–815. [CrossRef] [PubMed]
147. Stys, P.K. General mechanisms of axonal damage and its prevention. *J. Neurol. Sci.* **2005**, *233*, 3–13. [CrossRef]
148. Kornek, B.; Storch, M.K.; Bauer, J.; Djamshidian, A.; Weissert, R.; Wallstroem, E.; Stefferl, A.; Zimprich, F.; Olsson, T.; Linington, C.; et al. Distribution of a calcium channel subunit in dystrophic axons in multiple sclerosis and experimental autoimmune encephalomyelitis. *Brain* **2001**, *124*, 1114–1124. [CrossRef]
149. Strirling, D.P.; Stys, P.K. Mechanisms of axonal injury: Intermodal nanocomplexes and calcium deregulation. *Trends Mol. Med.* **2010**, *16*, 160–170. [CrossRef]
150. Khalil, M.; Teunissen, C.E.; Otto, M.; Piehl, F.; Sormani, M.P.; Gattringer, T.; Barro, C.; Kappos, L.; Comabella, M.; Fazekas, F.; et al. Neurofilaments as biomarkers in neurological disorders. *Nat. Rev. Neurol.* **2018**, *14*, 577–589. [CrossRef]
151. Lycke, J.N.; Karlsson, J.E.; Andersen, O.; Rosengren, L.E. Neurofilament protein in cerebrospinal fluid: A potential marker of activity in multiple sclerosis. *J. Neurol. Neurosurg. Psychiatry* **1998**, *64*, 402–404. [CrossRef] [PubMed]
152. Rosengren, L.E.; Karlsson, J.E.; Karlsson, J.O.; Persson, L.I.; Wikkelsø, C. Patients with amyotrophic lateral sclerosis and other neurodegenerative diseases have increased levels of neurofilament protein in CSF. *J. Neurochem.* **1996**, *67*, 2013–2018. [CrossRef] [PubMed]
153. Novakova, L.; Axelsson, M.; Khademi, M.; Zetterberg, H.; Blennow, K.; Malmeström, C.; Piehl, F.; Olsson, T.; Lycke, J. Cerebrospinal fluid biomarkers of inflammation and degeneration as measures of fingolimod efficacy in multiple Sclerosis. *Mult. Scler.* **2017**, *23*, 62–71. [CrossRef] [PubMed]
154. Gunnarsson, M.; Malmeström, C.; Axelsson, M.; Sundström, P.; Dahle, C.; Vrethem, M.; Olsson, T.; Piehl, F.; Norgren, N.; Rosengren, L.; et al. Axonal damage in relapsing multiple Sclerosis is markedly reduced by natalizumab. *Ann. Neurol.* **2011**, *69*, 83–89. [CrossRef] [PubMed]
155. Disanto, G.; Barro, C.; Benkert, P.; Naegelin, Y.; Schädelin, S.; Giardiello, A.; Zecca, C.; Blennow, K.; Zetterberg, H.; Leppert, D.; et al. Serum neurofialments light: A biomarker of neuronal damage in multiple Sclerosis. *Ann. Neurol.* **2017**, *81*, 857–870. [CrossRef] [PubMed]
156. Barro, C.; Benkert, P.; Disanto, G.; Tsagkas, C.; Amann, M.; Naegelin, Y.; Leppert, D.; Gobbi, C.; Granziera, C.; Yaldizli, Ö.; et al. Serum neurfilament as a predictor of disease worsening and brain and spinal cord atrophy in multiple Sclerosis. *Brain* **2018**. [CrossRef] [PubMed]
157. Simons, M.; Nave, K.A. Oligodendrocytes: Myelination and axonal support. *Cold Spring Harb. Perspect. Biol.* **2015**, *8*, a020479. [CrossRef] [PubMed]
158. Griffiths, I.; Klugmann, M.; Anderson, T.; Yool, D.; Thomson, C.; Schwab, M.H.; Schneider, A.; Zimmermann, F.; McCulloch, M.; Nadon, N.; et al. Axonal swellings and degeneration in mice lacking the major proteolipid protein. *Science* **1998**, *280*, 1610–1613. [CrossRef] [PubMed]

159. Lappe-Siefke, C.; Goebbels, S.; Gravel, M.; Nicksch, E.; Lee, J.; Braun, P.E.; Griffiths, I.R.; Nave, K.A. Dysruption of Cnp1 uncouples oligodendroglial functions in axonal support and myelination. *Nat. Gen.* **2003**, *33*, 366. [CrossRef] [PubMed]

160. Edgar, J.M.; McLaughlin, M.; Werner, H.B.; McCulloch, M.C.; Barrie, J.A.; Brown, A.; Faichney, A.B.; Snaidero, N.; Nave, K.A.; Griffiths, I.R. Early ultrastructural defects of axons and axon-glia junctions in mice lacking expression of Cnp1. *Glia* **2009**, *57*, 1815–1824. [CrossRef] [PubMed]

161. Oluich, L.J.; Stratton, J.A.; Xing, Y.L.; Ng, S.W.; Cate, H.S.; Sah, P.; Windels, F.; Kilpatrick, T.J.; Merson, T.D. Targeted ablation of oligodendrocytes induces axonal pathology independent of overt demyelination. *J. Neurosci.* **2012**, *32*, 8317–8330. [CrossRef] [PubMed]

162. Fünfschilling, U.; Supplie, L.M.; Mahad, D.; Boretius, S.; Saab, A.S.; Edgar, J.; Brinkmann, B.G.; Kassmann, C.M.; Tzvetanova, I.D.; Möbius, W.; et al. Glycolytic oligodendrocytes maintain myelin and long-term axonal integrity. *Nature* **2012**, *485*, 517–521. [CrossRef] [PubMed]

163. Correale, J.; Ysrraelit, M.C.; Benarroch, E.E. Metabolic coupling of axons and glial cells: Implications for multiple sclerosis progression. *Neurology* **2018**, *90*, 737–744. [CrossRef] [PubMed]

164. Philips, T.; Rothstein, J.D. Oligodendroglia: Metabolic supporters of neurons. *J. Clin. Investig.* **2017**, *127*, 3271–3280. [CrossRef] [PubMed]

165. Lee, Y.; Morrsion, B.M.; Li, Y.; Lengacher, S.; Farah, M.H.; Hoffman, P.N.; Liu, Y.; Tsingalia, A.; Jin, L.; Zhang, P.W.; et al. Oligodendroglia metabolically support axons and contribute to neurodegeneration. *Nature* **2012**, *487*, 443–448. [CrossRef] [PubMed]

166. Bélanger, M.; Allaman, I.; Magistretti, P.J. Barin metabolism: Focus on astrcoyte-neuron metabolic cooperation. *Cell Metab.* **2011**, *14*, 724–738. [CrossRef] [PubMed]

167. Brown, A.M.; Baltan Tekkök, S.; Ramson, B.R. Energy transfer from astrcoytes to axons: The role of CNS glycogen. *Neurochem. Int.* **2004**, *45*, 529–536. [CrossRef] [PubMed]

168. Menichella, D.M.; Goodenough, D.A.; Sirkowski, E.; Scherer, S.S.; Paul, D.L. COnnexins are critical for normal myelination in the CNS. *J. Neurosci.* **2003**, *23*, 5963–5973. [CrossRef] [PubMed]

169. Tress, O.; Maglione, M.; May, D.; Pivneva, T.; Richter, N.; Seyfarth, J.; Binder, S.; Zlomuzica, A.; Seifert, G.; Theis, M.; et al. Panglial gap junctional communication is essential for maintenance of myelin in the CNS. *J. Neurosci.* **2012**, *32*, 7499–7518. [CrossRef] [PubMed]

170. Niu, J.; Li, T.; Yi, C.; Huang, N.; Koulakoff, A.; Weng, C.; Li, C.; Zhao, C.J.; Giaume, C.; Xiao, L. Connexin-based channels contribute to metabolic pathways in the oligodendroglial lineage. *J. Cell Sci.* **2016**, *129*, 1902–1914. [CrossRef] [PubMed]

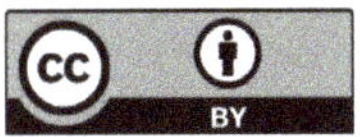

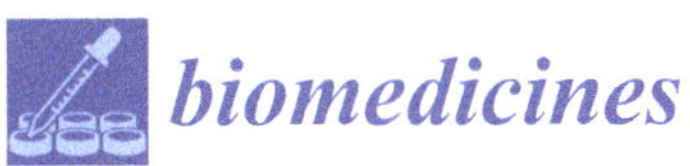 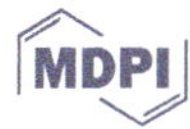

Review

Diagnosis and Management of Progressive Multiple Sclerosis

Gabrielle Macaron and Daniel Ontaneda *

Mellen Center for Multiple Sclerosis, Neurological Institute, Cleveland Clinic Foundation, Cleveland, OH 44195, USA
* Correspondence: ontaned@ccf.org; Tel.: +1-216-218-2841; Fax: +1-216-445-6259

Received: 8 July 2019; Accepted: 26 July 2019; Published: 29 July 2019

Abstract: Multiple sclerosis is a chronic autoimmune disease of the central nervous system that results in varying degrees of disability. Progressive multiple sclerosis, characterized by a steady increase in neurological disability independently of relapses, can occur from onset (primary progressive) or after a relapsing–remitting course (secondary progressive). As opposed to active inflammation seen in the relapsing–remitting phases of the disease, the gradual worsening of disability in progressive multiple sclerosis results from complex immune mechanisms and neurodegeneration. A few anti-inflammatory disease-modifying therapies with a modest but significant effect on measures of disease progression have been approved for the treatment of progressive multiple sclerosis. The treatment effect of anti-inflammatory agents is particularly observed in the subgroup of patients with younger age and evidence of disease activity. For this reason, a significant effort is underway to develop molecules with the potential to induce myelin repair or halt the degenerative process. Appropriate trial methodology and the development of clinically meaningful disability outcome measures along with imaging and biological biomarkers of progression have a significant impact on the ability to measure the efficacy of potential medications that may reverse disease progression. In this issue, we will review current evidence on the physiopathology, diagnosis, measurement of disability, and treatment of progressive multiple sclerosis.

Keywords: progressive multiple sclerosis; neurodegeneration; remyelination; outcome measures; biomarkers

1. Introduction

Multiple sclerosis (MS) is a chronic inflammatory disease of the central nervous system that affects over 2.3 million people globally, with an estimated prevalence of approximately 310 per 100,000 population in the United States [1,2]. Most patients (~90%) have relapsing–remitting disease at onset, which typically is followed by a secondary progressive course, while a minority of patients have a primary progressive course from onset (~10%). Relapsing–remitting MS (RRMS) is characterized by frequent formation of inflammatory lesions in the brain and spinal cord. Approved disease-modifying therapies (DMTs) target the inflammatory component of the disease, and strong evidence support their effectiveness in RRMS. However, trials evaluating their efficacy in slowing disease progression have shown mixed results, or have shown only modest effects in slowing progression. The goal of this review is to provide a comprehensive overview on the current knowledge of the pathogenesis, diagnosis, and treatment of progressive MS, as well as future directions in the field.

2. Pathogenesis

The pathogenesis of MS is incompletely elucidated. This is particularly the case for progressive MS, for which various and sometimes conflicting data have been proposed to explain the underlying pathogenic process of progression [3]. In RRMS, actively demyelinating plaques are the most prominent lesion type, and are characterized by inflammatory demyelination and axonal transection within the lesions [4–6]. However, active lesions are rare in progressive MS, and axonal transection is not seen as frequently within inactive lesions compared to highly inflammatory recently developed lesions [3–5]. Whole brain atrophy, smoldering and enlarging lesions, cortical demyelination (specifically subpial lesions), and diffuse axonal injury and microglial activation in normal appearing grey and white matter are prominent in patients with progressive MS compared to patients with early RRMS [6–10]. Disability in progressive MS is thought to be related to secondary neurodegeneration of chronically demyelinating axons, which is thought to be driven by a series of factors, including: (1) inflammation and lesion accumulation, with subsequent retrograde and anterograde degeneration, (2) mitochondrial damage and subsequently virtual hypoxia and oxidative stress, (3) iron accumulation in myelin sheath and oligodendrocytes with subsequent amplification of oxidative stress, (4) lymphoid follicle-like structures that might contribute to sustaining cortical pathology, and [5] age-related neurodegeneration and reduced neuronal reserve (loss of the ability to compensate for axonal loss) [3,11–15]. A recent paper by Brown et al. [16], among others, showed that the early use of DMTs, specifically highly-effective DMTs, decreases the odds of conversion to secondary progressive MS (SPMS), which supports the role of early disease activity in the development of long-term disability progression [16–21]. The role of age-related mechanisms is supported by the fact that children with MS rarely present with progressive disease and have a longer time to reach secondary progression and disability milestones compared to adult-onset MS, and that certain disability milestones are acquired at certain ages independently of the duration of the disease [22,23]. However, for primary progressive MS (PPMS), the time course of irreversible damage is not clearly affected by the presence or absence of superimposed relapses [24]. Recent observations support a change in the natural history of MS with earlier use of highly-effective DMTs; however, this effect seems to be more clearly evidenced in RRMS [25]. Despite the wide variability of clinical and radiological presentations and the inherent pathological differences between RRMS, SPMS, and PPMS, the consensus is that PPMS is biologically part of the MS spectrum [13].

3. Diagnostic Criteria and Disease Course Definitions

The diagnosis of progressive MS is based on patient-reported clinical history, and should be confirmed based on objective physical examination findings. Based on the 2017 McDonald diagnostic criteria, PPMS can be diagnosed in patients with a 1-year history of disability progression, which can be retrospectively or prospectively determined, independent of clinical relapses, plus two of the following criteria: (1) One or more T2 lesions characteristic of MS in one or more typical brain regions (periventricular, cortical or juxtacortical, infratentorial); (2) two or more T2 lesions in the spinal cord, and (3) the presence of CSF-specific oligoclonal bands. Unlike the 2010 McDonald criteria, both symptomatic and asymptomatic MRI lesions are taken into account [26,27]. The panel also recommends specifying a provisional disease course at the time of diagnosis, and whether disease activity and/or progression are present or not based on the previous year's history, which can then be revisited based on periodic re-evaluation [27]. Providing a clinical definition of disease progression, however, is somewhat harder. Progression is characterized by a steady increase in neurological disability occurring independently of relapses [27,28]. Symptoms can fluctuate (i.e., pseudo relapses), and bona fide superimposed relapses might occur. Detailed history taking is key in differentiating events suggestive of disease activity from worsening of previously experienced symptoms in the context of fatigue, heat, or stress. PPMS is defined by a progressive course from onset and SPMS by a progressive course following an initial relapsing–remitting course. The 2013 revisions of MS clinical course definitions aimed at standardizing the terminology across clinicians and researchers, for prognostication, design of clinical trials, and treatment decisions purposes [28]. These definitions included the presence or absence of clinical or radiological activity, and the presence or absence of disability progression into the phenotypic description of the disease. Figure 1 illustrates the currently used description of different progressive MS phenotypes. The distinction between "active" and "inactive" progressive disease, whether primary or secondary, has important therapeutic implications. This will be discussed in the treatment section of this manuscript.

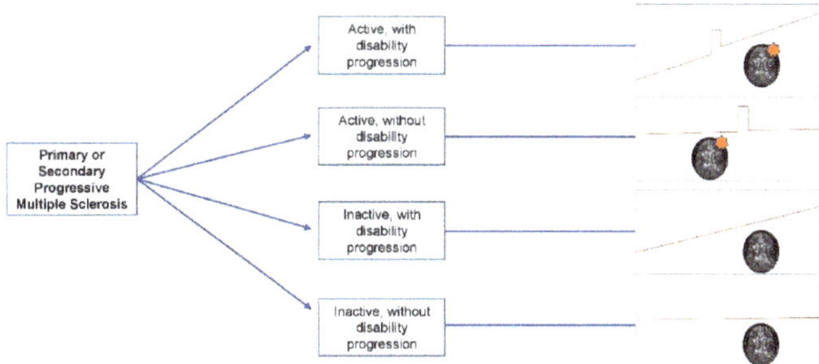

Figure 1. Clinical course of progressive multiple sclerosis. The orange star indicates the presence of radiological activity (new/enlarging T2 lesions or gadolinium enhancing lesions).

4. Disability Outcome Measures

Disability progression in MS affects multiple functional domains, occurs insidiously over time, and can be difficult to quantify in an objective, comprehensive, and reproducible manner. Reliable detection of clinical and sub-clinical progression is key to interpreting treatment efficacy in trials and in clinical practice of DMT and repair promoting strategies in progressive MS. The expanded disability status scale (EDSS) is the most commonly used clinical outcome measure in trials for quantification of physical disability in MS. However, the EDSS does not comprehensively reflect disability status, and is particularly restricted in assessing cognitive and upper extremity functions [29]. Other limitations of the EDSS include poor intra and inter-rater variability especially for lower scores. The test also shows little sensitivity to detect change, especially in patients with scores of 6.0 or more, and the EDSS is difficult to administer in routine care [30–32]. Since it is an ordinal scale, changes in EDSS scores are not equivalent across the range of the scale. Finally, the most commonly used outcome measure in progressive MS trials is the 3 or 6-month confirmed disability progression, which might be insufficient to predict long-term disability worsening [33]. Evaluating multiple functional domains improves the likelihood of observing a change in patients with MS. The multiple sclerosis functional composite (MSFC) [34,35] was developed as a quantitative clinical measure of neurologic disability to overcome some of the shortcomings of the EDSS. Cognitive function was evaluated originally using the paced auditory serial addition test (PASAT), but more recently using the symbol–digit modalities test (SDMT), and upper extremity function is evaluated using the 9-hole peg test (9HPT) [36,37]. Walking speed is usually evaluated using the timed-25-foot walk test (T25FW). The MSFC has proven to be more sensitive to change than the EDSS, and correlates with subsequent changes in EDSS [34] T1 and T2 lesion load on brain MRI [38], and patient reported physical and emotional functioning and quality of life [39]. In the interferon beta (IFN-β)-1a SPMS trial, there was some benefit of treatment on the MSFC z-scores but not on the EDSS [40]. This benefit was mainly driven by two of the components of the MSFC, the 9HPT and the PASAT, which further illustrates the importance of a comprehensive neurological evaluation to assess disability progression. The low contrast letter acuity testing using a low-contrast Sloan letter chart was later proposed as an additional component of the MSFC to capture visual dysfunction with a high sensitivity, and also correlates with other components of the MSFC and the EDSS [37,41,42]. In addition, internal consistency (reliability) is higher for the MSFC (Cronbach's alpha coefficient 0.93−0.96) than for the EDSS (Cronbach's alpha 0.7) [43,44]. Although the MSFC has been used as an outcome measure in clinical trials [40,45,46], administration in routine clinical practice is time consuming, and requires personnel to administer the test properly [47]. Recently, there has been increasing interest in developing tools to facilitate and standardize testing in MS patients. For example, a technology-enabled version of the MSFC has been developed and was incorporated into routine clinical practice. This tool, called the multiple sclerosis performance test (MSPT), comprises a battery of quantitative neuroperformance assessments administered using a suite of iPad® applications modeled after the MSFC approach, and has allowed the gathering of large-scale comprehensive and standardized measures of disability from routine care [48,49]. A limitation of these outcome measures is the uncertainty of what constitutes a clinically meaningful change, although a threshold of ± 20% change in T25FW [50,51] ±15–20% in the 9HPT [52,53] ±10% (or 4 points) in the SDMT [53,54] and ±7 letters in the low contrast letter acuity test [55] have been suggested as clinically meaningful in MS.

5. Measuring Disease Progression

Numerous imaging biomarkers that have been proposed for the monitoring of progressive disease in MS trials, whole brain atrophy being the most widely used. Monitoring of T1 hypointensity evolution over time on conventional imaging has also been suggested. Other more advanced MRI techniques that can reflect axonal loss in progressive MS include thalamic volume, spinal cord atrophy, hippocampal volume, gray matter fraction, cortical lesion quantification, and sodium imaging, among others [56,57]. Several additional advanced MRI measures have been used as exploratory outcomes [58] as well as neurophysiological measures, such as evoked potentials [59]. Optical coherence tomography (OCT) is a non-invasive tool that allows the measurements of retinal nerve fiber layer thickness, ganglion cell/inner plexiform layer thickness, and macular volume. Since these measurements correlate with whole brain and gray matter atrophy and physical disability, OCT can serve as an outcome measure of axonal loss in phase 2 proof of concept clinical trials of progressive MS [60]. Other imaging and non-imaging techniques are used in remyelination trials as biomarkers of myelin repair, and include magnetization transfer ratio, diffusion-weighted imaging, myelin water imaging, and visual evoked potentials [56].

There has been increasing interest in the use of serum neurofilament light chain (NfL) as a biomarker in MS over the past few years [61]. Serum NfL levels correlate with CSF NfL levels and reflect disease activity and response to therapy [61]. In progressive MS, NfL levels appear to be associated with superimposed clinical or radiological activity, as well as T1-hypointense lesion volume [62]. Recent data suggests that CSF NfL correlates with disease activity rather than progression, irrespective of the disease subtype, and does not reflect disease severity [63,64], whereas previous data report a strong correlation between NfL levels and future worsening on the EDSS and brain and cervical spinal volume loss [65,66]. Serum NfL levels can be easily obtained, and are being further investigated and used as an outcome measure in newer progressive MS trials.

6. Treatment

6.1. Anti-Inflammatory Disease-Modifying Therapies

6.1.1. Approved Therapies

Ocrelizumab (*Ocrevus*®) a humanized monoclonal antibody targeting the CD20 antigen on B-cells. Ocrelizumab exerts its anti-inflammatory effects by causing rapid and profound depletion of B cells. Ocrelizumab has been studied in patients with RRMS in two phase 3 double-blind, placebo-controlled randomized clinical trial (OPERA I and II) [67] and in patients with PPMS (ORATORIO trial) [68], but not in patients with SPMS. Participants with PPMS were required to have positive oligoclonal bands to enroll in the study. In the ORATORIO trial ocrelizumab significantly reduced the risk of 24-week confirmed disability progression compared to placebo (29.6% with ocrelizumab versus 35.7% with placebo). Treatment with ocrelizumab in PPMS also decreased worsening on the timed-25-foot walk, T2 lesion volume, and brain atrophy at 120 weeks compared to placebo. In a pre-specified subgroup analysis, the magnitude of the effect of ocrelizumab was larger in patients with baseline enhancing lesions and younger patients; however, older patients without enhancing lesions at baseline also derived benefit across primary and secondary endpoints [68]. The ENCORE study evaluated the effect of ocrelizumab on upper limb function in the ORATORIO cohort, and also showed positive results (reduction in time—to 12- and 24-week confirmed ≥15% increase on 9HPT by 37% (hazard ratio 0.627; $p = 0.001$) and 39% (HR = 0.607; $p = 0.002$) for both-hands) [69]. Ocrelizumab was approved by the FDA and the EMA to treat PPMS in 2017. Ongoing trials aim at evaluating the effect of ocrelizumab on hand function in patients with more advanced disability (ORATORIO-HAND, NCT03562975), and in a broader range of patients (with PPMS and SPMS, up to 65 years old) (CONSONNANCE, NCT03523858). It is important to note that previous trials using the chimeric monoclonal antibody rituximab, which has a similar mechanism of action as ocrelizumab, yielded results in one pivotal trial that shaped the inclusion criteria for the ORATORIO study. In the OLYMPUS trial of rituximab, the primary endpoint was negative but sub-group analysis found that younger patients with clinical or radiological evidence of disease activity did derive treatment benefit. The subgroup of patients who were older and did not have gadolinium-enhancing lesions had faster disability progression than those on placebo [70]. This indicates a potential harm of treating with a B-cell therapy in this population. Another recent observational study using retrospective data from three European centers and propensity score matching, analyzed the effect of rituximab treatment on disability progression in patients with SPMS. In this study, patients with SPMS treated with rituximab had significantly delayed confirmed progression compared with matched untreated controls at up to 10 years [71]. The difference in effects seen between ocrelizumab and rituximab are most likely related to trial design; however, biological differences may exist as well, given that ocrelizumab appears to promote cell death via greater antibody-dependent cellular cytotoxicity (ADCC) activity and less complement-dependent cytotoxicity (CDC) activity compared to rituximab, and has a more favorable antigenic profile compared to rituximab [72–74].

Siponimod (*Mayzent*®) is a selective sphingosine-1-phosphate receptor 1 and 5 modulator, which inhibits the egress of lymphocytes from lymph nodes, thus decreasing their entry into the CNS. In addition to its anti-inflammatory effects, siponimod has been found to have putative neuroprotective and repair properties in preclinical studies. It was recently approved for the treatment of SPMS based on the results of the EXPAND trial [75]. Compared to the placebo group, a significant reduction in time to 3 and 6-month confirmed disability progression (relative risk reductions of 21% and 26%, respectively) was observed in the siponimod group, and this trend was consistent in subgroup analysis with respect to pre-treatment relapse activity, disease progression rate, and disease severity. Significant reduction in markers of disease activity were also observed in the siponimod group, including annualized relapse rate, time to relapse, and gadolinium-enhancing lesions, and new/enlarging T2 lesions. Brain volume change from baseline was lower in the siponimod group at both months 12 and 24 compared to placebo [75]. Pre-clinical data also suggest that sphingosine-1-phosphate modulators cross the blood–brain barrier, and have the potential to improve morphological markers of remyelination [76]. In addition, modulation of sphingosine-1-phosphate receptor 5 has been shown to promote remyelination in vitro [76]. Interestingly, fingolimod, a sphingosine-1-phosphate receptor 1 to 5 modulator, failed to show significant reduction in confirmed disability worsening in patients with PPMS in the INFORMS trial [77]. The fact that other DMTs with a similar mechanism of action to siponimod and ocrelizumab failed to show benefit in PMS can be due to different patient population and sub-optimal trial designs, but also illustrates the lack of efficacy of anti-inflammatory strategies in the prevention of disability worsening in inactive PMS, and the need to develop molecules with a potential effect on neurodegeneration.

Mitoxantrone is a DNA intercalating agent that interferes with the replication and proliferation of B and T lymphocytes. Its use is nowadays limited due to the well-known serious adverse events (including cardio-toxicity, leukemia, amenorrhea, infections, alopecia, leucopenia, anemia, and hepatotoxicity) [78], and the availability of safer DMTs. The mitoxantrone in progressive multiple sclerosis (MIMS) trial was a double-blind, multicenter, phase 3 trial that randomized patients with worsening RRMS or SPMS to placebo or low (5 mg/m^2) or high (12 mg/m^2) dose mitoxantrone for 2 years [79]. About half of the participants had SPMS, with or without clinical activity in the year prior to enrollment. The primary outcome was a combination of five clinical measures: change from baseline EDSS at 24 months, change from baseline ambulation index at 24 months, number of relapses treated with corticosteroids, time to first treated relapse, and change from baseline standardized neurological status at 24 months [79]. In the cohort as a whole, a beneficial effect on the primary outcome clinical composite measure was observed for the mitoxantrone, with comparable treatment effects in patients with and without relapses in the year prior to enrollment. A few years later, the MIMS trial group analyzed the effect of low and high-dose mitoxantrone on measures of radiological activity in a subgroup of patients with worsening RRMS or SPMS, and surprisingly did not show a consistent effect of mitoxantrone on the presence of gadolinium-enhancing lesions for up to 24 months compared to placebo [80]. Mitoxantrone is approved by the FDA for the treatment of RRMS, SPMS, and what was previously referred to as "progressive relapsing MS". There is no evidence that supports a benefit of mitoxantrone in PPMS without clinical or radiological activity [81,82]. Single-nucleotide polymorphism in the ATP-binding cassette transporter genes may serve as pharmacogenetic markers associated with clinical response to mitoxantrone in RRMS and SPMS [83]; however, this association was not observed in patients with PPMS [81].

Cladibine produces rapid and long-lasting reductions in T-lymphocytes and rapid but transient reduction in B-lymphocytes, by disrupting cellular metabolism, inhibiting DNA synthesis and repair, and subsequent apoptosis of affected cells. The oral formulation of cladribine (*Mavenclad®*) has recently received FDA approval for the treatment of active RRMS and SPMS based on the results of the CLARITY and ORACLE MS trials, and post-hoc analysis of the ONWARD trial [84–87]. Intravenous formulations of cladribine have been mainly studied in progressive MS. An initial small trial (24 matched patients with clinically definite progressive MS as defined at the time of the study, baseline EDSS of 4.7, randomized to receive IV cladribine or placebo) showed a significant benefit of cladribine on EDSS worsening, with some patients even experiencing improvement on EDSS at month 12 [88]. There was also a positive effect on T2 lesion volume in this study. Another larger trial was then conducted in light of these results. Patients with SPMS or PPMS and a median baseline EDSS score of 6.0 were randomly assigned to receive either placebo or cladribine 0.07 mg/kg/day for 5 consecutive days every 4 weeks for 2 or 6 cycles, followed by placebo, for 8 cycles [89]. No benefit of cladribine on the primary outcome (mean change in EDSS at month 12) was observed compared to placebo. As expected, there was a significant effect of cladribine on gadolinium-enhancing lesions and T2 lesion accumulation, and a somewhat marginal benefit in a subgroup analysis of SPMS patients. Similarly, in another study, cladribine did not have a beneficial effect on whole brain volumes compared to placebo [90].

In the ONWARD trial, the effect of oral cladribine as an add-on to IFN-β in patients with active RRMS or SPMS was studied [87]. As expected, cladribine + IFN-β was superior to placebo + IFN-β in reducing annualized relapse rate and gadolinium-enhancing lesions. However, the confirmed EDSS progression over 96 weeks was similar between the two groups. In a post-hoc analysis of subgroups in the intention-to-treat population, cladribine + IFN-β was superior to placebo + IFN-β in reduction of annualized relapse rate (relative risk ratio of 0.11, 95% CI 0.01–0.94) in patients with active SPMS. Hence, oral cladribine was approved by the FDA for the treatment of active SPMS, but not for progressive MS without evidence of clinical or radiological activity.

6.1.2. Therapies with Negative or Weak Effect in Progressive MS

Studies of other anti-inflammatory DMTs in progressive MS have yielded deceiving results. Interferon-beta (IFN-β) has complex immunomodulatory effects (downregulation of pro-inflammatory and upregulation of anti-inflammatory cytokines). There is no robust evidence of the beneficial effect of IFN-β on progression, although early treatment in RRMS decreases conversion to SPMS, which is attributable to its anti-inflammatory properties [16–19]. In SPMS, IFN-β significantly delayed time to confirmed disability progression compared to those receiving placebo in the European SPMS IFN-β-1b trial [91]. However, discrepant results were observed in the North American SPMS IFN-β-1b trial, which did not show a difference in time to 6-month sustained EDSS progression compared to placebo [92]. A post hoc pooled analysis of the clinical trial data of both groups was performed to better clarify this discrepancy, and showed that patients in the European studies who benefited from treatment were significantly younger (41 vs. 46.9 years, $p < 0.001$), with shorter disease duration (13.1 vs. 14.7 years, $p < 0.001$), and more active disease (number of relapses in the last 2 years 1.7 vs. 0.8, contrast-enhancing lesions 2.6 vs. 1.5, $p < 0.001$) [93]. The lack of benefit of IFN-β-1b in patients with SPMS with less active disease was confirmed in other SPMS trials as well [94,95].

IFN-β trials in PPMS have also been largely mixed, with negative results on primary (confirmed disability progression) and most secondary endpoints [96–98], although significant differences in MSFC scores, MRI T2 lesion volume, and MRI T1 lesion volume after 2 years of treatment favoring IFN-β-1a was observed in one trial [98].

Glatiramer acetate (GA), a synthetic polypeptide with a complex and incompletely understood immunomodulatory mechanism of action, was studied in patients with PPMS in the PROMiSe trial, a multicenter, placebo-controlled, double-blind randomized clinical trial comparing GA to placebo over a 3-year period [99]. This trial was successful in including a large majority of patients without signs of disease activity. GA decreased markers of radiological activity (gadolinium enhancing lesions and accumulation of T2 lesions), and had some benefit on disability progression in males, but there was no effect on the primary outcome and the study was terminated early [99,100].

As discussed earlier in this manuscript, the INFORMS trial failed to show a positive effect of fingolimod (*Gilenya*®) on reduction in confirmed disability worsening in patients with PPMS [77]. The primary endpoint was defined by a composite of outcomes including the EDSS, T25FW, and 9HPT. There was no benefit of fingolimod on the disability composite (HR = 0.95, 95%FW CI 0.80–1.10, $p = 0.544$). Fingolimod has not been studied in SPMS.

Natalizumab (*Tysabri*®) is a monoclonal antibody that exerts its potent anti-inflammatory effect by inhibiting the alpha-4 integrin and subsequently preventing the migration of T-lymphocytes across the blood–brain barrier. The ASCEND trial evaluated the effect of natalizumab on a composite score including the EDSS, T25FW, and 9HPT in patients with SPMS [101]. No benefit was observed on the composite primary outcome, and individually on the EDSS and 9HPT, although in a post hoc analysis, there was a 44% reduction in hand function progression measured by the 9HPT (OR 0.56, 95% CI 0.40–0.80, $p = 0.001$).

Rituximab is a chimeric monoclonal antibody targeting the CD20 antigen on pre-B-cells and mature B-cells that has been used in many autoimmune neurological disorders of the central and peripheral nervous systems for decades [102]. Similarly to ocrelizumab, it causes rapid and profound depletion of B-cells via antibody-dependent cellular cytotoxicity (ADCC) and complement-dependent cytotoxicity (CDC) mechanisms leading to B-cell death [73,74]. Rituximab has been used off-label to treat progressive MS in certain countries, and there has been long-standing evidence of its efficacy to control inflammatory disease activity in observational studies [103]. Furthermore, as discussed above, a recent study also suggests that rituximab significantly delayed confirmed progression in SPMS [71]. The OLYMPUS trial evaluated the effect of rituximab on disability progression in patients with PPMS [70]. This was a phase 2/3 multicenter, placebo-controlled trial involving 439 patients with PPMS for 96 weeks. There were no differences in the primary endpoint in the overall cohort (time to 12-week confirmed disability progression using the EDSS at 96 weeks). There was a significant effect on T2 lesion volume, which was lower with rituximab. An important point of this trial is the result of the subgroup analysis, which showed a significant difference on the primary endpoint in the subgroup of patients who were <51 years old and who had baseline enhancing lesions (hazard ratio 0.52 ($p = 0.010$) and 0.41 ($p = 0.007$), respectively), whereas rituximab-treated patients who were older than 51 years and had no enhancing lesions at baseline had non-significant but worse outcomes than the placebo group (hazard ratio 1.27 ($p = 0.425$)). This highlights the predominantly anti-inflammatory effect of B-cell therapies in MS.

There has been evidence of the presence of lymphoid follicle-like structures in the cerebral meninges that are typically adjacent to large subpial lesions, and associated with more severe cortical pathology and accelerated disability progression in patients with SPMS [14,15]. Based on these observations, the eventual role of these lymphoid follicles in sustaining cortical injury and accelerating clinical worsening was hypothesized, and the effect of intrathecal rituximab was evaluated since IV rituximab does not cross the blood–brain barrier [104–107]. The RIVITALISE trial, a randomized, double-blind trial study of intravenous and intrathecal rituximab in patients with SPMS, showed that intrathecal rituximab transiently decreased the B cell counts in the CSF and did not induce consistent effects on CSF biomarkers [104].

A very recent trial evaluated the safety and efficacy of intrathecal rituximab in eight patients with progressive MS who had focal leptomeningeal contrast-enhancement on contrast-enhanced T2-FLAIR [105]. Transient reduction in CSF B cells and biomarkers (reduction in chemokine ligand 13 (CXCL-13) levels with an increase in B cell-activating factor belonging to the TNF family (BAFF) levels), along with profound peripheral B cell depletion was observed; however, the number of leptomeningeal lesions did not change.

Other immunomodulating and immunosuppressive therapies have been investigated in PMS. Examples include azathioprine [108–110], cyclophosphamide [111–114], intravenous immunoglobulins [110,115], methotrexate [116–118], cyclosporine [109,119], mycophenolate mofetil [120], laquinimod [121], and MBP8298 [122]. Results from these trials have been largely negative, with no or modest benefit on markers of disability progression.

6.2. Remyelination and Neuroprotection in Progressive MS

While some agents have shown to be beneficial on slowing disability progression, no molecules have shown to have an effect on halting progression or reversing neurological damage in well-powered clinical trials. There are two therapeutic approaches that are thought to be promising to achieve the latter: remyelination and neuroprotection. Remyelinating agents can theoretically repair damage and neuroprotective agents can theoretically prevent axonal loss. High-throughput methods have generated many promising remyelinating molecules to test in pre-clinical studies, to be followed by phase 1, 2, and 3 trials. Unfortunately, studies have been mostly negative or have shown only modest benefits on measures of brain atrophy for which clinical significance still needs to be better elucidated. Table 1 provides an overview of positive trials of molecules with a putative remyelinating and neuroprotective effect. Some agents such as biotin and mesenchymal stem cells may have both remyelinating and neuroprotective effects; these medications are discussed under neuroprotection.

Table 1. Potential remyelinating and neuroprotective molecules studied in multiple sclerosis.

Therapy	Potential Mechanism of Action	Trials	Primary Endpoint	Results
Remyelination strategies				
Clemastine fumarate	First-generation anti-histamine, promotes remyelination and oligodendrocyte differentiation via anti-muscarinic effect [123,124]	ReBUILD [125]	Shortening of P100 latency delay on visual-evoked potentials at 150 days	Improvement in P100 latency of 1.7 ms/eye (95% CI 0.5 to 2.9, $p = 0.0048$) with clemastine
Opicinumab	Anti-LINGO-1 antibody, promotes remyelination and oligodendrocyte differentiation via blocking of inhibitory adhesion molecule [126,127]	RENEW [128] (in acute unilateral optic neuritis)	24-week change in optic nerve conduction latency using full-field visual evoked potential	Non-significant trend towards improvement in the intention-to-treat analysis, modest but significant benefit at week 32 in the per-protocol analysis
		SYNERGY [129,130] (in RRMS and SPMS with active disease)	Percentage of participants with ≥3 month confirmed improvement of composite endpoint (EDSS, T25FW, 9HPT, PASAT) over 72 weeks	Benefit seen in those receiving the 30 mg/kg dose.
Neuroprotection strategies				
Ibudilast	Phosphodiesterase-inhibitor, inhibits macrophage migration inhibitory factor, and toll-like receptor 4 [131]	SPRINT-MS [132]	Progression of whole brain atrophy over 96 weeks	48% slowing in the rate of atrophy progression with ibudilast compared to placebo

Table 1. *Cont.*

Therapy	Potential Mechanism of Action	Trials	Primary Endpoint	Results
Simvastatin	HMG-CoA reductase inhibitor, inhibit MHCII-restricted antigen presentation, shifts cytokine production from a pro- to an anti-inflammatory response, decreases T-cell proliferation [133]	MS-STAT [134]	Progression of whole-brain atrophy, change in EDSS and total MS Impact Scale-29 at 24 months	Decrease in annualized rate of whole brain atrophy compared to placebo, benefit on EDSS and MS Impact Scale-29 as well
Lipoic acid	Endogenous antioxidant, various potential mechanisms, including free radical scavenging, oxidative damage repair, downregulation of inflammatory cytokines, T-cell migration in CNS inhibition [135,136]	Spain et al. [137].	Annual percent change of brain volume	68% reduction in the rate of brain atrophy compared to placebo over 24 months
Phenytoin	Selective sodium-channel inhibitor, reverses sodium influx, which drives calcium influx via reverse operation of the sodium/calcium exchanger after axonal injury [138]	Raftopoulos et al. [139].	RNFL thickness in the affected eye	30% reduction in the extent of RNFL loss with phenytoin compared with placebo at 6 months
Mesenchymal stem cells *	Pluripotent non-hematopoietic precursor cells (isolated from bone marrow or adipose tissue), release of soluble trophic factors that promote intrinsic tissue repair mechanisms [140]	Multiple small clinical trials and open label studies using variable route of administration and dosing regimens [141–149] Phase II randomized, double-blind trial, MESEMS (NCT01854957) [151] Open-label study, MSC-NTF Cells (NCT03799718)	Variable endpoints depending on trial Safety, reduction in the total number of contrast-gadolinium enhancing lesions Safety, T25FW change from baseline, changes in neurotrophic factors	Good safety and tolerability, efficacy not yet established [150] Ongoing Ongoing

Table 1. *Cont.*

Therapy	Potential Mechanism of Action	Trials	Primary Endpoint	Results
High-dose biotin (MD 1003) *	Essential co-factor for five carboxylases involved in fatty acid synthesis and energy production, promotes remyelination, and reduces axonal hypoxia [152]	Sedel et al. (pilot study) [153]	Shortening of P100 latency on visual-evoked potentials	Improvement or normalization of P100 latency
		Tourbah et al. (randomized, double-blind placebo-controlled trial) [154]	Proportion of patients with disability reversal on EDSS or T25FW at month 9, confirmed at month 12	2.6% of treated patients achieved the primary endpoint versus none of the placebo-treated patients ($p = 0.005$)
		Birnbaum et al. (open-label study of compound medication, not MD 1003) [155]	EDSS worsening or improvement while on treatment (3 to 12 months)	No benefits observed

* possibly dual effect on remyelination and neuroprotection. 9HPT: 9-hole-peg test, EDSS: Expanded disability status scale, LINGO-1: Leucine-rich repeat and immunoglobulin domain-containing neurite outgrowth inhibitor receptor interacting protein-1, PASAT: Paced auditory serial addition test, RRMS: Relapsing–remitting multiple sclerosis, RNFL: Retinal nerve fiber layer, SPMS: Secondary progressive multiple sclerosis, T25FW: Timed-25-foot walk.

In MS, progression secondary to neurodegeneration is thought to be secondary to chronic demyelination [3]. While neuronal cell bodies and axons have a low potential of regeneration, myelin may have a potential for repair. Remyelination can be seen in shadow plaques, which supports this potential repair property likely mediated by oligodendrocytes [3,6]. A few compounds promoting endogenous oligodendrocyte progenitor cell differentiation have been found in pre-clinical work to be promising remyelinating agents [156]. Out of thousands of compounds identified through high-volume screening of existing drugs [124], opicinumab [128–130], and clemastine [125] have been studied in phase 2 trials. Clemastine demonstrated improvement in P100 latency on visual evoked potential in patients with chronic optic neuropathy compared to placebo [125]. Opicinumab showed a similar effect in patients with acute optic neuritis [128,129] (Table 1). Other potentially effective molecules are currently being evaluated, including domperidone (in SPMS, NCT02308137), quetiapine (in RRMS and progressive MS, NCT02087631), liothyronine (in RRMS and progressive MS, NCT02760056), among others. Miconazole and clobetazol have recently been identified as agents with a potential to produce mature oligodendrocytes from progenitor cells [157].

Most of the trials of molecules with a potential for axonal repair have been deceiving. The SPRINT-MS study results were promising; however, phase 3 trials are needed to confirm this result before considering ibudilast as a therapy for progressive MS [132]. Similarly, lipoic acid and simvastatin [134] appear to be potentially beneficial in slowing brain atrophy, and further studies are needed to confirm the results of the phase 2 trials. In a randomized placebo-controlled phase 2 trial, phenytoin was found to have neuroprotective effects after acute optic neuritis compared to placebo [139]. The MS-SMART trial (NCT01910259) failed to show a benefit of amiloride, fluoxetine, or riluzole on brain atrophy in progressive MS (results presented at ECTRIMS 2018). High-dose biotin [153–155] and mesenchymal stem cells appear to have a dual effect on neuroprotection and remyelination, and have been studied in multiple small trials and open-label studies in progressive MS, with promising results (Table 1). It is important to note that treatment with autologous hematopoietic stem cell transplantation is reserved for patients with treatment-refractory highly active MS, specifically those who have poor prognostic factors of future disability, including ongoing clinical or radiological activity despite treatment with potent DMT [158], and is out of the scope of this review. Other compounds that are being investigated in phase 2 or 3 trials, include idebenone (NCT01854359), masitinib (NCT01433497), hormone-based therapies (ACTH (NCT01950234)), and erythropoietin (NCT01144117), lithium (NCT01259388), and T-cell receptor vaccines (NCT02057159), among others.

6.3. Symptomatic Management

Optimal symptom management is essential to improve quality of life of patients and to complement the beneficial effect of long-term maintenance therapies in MS. The most commonly encountered symptoms in MS include fatigue, spasticity-related symptoms, neuropathic pain, urinary dysfunction, sleep disturbances, and mood changes. A high number of patients complain of more than one symptom, many of which may be interrelated. For example, poor sleep and depression worsens diurnal fatigue, which can hence not solely be attributed to the disease. Routine evaluations should include screening for persistent symptoms, preferably using validated scales. A general rule in our experience is to start by treating the most disabling or consequential symptom, titrate medications up slowly, use molecules that have a potential to address more than one symptom, and avoid polypharmacy. Combining pharmacological and non-pharmacological approaches to address specific symptoms is important. For example, gait difficulties can be addressed with physical therapy (with a focus on improving ataxia or muscle strength depending on presentation), spasticity management (stretching, anti-spasticity medications, botulinum toxin injections, baclofen pump), and fatigue with dalfampridine. A significant emphasis should also be placed on physical, occupational, and speech therapy. Evaluation and treatment by a multi-disciplinary team is key to provide optimal care across the range of dysfunction in progressive MS. General wellness measures and management of comorbidities should always be discussed with patients, most importantly hyperlipidemia, hypertension, and diabetes control, consuming a healthy diet, weight loss, smoking cessation, vitamin D supplementation, osteoporosis management, and emotional wellness [159].

7. Challenges in Progressive MS Treatment and Research

There are many unmet needs in the field of progressive MS. First, our experience with anti-inflammatory medications like ocrelizumab and siponimod has shown positive but modest results. These medications work on the inflammatory component of the disease, and their potential mechanism of action on the neurodegenerative aspect of MS is probably minimal, if any. As discussed above, the rituximab/ocrelizumab and fingolimod/siponimod experiences in progressive MS provide evidence that therapeutic approaches for progressive MS should probably focus on a different pathophysiological aspect of the disease. Second, trial methodology has significant implications for the effect of agents in progressive MS. Study population selection and amount of disease activity (pre-trial and in-trial annualized relapse rates, presence or absence of baseline gadolinium enhancing lesions) in enrolled subjects are key in driving these efficacy differences between therapies. The definition of progressive MS also varies between trials, and often but not always, a minimum confirmed EDSS step of three at trial entry is required in progressive MS trials, which makes the study populations somewhat heterogeneous and trial results inconsistent and difficult to compare across studies [57].

Third, the selection of appropriate clinical outcome measures plays an important role in capturing treatment effects in progressive MS trials, as discussed earlier in this manuscript [160]. Non-ambulatory patients are typically excluded from progressive MS trials, and the benefit of different therapies on functional domains other than gait function could yield more promising results, specifically in this patient population. For example, studying hand and cognitive function or using composite outcomes like the MSFC rather than relying solely on ambulation as a primary endpoint could inform treatment effects in a more sensitive way. Hand function might be more amenable to treatment compared to lower extremity function in patients with more advanced disability. In the ASCEND trial for instance, natalizumab was associated with a 44% reduction in the relative risk of confirmed upper limb disability progression measured by the 9HPT (adjusted OR 0·56 (95% CI 0·40–0·80); $p = 0.001$), whereas no benefit was observed on other measures of disability like the EDSS and the T25FW [101]. In a pre-specified baseline subgroup analysis of patients with EDSS ≥6.0 and age >45 years from the OROTARIO trial, ocrelizumab also reduced disability progression as measured by the 12-week confirmed 9HPT in older non-ambulatory patients [161]. Moreover, despite the high prevalence of cognitive dysfunction in progressive MS, there are methodological gaps in outcome measures of cognition in MS, and cognitive function is not adequately and comprehensively evaluated in trials [57,162]. The use of composite outcome measures has been used increasingly in progressive MS trials, and appear to have higher sensitivity to changes. For example, the primary endpoint of the INFORMS trial was a novel composite outcome measure that was defined as a 3-month confirmed change from baseline of the EDSS, the T25FW, or the 9HPT, and although the trial was negative, this outcome measure detected changes with excellent sensitivity in this population [77] Trials evaluating therapies with a remyelinating or repair potential are expected to have a modest clinical effect and can particularly benefit from using composite measures to enhance detection of changes. This approach was used in the opicinimab (SYNERGY) [129] and ibudilast (SPRINT-MS) [132] trials. MRI outcome measures also have some limitations. For example, measures of whole brain atrophy are mostly used as primary endpoints, and have the issue of being variable, which is a concern for interpretability. Other measures like cortical atrophy or magnetization transfer ratio might be more useful depending on the population and mechanism of action of the investigational product.

Finally, the efficacy of molecules with a potential for remyelination and/or neuroprotection needs to be confirmed in large trials with clinically meaningful outcome measures, which will require time and resources. Ultimately, for FDA approval, an agent that can demonstrate clinically meaningful changes in disability measures in large multicenter phase 3 trials is needed. To be able to achieve that, research on the optimal outcome markers is needed. Moreover, many of these molecules are old drugs that do not generate interest in the pharmaceutical industry.

Overall, optimal and novel trial methodology and development of sensitive and clinically meaningful outcome measures and biomarkers are needed in the near-future. The International Progressive MS Alliance and the UK Expert Consortium for Progression in MS Clinical Trials have a mission to expedite development of therapies for progressive forms of MS, which includes the development of optimal trial designs and more responsive outcome measures.

8. Conclusions

A significant amount of effort is delivered to improve knowledge in the field of progressive MS. Future trials will incorporate lessons from previous trials, and hopefully, therapies that halt or even stop neurodegeneration in MS will be available in the future.

Author Contributions: G.M. drafted the manuscript. D.O. reviewed and edited the manuscript for scientific content.

Funding: This research received no external funding.

Conflicts of Interest: Gabrielle Macaron is currently supported by the National Multiple Sclerosis Society Institutional Clinician Training Award ICT 0002. Gabrielle Macaron received fellowship funding from the Biogen Fellowship Grant 6873-P-FEL. She also served in an advisory board for Genentech/Roche. Daniel Ontaneda received research support from the National Multiple Sclerosis Society, National Institutes of Health, Patient Centered Research Institute, Race to Erase MS Foundation, Genentech, and Genzyme. He also received consulting fees from Biogen Idec, Genentech/Roche, Genzyme, Novartis, and Merck.

References

1. Wallin, M.T.; Culpepper, W.J.; Campbell, J.D.; Nelson, M.L.; Langer-Gould, A.; Marrie, R.A.; Cutter, G.R.; Kaye, W.E.; Wagner, L.; Tremlett, H.; et al. The prevalence of MS in the United States: A population-based estimate using health claims data. *Neurology* **2019**, *92*, e1019–e1024. [CrossRef] [PubMed]
2. Browne, P.; Chandraratna, D.; Angood, C.; Tremlett, H.; Baker, C.; Taylor, B.V.; Thompson, A.J. Atlas of Multiple Sclerosis 2013: A growing global problem with widespread inequity. *Neurology* **2014**, *83*, 1022–1024. [CrossRef] [PubMed]
3. Mahad, D.H.; Trapp, B.D.; Lassmann, H. Pathological mechanisms in progressive multiple sclerosis. *Lancet Neurol.* **2015**, *14*, 183–193. [CrossRef]
4. Trapp, B.D.; Peterson, J.; Ransohoff, R.M.; Rudick, R.; Mörk, S.; Bö, L. Axonal Transection in the Lesions of Multiple Sclerosis. *N. Engl. J. Med.* **1998**, *338*, 278–285. [CrossRef] [PubMed]
5. Kornek, B.; Storch, M.K.; Weissert, R.; Wallstroem, W.; Stefferl, A.; Olsson, T.; Linington, C.; Schmidbauer, M.; Lassmann, H. Multiple sclerosis and chronic autoimmune encephalomyelitis: A comparative quantitative study of axonal injury in active, inactive, and remyelinated lesions. *Am. J. Pathol.* **2000**, *157*, 267–276. [CrossRef]
6. Frischer, J.M.; Weigand, S.D.; Guo, Y.; Kale, N.; Parisi, J.E.; Pirko, I.; Mandrekar, J.; Bramow, S.; Metz, I.; Bruck, W.; et al. Clinical and Pathological Insights into the Dynamic Nature of the White Matter Multiple Sclerosis Plaque. *Ann. Neurol.* **2015**, *78*, 710–721. [CrossRef]
7. De Stefano, N.; Giorgio, A.; Battaglini, M.; Rovaris, M.; Sormani, M.P.; Barkhof, F.; Korteweg, T.; Enzinger, C.; Fazekas, F.; Calabrese, M.; et al. Assessing brain atrophy rates in a large population of untreated multiple sclerosis subtypes. *Neurology* **2010**, *74*, 1868–1876. [CrossRef] [PubMed]
8. Lucchinetti, C.F.; Rauschka, H.; Bergmann, M.; Schmidbauer, M.; Kutzelnigg, A.; Parisi, J.E.; Stadelmann, C.; Brück, W.; Lassmann, H. Cortical demyelination and diffuse white matter injury in multiple sclerosis. *Brain* **2005**, *128*, 2705–2712.
9. Amato, M.P.; Portaccio, E.; Goretti, B.; Zipoli, V.; Battaglini, M.; Bartolozzi, M.L.; Stromillo, M.L.; Guidi, L.; Siracusa, G.; Sorbi, S.; et al. Association of Neocortical Volume Changes with Cognitive Deterioration in Relapsing-Remitting Multiple Sclerosis. *Arch. Neurol.* **2007**, *64*, 1157–1161. [CrossRef]

10. Calabrese, M.; Agosta, F.; Rinaldi, F.; Mattisi, I.; Grossi, P.; Favaretto, A.; Atzori, M.; Bernardi, V.; Barachino, L.; Rinaldi, L.; et al. Cortical Lesions and Atrophy Associated with Cognitive Impairment in Relapsing-Remitting Multiple Sclerosis. *Arch. Neurol.* **2009**, *66*, 1144–1150. [CrossRef]

11. Mahad, D.J.; Ziabreva, I.; Campbell, G.; Lax, N.; White, K.; Hanson, P.S.; Lassmann, H.; Turnbull, D.M. Mitochondrial changes within axons in multiple sclerosis. *Brain* **2009**, *132*, 1161–1174. [CrossRef] [PubMed]

12. Trapp, B.D.; Stys, P.K. Virtual hypoxia and chronic necrosis of demyelinated axons in multiple sclerosis. *Lancet Neurol.* **2009**, *8*, 280–291. [CrossRef]

13. Ontaneda, D.; Thompson, A.J.; Fox, R.J.; ACohen, J. Progressive multiple sclerosis: Prospects for disease therapy, repair, and restoration of function. *Lancet* **2017**, *389*, 1357–1366. [CrossRef]

14. Howell, O.W.; Reeves, C.A.; Nicholas, R.; Carassiti, D.; Radotra, B.; Gentleman, S.M.; Serafini, B.; Aloisi, F.; Roncaroli, F.; Magliozzi, R.; et al. Meningeal inflammation is widespread and linked to cortical pathology in multiple sclerosis. *Brain* **2011**, *134*, 2755–2771. [CrossRef] [PubMed]

15. Magliozzi, R.; Howell, O.; Vora, A.; Serafini, B.; Nicholas, R.; Puopolo, M.; Reynolds, R.; Aloisi, F. Meningeal B-cell follicles in secondary progressive multiple sclerosis associate with early onset of disease and severe cortical pathology. *Brain* **2007**, *130*, 1089–1104. [CrossRef]

16. Brown, J.W.L.; Coles, A.; Horakova, D.; Havrdova, E.; Izquierdo, G.; Prat, A.; Girard, M.; Duquette, P.; Trojano, M.; Lugaresi, A.; et al. Association of Initial Disease-Modifying Therapy with Later Conversion to Secondary Progressive Multiple Sclerosis. *JAMA* **2019**, *321*, 175–187. [CrossRef] [PubMed]

17. Bergamaschi, R.; Quaglini, S.; Tavazzi, E.; Amato, M.P.; Paolicelli, D.; Zipoli, V.; Romani, A.; Tortorella, C.; Portaccio, E.; D'Onghia, M.; et al. Immunomodulatory therapies delay disease progression in multiple sclerosis. *Mult. Scler. J.* **2016**, *22*, 1732–1740. [CrossRef]

18. Trojano, M.; Pellegrini, F.; Paolicelli, D.; Fuiani, A.; Zimatore, G.B.; Tortorella, C.; Simone, I.L.; Patti, F.; Ghezzi, A.; Zipoli, V.; et al. Real-life impact of early interferon beta therapy in relapsing multiple sclerosis. *Ann. Neurol.* **2009**, *66*, 513–520. [CrossRef]

19. Trojano, M.; Pellegrini, F.; Fuiani, A.; Paolicelli, D.; Zipoli, V.; Zimatore, G.B.; Monte, E.D.; Portaccio, C.; Lepore, V.; Livrea, P.; et al. New natural history of interferon-beta-treated relapsing multiple sclerosis. *Ann. Neurol.* **2007**, *61*, 300–306. [CrossRef]

20. Haider, L.; Simeonidou, C.; Steinberger, G.; Hametner, S.; Grigoriadis, N.; Deretzi, G.; Kovacs, G.G.; Kutzelnigg, A.; Lassmann, H.; Frischer, J.M. Multiple sclerosis deep grey matter: The relation between demyelination, neurodegeneration, inflammation and iron. *J. Neurol. Neurosurg. Psychiatry* **2014**, *85*, 1386–1395. [CrossRef]

21. Hametner, S.; Wimmer, I.; Haider, L.; Pfeifenbring, S.; Brück, W.; Lassmann, H. Iron and neurodegeneration in the multiple sclerosis brain. *Ann. Neurol.* **2013**, *74*, 848–861. [CrossRef]

22. Harding, K.E.; Liang, K.; Cossburn, M.D.; Ingram, G.; Hirst, C.; Pickersgill, T.; Te Water, N.; Johann, W.; Ben-Shlomo, M.; Robertson, Y.; et al. Long-term outcome of paediatric-onset multiple sclerosis: A population-based study. *J Neurol. Neurosurg. Psychiatry* **2013**, *84*, 141–147. [CrossRef]

23. Leray, E.; Yaouanq, J.; Le Page, E.; Coustans, M.; Laplaud, D.; Oger, J.; Edan, G. Evidence for a two-stage disability progression in multiple sclerosis. *Brain* **2010**, *133*, 1900–1913. [CrossRef]

24. Confavreux, C.; Moreau, T.; Vukusic, S.; Adeleine, P. Relapses and Progression of Disability in Multiple Sclerosis. *N. Engl. J. Med.* **2000**, *343*, 1430–1438. [CrossRef]

25. Beiki, O.; Frumento, P.; Bottai, M.; Manouchehrinia, A.; Hillert, J. Changes in the Risk of Reaching Multiple Sclerosis Disability Milestones in Recent Decades: A Nationwide Population-Based Cohort Study in Sweden. *JAMA Neurol.* **2019**, 1–7. [CrossRef]

26. Polman, C.H.; Reingold, S.C.; Banwell, B.; Clanet, M.; Cohen, J.A.; Filippi, M.; Fujihara, K.; Havrdova, E.K.; Hutchinson, M.; Kappos, L.; et al. Diagnostic criteria for multiple sclerosis: 2010 Revisions to the McDonald criteria. *Ann. Neurol.* **2011**, *69*, 292–302. [CrossRef]

27. Thompson, A.J.; Banwell, B.L.; Barkhof, F.; Carroll, W.; Coetzee, T.; Comi, G.; Correale, J.; Fazekas, F.; Filippi, M.; Freedman, M.; et al. Diagnosis of multiple sclerosis: 2017 revisions of the McDonald criteria. *Lancet Neurol.* **2018**, *17*, 162–173. [CrossRef]

28. Lublin, F.; Stephen, C.; Reingold, P.; Cohen, J.A.; Cutter, G.; Sørensen, P.S.; Thompson, A.J.; Wolinsky, J.S.; Balcer, L.J.; Banwell, B.; et al. Defining the clinical course of multiple sclerosis: The 2013 revisions. *Neurology* **2014**, *83*, 278–286. [CrossRef]

29. Whitaker, J.N.; McFarland, H.F.; Rudge, P.; Reingold, R.S. Outcomes assessment in multiple sclerosis trials. *Mult. Scler.* **1995**, *1*, 37–47. [CrossRef]

30. Noseworthy, J.H.; Vandervoort, M.K.; Wong, C.J.; Ebers, G.C. Interrater variability with the Expanded Disability Status Scale (EDSS) and Functional Systems (FS) in a multiple sclerosis clinical trial. *Neurology* **1990**, *40*, 971. [CrossRef]

31. Goodkin, D.E.; Cookfair, D.; Wende, K.; Bourdette, D.; Pullicino, P.; Scherokman, B.; Whitham, R. Inter- and intrarater scoring agreement using grades 1.0 to 3.5 of the Kurtzke Expanded Disability Status Scale (EDSS). *Neurology* **1992**, *42*, 859. [CrossRef]

32. Kragt, J.J.; Nielsen, J.M.; Van Der Linden, F.A.; Uitdehaag, B.M.; Polman, C.H. How similar are commonly combined criteria for EDSS progression in multiple sclerosis? *Mult. Scler. J.* **2006**, *12*, 782–786. [CrossRef]

33. Ontaneda, D.; ACohen, J.; Amato, M.P. Clinical outcome measures for progressive MS trials. *Mult. Scler. J.* **2017**, *23*, 1627–1635. [CrossRef]

34. Cutter, G.R.; Baier, M.L.; Rudick, R.A.; Cookfair, D.L.; Fischer, J.S.; Petkau, J.; Syndulko, K.; Weinshenker, B.G.; Antel, J.P.; Confavreux, C.; et al. Development of a multiple sclerosis functional composite as a clinical trial outcome measure. *Brain* **1999**, *122*, 871–882. [CrossRef]

35. Fischer, J.; Rudick, R.; Cutter, G.; Reingold, S. The Multiple Sclerosis Functional Composite measure (MSFC): An integrated approach to MS clinical outcome assessment. *Mult. Scler. J.* **1999**, *5*, 244–250. [CrossRef]

36. Cohen, J.A.; Cutter, G.R.; Fischer, J.S.; Goodman, A.D.; Heidenreich, F.R.; Jak, A.J.; Kniker, J.E.; Kooijmans, M.F.; Lull, J.M.; Sandrock, A.W.; et al. Use of the Multiple Sclerosis Functional Composite as an Outcome Measure in a Phase 3 Clinical Trial. *Arch. Neurol.* **2001**, *58*, 961–967. [CrossRef]

37. Polman, C.H.; Rudick, R.A. The Multiple Sclerosis Functional Composite: A clinically meaningful measure of disability. *Neurology* **2010**, *74*, 8–15. [CrossRef]

38. Kalkers, N.; Bergers, L.; De Groot, V.; Lazeron, R.; Van Walderveen, M.; Uitdehaag, B.; Polman, C.; Barkhof, F. Concurrent validity of the MS Functional Composite using MRI as a biological disease marker. *Neurology* **2001**, *56*, 215–219. [CrossRef]

39. Miller, D.M.; Rudick, R.A.; Cutter, G.; Baier, M.; Fischer, J.S. Clinical Significance of the Multiple Sclerosis Functional Composite. *Arch. Neurol.* **2000**, *57*, 1319–1324. [CrossRef]

40. Cohen, J.A.; Cutter, G.R.; Fischer, J.S.; Goodman, A.; Heidenreich, F.R.; Kooijmans, M.F.; Sandrock, A.W.; Rudick, R.A.; Simon, J.H.; Simonian, N.A.; et al. Benefit of interferon -1a on MSFC progression in secondary progressive multiple sclerosis. *Neurology* **2002**, *59*, 679–687. [CrossRef]

41. Baier, M.L.; Cutter, G.R.; Rudick, R.A.; Miller, D.; Cohen, J.A.; Weinstock-Guttman, B.; Mass, M.; Balcer, L.J. Low-contrast letter acuity testing captures visual dysfunction in patients with multiple sclerosis. *Neurology* **2005**, *64*, 992–995. [CrossRef]

42. Balcer, L.J.; Baier, M.L.; Cohen, J.A.; Kooijmans, M.F.; Sandrock, A.W.; Nano-Schiavi, M.L.; Pfohl, D.C.; Mills, M.; Bowen, J.; Ford, C.; et al. Contrast letter acuity as a visual component for the Multiple Sclerosis Functional Composite. *Neurology* **2003**, *61*, 1367–1373. [CrossRef]

43. Freeman, J.; Hobart, J.; Thompson, A. Kurtzke scales revisited: The application of psychometric methods to clinical intuition. *Brain* **2000**, *123*, 1027–1040.

44. Rasova, K.; Martinkova, P.; Vyskotova, J.; Sedova, M. Assessment set for evaluation of clinical outcomes in multiple sclerosis: Psychometric properties. *Patient Relat. Outcome Meas.* **2012**, *3*, 59–70. [CrossRef]

45. ACohen, J.; Coles, A.J.; Arnold, D.L.; Confavreux, C.; Fox, E.J.; Hartung, H.-P.; Havrdova, E.K.; Selmaj, K.W.; Weiner, H.L.; Fisher, E.; et al. Alemtuzumab versus interferon beta 1a as first-line treatment for patients with relapsing-remitting multiple sclerosis: A randomised controlled phase 3 trial. *Lancet* **2012**, *380*, 1819–1828.

46. Polman, C.; Hohlfeld, R.; Agoropoulou, C.; Leyk, M.; Zhang-Auberson, L.; Burtin, P.; Kappos, L.; Radue, E.-W.; O'Connor, P.; Calabresi, P.; et al. A Placebo-Controlled Trial of Oral Fingolimod in Relapsing Multiple Sclerosis. *N. Engl. J. Med.* **2010**, *362*, 387–401.

47. Meyer-Moock, S.; Feng, Y.-S.; Maeurer, M.; Dippel, F.-W.; Kohlmann, T. Systematic literature review and validity evaluation of the Expanded Disability Status Scale (EDSS) and the Multiple Sclerosis Functional Composite (MSFC) in patients with multiple sclerosis. *BMC Neurol.* **2014**, *14*, 58. [CrossRef]

48. Rudick, R.A.; Miller, D.; Bethoux, F.; Rao, S.M.; Lee, J.-C.; Stough, D.; Reece, C.; Schindler, D.; Mamone, B.; Alberts, J. The Multiple Sclerosis Performance Test (MSPT): An iPad-Based Disability Assessment Tool. *J. Vis. Exp.* **2014**, e51318. [CrossRef]

49. Macaron, G.; Moss, B.P.; Li, H.; Baldassari, L.; Rao, S.; Schindler, D.; Alberts, J.; Weber, M.; Ayers, M.; Bethoux, F.; et al. Technology-enabled assessments to enhance multiple sclerosis clinical care and research. *Neurol. Clin. Pract.* **2019**, in press.

50. Motl, R.W.; A Cohen, J.; Benedict, R.; Phillips, G.; LaRocca, N.; Hudson, L.D.; Rudick, R. Multiple Sclerosis Outcome Assessments Consortium Validity of the timed 25-foot walk as an ambulatory performance outcome measure for multiple sclerosis. *Mult. Scler. J.* **2017**, *23*, 704–710. [CrossRef]

51. Feng, J.; Qu, J.; Felix, C.; McGinley, M.; Nakamura, K.; Macaron, G.; Moss, B.; Li, H.; Jones, S.; Rao, S.; et al. Quantitative MRI and patient-reported outcomes validate clinically meaningful changes on tests of ambulation and hand function. *ACTRIMS* **2019**, P050.

52. Feys, P.; Lamers, I.; Francis, G.; Benedict, R.; Phillips, G.; LaRocca, N.; Hudson, L.D.; Rudick, R. Multiple Sclerosis Outcome Assessments Consortium the Nine-Hole Peg Test as a manual dexterity performance measure for multiple sclerosis. *Mult. Scler. J.* **2017**, *23*, 711–720. [CrossRef]

53. Benedict, R.H.; DeLuca, J.; Phillips, G.; LaRocca, N.; Hudson, L.D.; Rudick, R. Multiple Sclerosis Outcome Assessments Consortium Validity of the Symbol Digit Modalities Test as a cognition performance outcome measure for multiple sclerosis. *Mult. Scler. J.* **2017**, *23*, 721–733. [CrossRef]

54. Macaron, G.; Moss, B.; Baldassari, L.E.; Conway, D.; McGinley, M.; Alshehri, E.; Feng, J.; Bermel, R.; Boissy, A.; Cohen, J.A.; et al. Cross-sectional predictive value of clinically meaningful change in processing speed on self-reported cognition and MRI metrics. *ACTRIMS* **2019**, P034.

55. Balcer, L.J.; Raynowska, J.; Nolan, R.; Galetta, S.L.; Kapoor, R.; Benedict, R.; Phillips, G.; LaRocca, N.; Hudson, L.; Rudick, R.; et al. Validity of low-contrast letter acuity as a visual performance outcome measure for multiple sclerosis. *Mult. Scler. J.* **2017**, *23*, 734–747. [CrossRef]

56. Oh, J.; Ontaneda, D.; Azevedo, C.; Klawiter, E.; Absinta, M.; Arnold, D.; Bakshi, R.; Calabresi, P.; Crainiceanu, C.; Dewey, B.; et al. Imaging outcome measures of neuroprotection repair in MS: A consensus statement from NAIMS. *Neurology* **2019**, *92*, 519–533. [CrossRef]

57. Ontaneda, D.; Fox, R.J.; Chataway, J. Clinical trials in progressive multiple sclerosis: Lessons learned and future perspectives. *Lancet Neurol.* **2015**, *14*, 208–223. [CrossRef]

58. Mahajan, K.R.; Ontaneda, D. The Role of Advanced Magnetic Resonance Imaging Techniques in Multiple Sclerosis Clinical Trials. *Neurotherapeutics* **2017**, *14*, 905–923. [CrossRef]

59. Hardmeier, M.; Leocani, L.; Fuhr, P. A new role for evoked potentials in MS? Repurposing evoked potentials as biomarkers for clinical trials in MS. *Mult. Scler. J.* **2017**, *23*, 1309–1319. [CrossRef]

60. Saidha, S.; Al-Louzi, O.; Ratchford, J.N.; Bhargava, P.; Oh, J.; Newsome, S.D.; Prince, J.L.; Pham, D.; Roy, S.; Van Zijl, P.; et al. Optical Coherence Tomography Reflects Brain Atrophy in Multiple Sclerosis: A Four-Year Study. *Ann. Neurol.* **2015**, *78*, 801–813. [CrossRef]

61. Novakova, L.; Zetterberg, H.; Sundström, P.; Axelsson, M.; Khademi, M.; Gunnarsson, M.; Malmeström, C.; Svenningsson, A.; Olsson, T.; Piehl, F.; et al. Monitoring disease activity in multiple sclerosis using serum neurofilament light protein. *Neurology* **2017**, *89*, 2230–2237. [CrossRef]

62. Damasceno, A.; Dias-Carneiro, R.P.C.; Moraes, A.S.; Boldrinib, V.O.; Quintilianob, R.P.S.; de Paula Galdino da Silvab, V.A.; Fariasb, A.S.; Brandãob, C.O.; Damascenoa, B.P.; dos Santos, L.M.B.; et al. Clinical MRI correlates of CSF neurofilament light chain levels in relapsing progressive multiple sclerosis. *Mult. Scler. Relat. Disord.* **2019**, *30*, 149–153. [CrossRef]

63. Martin, S.J.; McGlasson, S.; Hunt, D.; Overell, J. Cerebrospinal fluid neurofilament light chain in multiple sclerosis and its subtypes: A meta-analysis of case-control studies. *J. Neurol. Neurosurg. Psychiatry* **2019**. [CrossRef]

64. Pawlitzki, M.; Schreiber, S.; Bittner, D.; Kreipe, J.; Leypoldt, F.; Rupprecht, K.; Carare, R.O.; Meuth, S.G.; Vielhaber, S.; Körtvélyessy, P. CSF Neurofilament Light Chain Levels in Primary Progressive MS: Signs of Axonal Neurodegeneration. *Front. Neurol.* **2018**, *9*, 9. [CrossRef]

65. Barro, C.; Naegelin, Y.; Schädelin, S.; Giardiello, A.; Zecca, C.; Blennow, K.; Zetterberg, H.; Leppert, D.; Gobbi, C.; Kuhle, J.; et al. Serum Neurofilament light: A biomarker of neuronal damage in multiple sclerosis. *Ann. Neurol.* **2017**, *81*, 857–870.

66. Barro, C.; Benkert, P.; Disanto, G.; Tsagkas, C.; Amann, M.; Naegelin, Y.; Leppert, D.; Gobbi, C.; Granziera, C.; Yaldizli, O.; et al. Serum neurofilament as a predictor of disease worsening and brain and spinal cord atrophy in multiple sclerosis. *Brain* **2018**, *141*, 2382–2391. [CrossRef]

67. Hauser, S.L.; Bar-Or, A.; Comi, G.; Giovannoni, G.; Hartung, H.-P.; Hemmer, B.; Lublin, F.; Montalban, X.; Rammohan, K.W.; Selmaj, K.; et al. Ocrelizumab versus Interferon Beta-1a in Relapsing Multiple Sclerosis. *N. Engl. J. Med.* **2017**, *376*, 221–234. [CrossRef]

68. Montalban, X.; Hauser, S.L.; Kappos, L.; Arnold, D.L.; Bar-Or, A.; Comi, G.; De Seze, J.; Giovannoni, G.; Hartung, H.-P.; Hemmer, B.; et al. Ocrelizumab versus Placebo in Primary Progressive Multiple Sclerosis. *N. Engl. J. Med.* **2017**, *376*, 209–220. [CrossRef]

69. Fox, E.; Markowitz, C.; Applebee, A.; Montalban, X.; Wolinsky, J.S.; Belachew, S.; Damian, F.; Han, J.; Musch, B.; Giovannoni, G. Effect of ocrelizumab on upper limb function in patients with primary progressive multiple sclerosis (PPMS) in the oratorio study (ENCORE). *J. Neurol. Neurosurg. Psychiatry* **2018**, *89*, A14. [CrossRef]

70. Hawker, K.; O'Connor, P.; Freedman, M.S.; Calabresi, P.A.; Antel, J.; Simon, J.; Hauser, S.; Waubant, E.; Vollmer, T.; Panitch, H.; et al. Rituximab in patients with primary progressive multiple sclerosis: Results of a randomized double-blind placebo-controlled multicenter trial. *Ann. Neurol.* **2009**, *66*, 460–471. [CrossRef]

71. Naegelin, Y.; Naegelin, P.; Von Felten, S.; Lorscheider, J.; Sonder, J.; Uitdehaag, B.M.J.; Scotti, B.; Zecca, C.; Gobbi, C.; Kappos, L.; et al. Association of Rituximab Treatment with Disability Progression Among Patients With Secondary Progressive Multiple Sclerosis. *JAMA Neurol.* **2019**, *76*, 274. [CrossRef]

72. Gelfand, J.M.; Cree, B.A.C.; Hauser, S.L. Ocrelizumab and Other CD20+ B-Cell-Depleting Therapies in Multiple Sclerosis. *Neurotherapeutics* **2017**, *14*, 835–841. [CrossRef]

73. Klein, C.; Lammens, A.; Schäfer, W.; Georges, G.; Schwaiger, M.; Mössner, E.; Hopfner, K.-P.; Umana, P.; Niederfellner, G. Epitope interactions of monoclonal antibodies targeting CD20 and their relationship to functional properties. *mAbs* **2013**, *5*, 22–33. [CrossRef]

74. Feng, J.J.; Ontaneda, D. Treating primary-progressive multiple sclerosis: Potential of ocrelizumab and review of B-cell therapies. *Degener. Neurol. Neuromuscul. Dis.* **2017**, *7*, 31–45. [CrossRef]

75. Kappos, L.; Bar-Or, A.; Cree, B.A.C.; Fox, R.J.; Giovannoni, G.; Gold, R.; Vermersch, P.; Arnold, D.L.; Arnould, S.; Scherz, T.; et al. Siponimod versus placebo in secondary progressive multiple sclerosis (EXPAND): A double-blind, randomised, phase 3 study. *Lancet* **2018**, *391*, 1263–1273. [CrossRef]

76. Jackson, S.J.; Giovannoni, G.; Baker, D. Fingolimod modulates microglial activation to augment markers of remyelination. *J. Neuroinflamm.* **2011**, *8*, 76. [CrossRef]

77. Lublin, F.; Miller, D.H.; Freedman, M.S.; Cree, B.A.C.; Wolinsky, J.S.; Weiner, H.; Lubetzki, C.; Hartung, H.-P.; Montalban, X.; Uitdehaag, B.M.J.; et al. Oral fingolimod in primary progressive multiple sclerosis (INFORMS): A phase 3, randomised, double-blind, placebo-controlled trial. *Lancet* **2016**, *387*, 1075–1084. [CrossRef]

78. Martinelli Boneschi, F.; Vacchi, L.; Rovaris, M.; Capra, R.; Comi, G. Mitoxantrone for multiple sclerosis. *Cochrane Database Syst. Rev.* **2013**, *5*, CD002127. [CrossRef]

79. Hartung, H.P.; Gonsette, R.; König, N.; Kwiecinski, H.; Guseo, A.; Morrissey, S.; Krapf, S.; Zwingers, T. Mitoxantrone in Multiple Sclerosis Study Group. Mitoxantrone in progressive multiple sclerosis: A placebo-controlled, double-blind, randomised, multicentre trial. *Lancet* **2002**, *28*, 2018–2025. [CrossRef]

80. Krapf, H.; Morrissey, S.P.; Zenker, O.; Zwingers, T.; Gonsette, R.; Hartung, H.-P. Effect of mitoxantrone on MRI in progressive MS: Results of the MIMS trial. *Neurology* **2005**, *65*, 690–695. [CrossRef]

81. Grey Née Cotte, S.; Salmen Née Stroet, A.; Von Ahsen, N.; Starck, M.; Winkelmann, A.; Zettl, U.K.; Comabella, M.; Montalban, X.; Zipp, F.; Fleischer, V.; et al. Lack of efficacy of mitoxantrone in primary progressive Multiple Sclerosis irrespective of pharmacogenetic factors: A multi-center, retrospective analysis. *J. Neuroimmunol.* **2015**, *278*, 277–279. [CrossRef]

82. Pelfrey, C.M.; Cotleur, A.C.; Zamor, N.; Lee, J.C.; Robert, R.J. Immunological studies of mitoxantrone in primary progressive multiple sclerosis. *J. Neuroimmunol.* **2006**, *175*, 192–199. [CrossRef]

83. Cotte, S.; Von Ahsen, N.; Kruse, N.; Huber, B.; Winkelmann, A.; Zettl, U.K.; Starck, M.; König, N.; Téllez, N.; Dorr, J.; et al. ABC-transporter gene-polymorphisms are potential pharmacogenetic markers for mitoxantrone response in multiple sclerosis. *Brain* **2009**, *132*, 2517–2530. [CrossRef]

84. US Food and Drug Administration. Press Announcement–FDA Approves New Oral Drug to Treat Multiple Sclerosis. Office of the Commissioner. Available online: https://www.fda.gov/NewsEvents/Newsroom/PressAnnouncements/ucm634469.htm (accessed on 2 April 2019).

85. Giovannoni, G.; Comi, G.; Cook, S.; Rammohan, K.; Rieckmann, P.; Sørensen, P.S.; Vermersch, P.; Chang, P.; Hamlett, A.; Musch, B.; et al. A Placebo-Controlled Trial of Oral Cladribine for Relapsing Multiple Sclerosis. *N. Engl. J. Med.* **2010**, *362*, 416–426. [CrossRef]

86. Montalban, X.; Leist, T.P.; Cohen, B.A.; Moses, H.; Campbell, J.; Hicking, C.; Dangond, F. Cladribine tablets added to IFN-β in active relapsing multiple sclerosis. *Neurol. Neuroimmunol. NeuroInflamm.* **2018**, *5*, 477. [CrossRef]

87. Leist, T.P.; Comi, G.; Cree, B.A.C.; Coyle, P.K.; Freedman, M.S.; Hartung, H.-P.; Vermersch, P.; Casset-Semanaz, F.; Scaramozza, M. Effect of oral cladribine on time to conversion to clinically definite multiple sclerosis in patients with a first demyelinating event (ORACLE MS): A phase 3 randomised trial. *Lancet Neurol.* **2014**, *13*, 257–267. [CrossRef]

88. Sipe, J. Cladribine in treatment of chronic progressive multiple sclerosis. *Lancet* **1994**, *344*, 9–13. [CrossRef]

89. Rice, G.P.A.; Filippi, M.; Comi, G. Cladribine and progressive MS: Clinical and MRI outcomes of a multicenter controlled trial. *Neurology* **2000**, *54*, 1145–1155. [CrossRef]

90. Filippi, M.; Rovaris, M.; Iannucci, G.; Mennea, S.; Sormani, M.P.; Comi, G. Whole brain volume changes in patients with progressive multiple sclerosis treated with cladribine. *Neurology* **2000**, *55*, 1714–1718. [CrossRef]

91. Polman, C.; Pozzilli, C.; Thompson, A.; Beckmann, K.; Dahlke, F. Final analysis of the European multicenter trial on IFNbeta-1b in secondary-progressive multiple sclerosis. *Neurology* **2001**, *57*, 1969–1975.

92. The North American Study Group. Interferon beta-1b in secondary progressive MS: Results from a 3-year controlled study. *Neurology* **2004**, *63*, 1788–1795. [CrossRef]

93. Kappos, L.; Weinstock-Guttman, B.; Pozzilli, C.; Thompson, A.J.; Dahlke, F.; Beckmann, K.; Polman, C.; McFarland, H.; European (EU-SPMS) Interferon beta-1b in Secondary Progressive Multiple Sclerosis Trial Steering Committee and Independent Advisory Board; North American (NA-SPMS) Interferon beta-1b in Secondary Progressive Multiple Sclerosis Trial Steering Committee and Independent Advisory Board. Interferon beta-1b in secondary progressive multiple sclerosis. A combined analysis of the two trials. *Neurology* **2004**, *63*, 1779–1787. [CrossRef]

94. Secondary Progressive Efficacy Clinical Trial of Recombinant Interferon-Beta-1a in MS (SPECTRIMS) Study Group. Randomized controlled trial of interferon- beta-1a in secondary progressive MS: Clinical results. *Neurology* **2001**, *56*, 1496–1504. [CrossRef]

95. Andersen, O.; Elovaara, I.; Färkkilä, M.; Hansen, H.J.; Mellgren, S.; Myhr, K.-M.; Sandberg-Wollheim, M.; Soelberg, S. Multicentre, randomised, double blind, placebo controlled, phase III study of weekly, low dose, subcutaneous interferon beta-1a in secondary progressive multiple sclerosis. *J. Neurol. Neurosurg. Psychiatry* **2004**, *75*, 706–710. [CrossRef]

96. Leary, S.M.; Miller, D.H.; Stevenson, V.L.; Brex, P.A.; Chard, D.T.; Thompson, A.J. Interferon beta-1a in primary progressive MS: An exploratory, randomized, controlled trial. *Neurology* **2003**, *60*, 44–51. [CrossRef]

97. Montalban, X. Overview of European pilot study of interferon beta-Ib in primary progressive multiple sclerosis. *Mult. Scler.* **2004**, *10*, S62–S64.

98. Montalban, X.; Garriga, J.S.; Tintoré, M.; Brieva, L.; Aymerich, F.; Rio, J.; Porcel, J.; Borràs, C.; Nos, C.; Rovira, À.; et al. A single-center, randomized, double-blind, placebo-controlled study of interferon beta-1b on primary progressive and transitional multiple sclerosis. *Mult. Scler. J.* **2009**, *15*, 1195–1205. [CrossRef]

99. Wolinsky, J.S.; Narayana, P.A.; O'Connor, P.; Coyle, P.K.; Ford, C.; Johnson, K.; Miller, A.; Pardo, L.; Kadosh, S.; Ladkani, D.; et al. Glatiramer acetate in primary progressive multiple sclerosis: Results of a multinational, multicenter, double-blind, placebo-controlled trial. *Ann. Neurol.* **2007**, *61*, 14–24. [CrossRef]

100. Wolinsky, J.S.; Shochat, T.; Weiss, S.; Ladkani, D. Glatiramer acetate treatment in PPMS: Why males appear to respond favorably. *J. Neurol. Sci.* **2009**, *286*, 92–98. [CrossRef]

101. Ho, P.-R.; Campbell, N.; Chang, I.; Deykin, A.; Forrestal, F.; Lucas, N.; Yu, B.; Arnold, D.L.; Hartung, H.-P.; Miller, A.; et al. Effect of natalizumab on disease progression in secondary progressive multiple sclerosis (ASCEND): A phase 3, randomised, double-blind, placebo-controlled trial with an open-label extension. *Lancet Neurol.* **2018**, *17*, 405–415.

102. Graves, D.; Vernino, S. Immunotherapies in Neurologic Disorders. *Med. Clin. N. Am.* **2012**, *96*, 497–523. [CrossRef]

103. Salzer, J.; Svenningsson, R.; Alping, P.; Novakova, L.; Bjorck, A.; Fink, K.; Islam-Jakobsson, P.; Malmestrom, C.; Axelsson, M.; Vagberg, M. Rituximab in multiple sclerosis: A retrospective observational study on safety and efficacy. *Neurology* **2016**, *87*, 2074–2081. [CrossRef]

104. Komori, M.; Lin, Y.C.; Cortese, I.; Blake, A.; Ohayon, J.; Cherup, J.; Maric, D.; Kosa, P.; Wu, T.; Bielekova, B. Insufficient disease inhibition by intrathecal rituximab in progressive multiple sclerosis. *Ann. Clin. Transl. Neurol.* **2016**, *3*, 166–179. [CrossRef]

105. Bhargava, P.; Wicken, C.; Smith, M.D.; Strowd, R.E.; Cortese, I.; Reich, D.S.; Calabresi, P.A.; Mowry, E.M. Trial of intrathecal rituximab in progressive multiple sclerosis patients with evidence of leptomeningeal contrast enhancement. *Mult. Scler. Relat. Disord.* **2019**, *30*, 136–140. [CrossRef]

106. Bergman, J.; Burman, J.; Gilthorpe, J.D.; Zetterberg, H.; Jiltsova, E.; Bergenheim, T.; Svenningsson, A. Intrathecal treatment trial of rituximab in progressive MS: An open-label phase 1b study. *Neurology* **2018**, *91*, e1893–e1901. [CrossRef]

107. Topping, J.; Dobson, R.; Lapin, S.; Maslyanskiy, A.; Kropshofer, H.; David, L.; Giovannoni, G.; Evdoshenko, E. The effects of intrathecal rituximab on biomarkers in multiple sclerosis. *Mult. Scler. Relat. Disord.* **2016**, *6*, 49–53. [CrossRef]

108. British and Dutch Multiple Sclerosis Azathioprine Trial Group. Double-masked trial of azathioprine in multiple sclerosis. *Lancet* **1988**, *2*, 179–183.

109. Kappos, L.; Pätzold, U.; Dommasch, D.; Poser, S.; Haas, J.; Krauseneck, P.; Malin, J.-P.; Fierz, W.; Graffenried, B.U.; Gugerli, U.S. Cyclosporine versus azathioprine in the long-term treatment of multiple sclerosis? results of the german multicenter study. *Ann. Neurol.* **1988**, *23*, 56–63. [CrossRef]

110. Uccelli, A.; Capello, E.; Fenoglio, D.; Incagliato, M.; Valbonesi, M.; Mancardi, G.L. Intravenous immunoglobulin, plasmalymphocytapheresis and azathioprine in chronic progressive multiple sclerosis. *Neurol. Sci.* **1994**, *15*, 49–53. [CrossRef]

111. Perini, P.; Calabrese, M.; Tiberio, M.; Ranzato, F.; Battistin, L.; Gallo, P. Mitoxantrone versus cyclophosphamide in secondary-progressive multiple sclerosis: A comparative study. *J. Neurol.* **2006**, *253*, 1034–1040. [CrossRef]

112. Zephir, H.; De Seze, J.; Duhamel, A.; Debouverie, M.; Hautecoeur, P.; Lebrun, C.; Malíková, I.; Pelletier, J.; Sénéchal, O.; Vermersch, P. Treatment of progressive forms of multiple sclerosis by cyclophosphamide: A cohort study of 490 patients. *J. Neurol. Sci.* **2004**, *218*, 73–77. [CrossRef]

113. Brochet, B.; Deloire, M.S.A.; Perez, P.; Loock, T.; Baschet, L.; Debouverie, M.; Pittion, S.; Ouallet, J.-C.; Clavelou, P.; De Seze, J.; et al. Double-Blind Controlled Randomized Trial of Cyclophosphamide versus Methylprednisolone in Secondary Progressive Multiple Sclerosis. *PLoS ONE* **2017**, *12*, e0168834. [CrossRef]

114. Weiner, H.L.; Mackin, G.A.; Orav, E.J.; Hafler, D.A.; Dawson, D.M.; Lapierre, Y.; Herndon, R.; Lehrich, J.R.; Hauser, S.L.; Turel, A.; et al. Intermittent cyclophosphamide pulse therapy in progressive multiple sclerosis: Final report of the Northeast Cooperative Multiple Sclerosis Treatment Group. *Neurology* **1993**, *43*, 910. [CrossRef]

115. Hommes, O.R.; Sørensen, P.S.; Fazekas, F.; Enriquez, M.M.; Koelmel, H.W.; Fernández, Ó.; Pozzilli, C.; O'Connor, P. Intravenous immunoglobulin in secondary progressive multiple sclerosis: Randomised placebo-controlled trial. *Lancet* **2004**, *364*, 1149–1156. [CrossRef]

116. Goodkin, D.; Rudick, R.; Medendorp, S.V.; Daughtry, M.; Van Dyke, C. Low-dose oral methotrexate in chronic progressive multiple sclerosis: Analyses of serial MRIs. *Neurology* **1996**, *47*, 1153–1157. [CrossRef]

117. Goodkin, D.E.; Rudick, R.A.; Medendorp, S.V.; Daughtry, M.M.; Schwetz, K.M.; Fischer, J.; Van Dyke, C. Low-dose (7.5 mg) oral methotrexate reduces the rate of progression in chronic progressive multiple sclerosis. *Ann. Neurol.* **1995**, *37*, 30–40. [CrossRef]

118. Lugaresi, A.; Caporale, C.; Farina, D.; Marzoli, F.; Bonanni, L.; Muraro, P.A.; De Luca, G.; Iarlori, C.; Gambi, D. Low-dose oral methotrexate treatment in chronic progressive multiple sclerosis. *Neurol. Sci. Off. J. Ital. Neurol. Soc. Ital. Soc. Clin. Neurophysiol.* **2001**, *22*, 209–210. [CrossRef]

119. The Multiple Sclerosis Study Group. Efficacy and toxicity of cyclosporine in chronic progressive multiple sclerosis: A randomized, double-blinded, placebo-controlled clinical trial. *Ann Neurol.* **1990**, *27*, 591–605. [CrossRef]

120. Fakih, R.; Matiello, M.; Chitnis, T.; Stankiewicz, J.M. Efficacy and safety of mycophenolate mofetil in progressive multiple sclerosis patients. *J. Neurol.* **2018**, *265*, 2688–2694. [CrossRef]

121. Barkhof, F.; Giovannoni, G.; Hartung, H.P.; Cree, B.; Uccelli, A.; Sormani, M.P.; Krieger, S.; Uitdehaag, B.; Vollmer, T.; Montalban, X. ARPEGGIO: A randomized, placebo-controlled study to evaluate oral laquinimod in patients with primary progressive multiple sclerosis (PPMS) (P7.210). *Neurology* **2015**, *84*, P7.210.

122. Freedman, M.S.; Bar-Or, A.; Oger, J.; Traboulsee, A.; Patry, D.; Young, C.; Olsson, T.; Li, D.; Hartung, H.P.; Krantz, M.; et al. A phase III study evaluating the efficacy safety of MBP8298 in secondary progressive multiple sclerosis. *Neurology* **2011**, *77*, 1551–1560. [CrossRef]

123. Deshmukh, V.A.; Tardif, V.; Lyssiotis, C.A.; Green, C.C.; Kerman, B.; Kim, H.J.; Padmanabhan, K.; Swoboda, J.G.; Ahmad, I.; Kondo, T.; et al. A regenerative approach to the treatment of multiple sclerosis. *Nature* **2013**, *502*, 327–332. [CrossRef]

124. Mei, F.; Fancy, S.P.J.; Shen, Y.A.; Niu, J.; Zhao, C.; Presley, B.; Miao, E.; Lee, S.; Mayoral, S.R.; Redmond, S.A.; et al. Micropillar arrays as a high-throughput screening platform for therapeutics in multiple sclerosis. *Nat. Med.* **2014**, *20*, 954–960. [CrossRef]

125. Green, A.J.; Gelfand, J.M.; Cree, B.A.; Bevan, C.; Boscardin, W.J.; Mei, F.; Inman, J.; Arnow, S.; Devereux, M.; Abounasr, A.; et al. Clemastine fumarate as a remyelinating therapy for multiple sclerosis (ReBUILD): A randomised, controlled, double-blind, crossover trial. *Lancet* **2017**, *390*, 2481–2489. [CrossRef]

126. Jepson, S.; Vought, B.; Gross, C.H.; Gan, L.; Austen, D.; Frantz, J.D.; Zwahlen, J.; Lowe, D.; Markland, W.; Krauss, R. LINGO-1, a Transmembrane Signaling Protein, Inhibits Oligodendrocyte Differentiation and Myelination through Intercellular Self-interactions. *J. Boil. Chem.* **2012**, *287*, 22184–22195. [CrossRef]

127. Mi, S.; Miller, R.H.; Lee, X.; Scott, M.L.; Shulag-Morskaya, S.; Shao, Z.; Chang, J.; Thill, G.; Levesque, M.; Zhang, M.; et al. LINGO-1 negatively regulates myelination by oligodendrocytes. *Nat. Neurosci.* **2005**, *8*, 745–751. [CrossRef]

128. Cadavid, D.; Balcer, L.; Galetta, S.; Aktas, O.; Ziemssen, T.; Vanopdenbosch, L.; Frederiksen, J.; Skeen, M.; Jaffe, G.J.; Butzkueven, H.; et al. Safety and efficacy of opicinumab in acute optic neuritis (RENEW): A randomised, placebo-controlled, phase 2 trial. *Lancet Neurol.* **2017**, *16*, 189–199. [CrossRef]

129. Mellion, M.; Edwards, K.R.; Hupperts, R.; Drulović, J.; Montalban, X.; Hartung, H.P.; Brochet, B.; Calabresi, P.A.; Rudick, R.; Ibrahim, A. Efficacy Results from the Phase 2b SYNERGY Study: Treatment of Disabling Multiple Sclerosis with the Anti-LINGO-1 Monoclonal Antibody Opicinumab (S33.004). *Neurology* **2017**, *88*, S33.004.

130. .McCroskery, P.; Selmaj, K.; Fernandez, O.; Grimaldi, L.; Silber, E.; Pardo, G.; Freedman, M.S.; Zhang, Y.; Xu, L.; Cadavid, D. Safety and Tolerability of Opicinumab in Relapsing Multiple Sclerosis. *Neurology* **2017**, *88*, P5.369.

131. Cho, Y.; Crichlow, G.V.; Vermeire, J.J.; Leng, L.; Du, X.; Hodsdon, M.E.; Bucala, R.; Cappello, M.; Gross, M.; Gaeta, F.; et al. Allosteric inhibition of macrophage migration inhibitory factor revealed by ibudilast. *Proc. Natl. Acad. Sci. USA* **2010**, *107*, 11313–11318. [CrossRef]

132. Fox, R.J.; Coffey, C.S.; Conwit, R.; Cudkowicz, M.E.; Gleason, T.; Goodman, A.; Klawiter, E.C.; Matsuda, K.; McGovern, M.; Naismith, R.T.; et al. Phase 2 Trial of Ibudilast in Progressive Multiple Sclerosis. *N. Engl. J. Med.* **2018**, *379*, 846–855. [CrossRef]

133. Greenwood, J.; Steinman, L.; Zamvil, S.S. Statin therapy and autoimmune disease: From protein prenylation to immunomodulation. *Nat. Rev. Immunol.* **2006**, *6*, 358–370. [CrossRef]

134. Chataway, J.; Schuerer, N.; Alsanousi, A.; Chan, D.; MacManus, D.; Hunter, K.; Anderson, V.; Bangham, C.R.M.; Clegg, S.; Nielsen, C.; et al. Effect of high-dose simvastatin on brain atrophy and disability in secondary progressive multiple sclerosis (MS-STAT): A randomised, placebo-controlled, phase 2 trial. *Lancet* **2014**, *383*, 2213–2221. [CrossRef]

135. Rocamonde, B.; Paradells, S.; Barcia, J.; Barcia, C.; García-Verdugo, J.M.; Miranda, M.; Gómez, F.R.; Soria, J. Neuroprotection of lipoic acid treatment promotes angiogenesis and reduces the glial scar formation after brain injury. *Neuroscience* **2012**, *224*, 102–115. [CrossRef]

136. Rochette, L.; Ghibu, S.; Richard, C.; Zeller, M.; Cottin, Y.; Vergely, C. Direct and indirect antioxidant properties of alpha-lipoic acid and therapeutic potential. *Mol. Nutr. Food Res.* **2013**, *57*, 114–125. [CrossRef]

137. Spain, R.; Powers, K.; Murchison, C.; Heriza, E.; Winges, K.; Yadav, V.; Cameron, M.; Kim, E.; Horak, F.; Simon, J.; et al. Lipoic acid in secondary progressive multiple sclerosis: A randomized controlled pilot trial. *Neur. Neuroimmunol. Neuroinflamm.* **2017**, *4*, e374. [CrossRef]

138. Lo, A.C.; Saab, C.Y.; Black, J.A.; Waxman, S.G. Phenytoin Protects Spinal Cord Axons and Preserves Axonal Conduction and Neurological Function in a Model of Neuroinflammation in Vivo. *J. Neurophysiol.* **2003**, *90*, 3566–3571. [CrossRef]

139. Raftopoulos, R.; Hickman, S.J.; Toosy, A.; Sharrack, B.; Mallik, S.; Paling, D.; Altmann, D.R.; Yiannakas, M.C.; Malladi, P.; Sheridan, R.; et al. Phenytoin for neuroprotection in patients with acute optic neuritis: A randomised, placebo-controlled, phase 2 trial. *Lancet Neurol.* **2016**, *15*, 259–269. [CrossRef]

140. Cohen, J.A. Mesenchymal Stem Cell Transplantation in Multiple Sclerosis. *J. Neurol. Sci.* **2013**, *333*, 43–49. [CrossRef]

141. Bonab, M.M.; Yazdanbakhsh, S.; Lotfi, J.; Alimoghaddom, K.; Talebian, F.; Hooshmand, F.; Ghavamzadeh, A.; Nikbin, B. Does mesenchymal stem cell therapy help multiple sclerosis patients? Report of a pilot study. *Iran. J. Immunol. IJI* **2007**, *4*, 50–57.

142. Bonab, M.M.; Sahraian, M.A.; Aghsaie, A.; Karvigh, S.A.; Hosseinian, S.M.; Nikbin, B.; Lotfi, J.; Khorramnia, S.; Motamed, M.R.; Togha, M.; et al. Autologous mesenchymal stem cell therapy in progressive multiple sclerosis: An open label study. *Curr. Stem Cell Res. Ther.* **2012**, *7*, 407–414. [CrossRef]

143. Yamout, B.; Hourani, R.; Salti, H.; Barada, W.; El-Hajj, T.; Al-Kutoubi, A.; Herlopian, A.; Baz, E.K.; Mahfouz, R.; Khalil-Hamdan, R.; et al. Bone marrow mesenchymal stem cell transplantation in patients with multiple sclerosis: A pilot study. *J. Neuroimmunol.* **2010**, *227*, 185–189. [CrossRef]

144. Lublin, F.D.; Bowen, J.D.; Huddlestone, J.; Kremenchutzky, M.; Carpenter, A.; Corboy, J.R.; Freedman, M.S.; Krupp, L.; Paulo, C.; Hariri, R.J.; et al. Human placenta-derived cells (PDA-001) for the treatment of adults with multiple sclerosis: A randomized, placebo-controlled, multiple-dose study. *Mult. Scler. Relat. Disord.* **2014**, *3*, 696–704. [CrossRef]

145. Karussis, D.; Karageorgiou, C.; Vaknin-Dembinsky, A.; Gowda-Kurkalli, B.; Gomori, J.M.; Kassis, I.; Bulte, J.W.M.; Petrou, P.; Ben-Hur, T.; Abramsky, O.; et al. Safety and Immunological Effects of Mesenchymal Stem Cell Transplantation in Patients with Multiple Sclerosis and Amyotrophic Lateral Sclerosis. *Arch. Neurol.* **2010**, *67*, 1187–1194. [CrossRef]

146. Harris, V.K.; Vyshkina, T.; Sadiq, S.A. Clinical safety of intrathecal administration of mesenchymal stromal cell–derived neural progenitors in multiple sclerosis. *Cytotherapy* **2016**, *18*, 1476–1482. [CrossRef]

147. Harris, V.K.; Stark, J.; Vyshkina, T.; Blackshear, L.; Joo, G.; Stefanova, V.; Sara, G.; Sadiq, S.A. Phase I Trial of Intrathecal Mesenchymal Stem Cell-derived Neural Progenitors in Progressive Multiple Sclerosis. *EBioMedicine* **2018**, *29*, 23–30. [CrossRef]

148. Li, J.-F.; Zhang, D.-J.; Geng, T.; Chen, L.; Huang, H.; Yin, H.-L.; Zhang, Y.-Z.; Lou, J.-Y.; Cao, B.; Wang, Y.-L. The Potential of Human Umbilical Cord-Derived Mesenchymal Stem Cells as a Novel Cellular Therapy for Multiple Sclerosis. *Cell Transplant.* **2014**, *23*, 113–122. [CrossRef]

149. Liang, J.; Zhang, H.; Hua, B.; Wang, H.; Wang, J.; Han, Z.; Sun, L. Allogeneic mesenchymal stem cells transplantation in treatment of multiple sclerosis. *Mult. Scler. J.* **2009**, *15*, 644–646. [CrossRef]

150. Cohen, J.A.; Atkins, H.; Banwell, B.; Bar-Or, A.; Bebo, B.; Bowen, J.; Burt, R.; Calabresi, P.; Cohen, J.; Comi, G.; et al. Cell-based therapeutic strategies for multiple sclerosis. *Brain* **2017**, *140*, 2776–2796.

151. Uccelli, A.; Brundin, L.; Clanet, M.; Fernandez, O.; Nabavi, S.M.; Muraro, P.A.; Oliveri, R.S.; Radue, E.W.; Sellner, J.; Sorensen, P.S.; et al. MEsenchymal StEm cells for Multiple Sclerosis (MESEMS): A randomized, double blind, cross-over phase I/II clinical trial with autologous mesenchymal stem cells for the therapy of multiple sclerosis. *Trials* **2019**, *20*, 263. [CrossRef]

152. Sedel, F.; Bernard, D.; Mock, D.M.; Tourbah, A. Targeting demyelination and virtual hypoxia with high-dose biotin as a treatment for progressive multiple sclerosis. *Neuropharmacology* **2016**, *110*, 644–653. [CrossRef]

153. Sedel, F.; Papeix, C.; Bellanger, A.; Touitou, V.; Lebrun-Frenay, C.; Galanaud, D.; Gout, O.; Lyon-Caen, O.; Tourbah, A. High doses of biotin in chronic progressive multiple sclerosis: A pilot study. *Mult. Scler. Relat. Disord.* **2015**, *4*, 159–169. [CrossRef]

154. Tourbah, A.; Lebrun-Frenay, C.; Edan, G.; Clanet, M.; Papeix, C.; Vukusic, S.; De Sèze, J.; Debouverie, M.; Gout, O.; Clavelou, P.; et al. MD1003 (high-dose biotin) for the treatment of progressive multiple sclerosis: A randomised, double-blind, placebo-controlled study. *Mult. Scler. J.* **2016**, *22*, 1719–1731. [CrossRef]

155. Birnbaum, G.; Stulc, J. High dose biotin as treatment for progressive multiple sclerosis. *Mult. Scler. Relat. Disord.* **2017**, *18*, 141–143. [CrossRef]

156. Baldassari, L.E.; Feng, J.; Clayton, B.L.; Oh, S.-H.; Sakaie, K.; Tesar, P.J.; Wang, Y.; Cohen, J.A. Developing therapeutic strategies to promote myelin repair in multiple sclerosis. *Expert Rev. Neurother.* **2019**, 1–17. [CrossRef]

157. Najm, F.J.; Madhavan, M.; Zaremba, A.; Shick, E.; Karl, R.T.; Factor, D.C.; Miller, T.E.; Nevin, Z.S.; Kantor, C.; Sargent, A.; et al. Drug-based modulation of endogenous stem cells promotes functional remyelination in vivo. *Nature* **2015**, *522*, 216–220. [CrossRef]

158. Cohen, J.A.; Baldassari, L.E.; Atkins, H.L.; Bowen, J.D.; Bredeson, C.; Carpenter, P.A.; Corboy, J.R.; Freedman, M.S.; Griffith, L.M.; Lowsky, R.; et al. Autologous Hematopoietic Cell Transplantation for Treatment-Refractory Relapsing Multiple Sclerosis: Position Statement from the American Society for Blood and Marrow Transplantation. *Boil. Blood Marrow Transplant.* **2019**, *25*, 845–854. [CrossRef]

159. Marrie, R.A.; Hanwell, H. General health issues in multiple sclerosis: Comorbidities, secondary conditions, and health behaviors. *Continuum* **2013**, *19*, 1046–1057. [CrossRef]
160. Ontaneda, D. Inadequate outcome measures are the biggest impediment to successful clinical trials in progressive MS-Commentary. *Mult. Scler.* **2017**, *23*, 508–509. [CrossRef]
161. Giovannoni, G.; Airas, L.; Bove, R.; Boyko, A.; Cutter, G.; Hobart, J.; Kuhle, J.; Oh, J.; Tur, C.; Garas, M.; et al. *Ocrelizumab Treatment Effect on Upper Limb Function in PPMS Patients with Disability: Subgroup Results of the ORATORIO Study to Inform the ORATORIO-HAND Study Design*; ECTRIMS Online Library: London, UK, 2018; p. 619.
162. Sumowski, J.F.; Benedict, R.; Enzinger, C.; Filippi, M.; Geurts, J.J.; Hamalainen, P.; Hulst, H.; Inglese, M.; Leavitt, V.M.; Rocca, M.A.; et al. Cognition in multiple sclerosis State of the field and priorities for the future. *Neurology* **2018**, *90*, 278–288. [CrossRef]

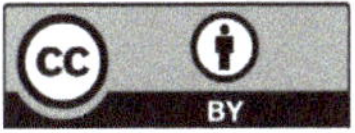

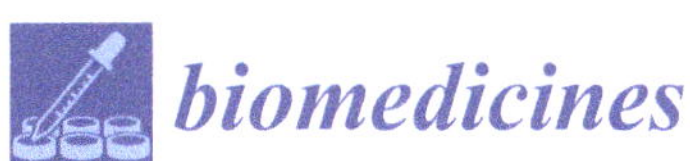 *biomedicines*

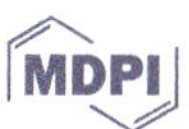

Review

Neuromyelitis Optica Spectrum Disorder and Anti-MOG Syndromes

Marco A. Lana-Peixoto * and Natália Talim

CIEM MS Research Center, Federal University of Minas Gerais Medical School, Belo Horizonte, MG 30130-090, Brazil; talim.fono@gmail.com
* Correspondence: marco.lanapeixoto@gmail.com; Tel.: +55-31-32223935

Received: 20 May 2019; Accepted: 2 June 2019; Published: 12 June 2019

Abstract: Neuromyelitis optica spectrum disorder (NMOSD) and anti-myelin oligodendrocyte glycoprotein (anti-MOG) syndromes are immune-mediated inflammatory conditions of the central nervous system that frequently involve the optic nerves and the spinal cord. Because of their similar clinical manifestations and habitual relapsing course they are frequently confounded with multiple sclerosis (MS). Early and accurate diagnosis of these distinct conditions is relevant as they have different treatments. Some agents used for MS treatment may be deleterious to NMOSD. NMOSD is frequently associated with antibodies which target aquaporin-4 (AQP4), the most abundant water channel in the CNS, located in the astrocytic processes at the blood-brain barrier (BBB). On the other hand, anti-MOG syndromes result from damage to myelin oligodendrocyte glycoprotein (MOG), expressed on surfaces of oligodendrocytes and myelin sheaths. Acute transverse myelitis with longitudinally extensive lesion on spinal MRI is the most frequent inaugural manifestation of NMOSD, usually followed by optic neuritis. Other core clinical characteristics include area postrema syndrome, brainstem, diencephalic and cerebral symptoms that may be associated with typical MRI abnormalities. Acute disseminated encephalomyelitis and bilateral or recurrent optic neuritis are the most frequent anti-MOG syndromes in children and adults, respectively. Attacks are usually treated with steroids, and relapses prevention with immunosuppressive drugs. Promising emerging therapies for NMOSD include monoclonal antibodies and tolerization.

Keywords: neuromyelitis optica spectrum disorders; anti-MOG syndrome; aquaporin 4-IgG; myelin oligodendrocyte glycoprotein; multiple sclerosis

---

1. Introduction

Neuromyelitis optica spectrum disorders (NMOSD) and anti-myelin oligodendrocyte glycoprotein (anti-MOG) syndromes are immune-mediated inflammatory conditions of the central nervous system (CNS) that frequently involve the optic nerves and the spinal cord. Because of their clinical manifestations and habitual relapsing course, they are frequently confounded with multiple sclerosis (MS). Early and accurate diagnosis of these distinct conditions is very relevant as they have different therapeutic approaches. Even a more important reason is the observation that some agents used in MS treatment may be deleterious to patients with NMOSD [1–3].

Although NMOSD and anti-MOG syndromes share a number of clinical manifestations, they are independent nosological entities with distinct pathophysiological mechanisms and histopathological features [4–7].

Whereas NMOSD is most frequently associated with antibodies which target aquaporin-4 (AQP4), the most abundant water channel in the CNS, particularly expressed in the astrocytic processes at the blood-brain barrier (BBB) [8], anti-MOG syndromes result from damage to myelin oligodendrocyte glycoprotein (MOG), a membrane protein expressed on oligodendrocyte cell surfaces and on the outermost surface of myelin sheaths. Because of this particular location, MOG is a good antigen candidate for autoimmune demyelination [6,7,9–11]. Moreover, three fourths of NMOSD patients test positive for AQP4 antibody, while serum MOG antibody is only detected in a minority of seronegative AQP4-IgG NMOSD patients [12–14].

The lack of coexistence of AQP4-IgG and MOG-IgG in the serum of a same patient further suggests that AQP4-IgG NMOSD and anti-MOG syndromes are distinct diseases [15]. On the other hand, failure to identify either AQP4-IgG or MOG-IgG in a proportion of patients with NMOSD phenotype supports the view that other autoantibodies or factors may also play a role in NMOSD pathogenesis. In line with that, N-methyl-D-aspartate receptor-IgG and CV2/CRMP5-IgG have been described in association with NMOSD phenotype [16–19].

2. Neuromyelitis Optica Spectrum Disorders

The term *neuromyelitis optica* was introduced by Eugène Devic and Fernand Gault in 1894, who first recognized the association of amaurosis and myelitis as a new clinical entity. Devic [20] reported the case of a 45-year-old French woman who was seen at the Hôtel-Dieu hospital of Lyon because of an intractable headache and depression in addition to general asthenia. One month later, she developed urinary retention, complete paraplegia and blindness, and died few weeks later. Autopsy disclosed severe demyelinating and necrotic lesions extending 4–5 cm length in the lower thoracic and lumbar spinal cord. There was demyelination of the optic nerves, but a gross examination of the brain was unrevealing. In this paper, Devic emphasized the similarity of the pathological process involving the spinal cord and the optic nerves, named the syndrome "neuro-myélite optique", or "neuroptico-myélite", and discussed its relationship with MS. Fernand Gault, a disciple of Devic's, reviewed in detail 17 cases of this condition in his doctoral thesis named "De la neuromyélite optique aiguë" [21]. The eponym "Devic's disease" was suggested by Acchiote [22]. However, the association of myelitis and blindness had already been reported by other authors in the early and mid 19th century. The *case of Marquis de Causan*—known as the first description of this association by the French anatomist and pathologist Antoine Portal in 1803–1804—was characterized by relapsing myelitis followed by amaurosis and signs of brainstem involvement [23]. Other previously reported cases included those by Giovanni Battista Pescetto in 1844 [24], Christopher Mercer Durrant in 1850 [25], Jacob Augustus Lockhart Clarke in 1862 [26], Thomas Clifford Albutt in 1870 [27], and Wilhelm Heinrich Erb in 1879–1880 [28]. Also, in the American continent, the association of optic neuritis and myelitis was identified by Seguin (1880) [29] prior to Devic and Gault's pioneering publication. None of these previous authors however, had used the term "neuromyelitis optica", or considered their cases as expression of a new nosological entity. It was only in 1943 that the disease was first identified in Latin America, when Aluizio Marques, in Rio de Janeiro, described two female patients who developed bilateral blindness and acute transverse myelitis [30].

2.1. Pathophysiology

The discovery of NMO-IgG and AQP4 as its targeted antigen unequivocally confirmed neuromyelitis optica as a disease distinct from MS and allowed its early laboratorial recognition [31,32]. The serum identification of AQP4-IgG expanded the clinical spectrum of the disease to include its limited forms (single or recurrent longitudinally extensive transverse myelitis [LETM], defined by MRI as a lesion extending for three or more vertebral segments, or recurrent isolated optic neuritis) [33], along with a wide variety of brainstem, diencephalic, and cerebral manifestations [34,35].

Aquaporin-4 monomers assemble to form tetramers which further aggregate in cell plasma membranes to form supramolecular arrays called orthogonal arrays of particles (OAP). There are two major forms of AQP-4: the full-length 323 amino acid M1 isoform, and the shorter 301 amino acid M23 isoform. Only the M23 isoform forms large OAPs [14]. It has been shown that M1 isoform does not form OAPs on its own, but can co-assemble with M23 in heterotetramers that limit OAP size [36,37].

Aquaporin-4 is widely expressed throughout the CNS. It is also highly expressed in the optic nerves and spinal cord, explaining their preferential involvement in the disease. Other CNS sites expressing AQP-4 include the supraoptic nucleus of the hypothalamus, the periventricular structures such as area postrema and the vascular organ of lamina terminalis, which lack BBB and contain osmo-sensitive neurons that regulate fluid homeostasis and release arginine-vasopressin, which facilitates this process. Aquaporin-4 is also expressed in non-neural tissues including skeletal muscle cells, lung airway cells, gastric parietal cells, renal collecting duct cells, inner ear, retinal Muller cells, lacrimal gland and salivary duct cells, and olfactory epithelial cells [38]. Human and experimental studies have shown that AQP4-IgG belongs mainly to IgG1 class, a potent activator of complement. The antibody enters the CNS, binds the antigen at astrocyte processes, induces complement-mediated inflammation, granulocyte infiltration, and astrocyte death [37,39]. Complement-mediated inflammation with secondary neutrophils and eosinophil infiltration plays a key role in the pathophysiology of NMOSD attacks [40].

Aquaporin-4 antibodies are more abundant in the peripheral blood than in the cerebrospinal fluid (CSF) [41]. In the periphery, they are produced by a number of B cell subpopulations which are vulnerable to interleukin-6 (IL-6), which enhances their survival and AQP4-IgG secretion [42]. Although AQP4-IgG can gain direct access to AQP4 on astrocytes located at circumventricular organs where the endothelia lack tight junction, the mechanisms of its penetration into other CNS sites that are protected byBBB are still unclear. Recent findings have shown that AQP4-IgG is not sufficient or even necessary to cause BBB disruption [43]. Sera from NMO patients contain non-reactive AQP4 antibodies, identified as recombinant antibodies (rAb) ON-12-2-46 and ON-07-5-31 which target glucose-regulated protein 78 (GRP78) on the cell surface of brain microvascular endothelial cells (BMEC). GRP78 is a stress protein of the heat shock 70 family expressed in all CNS cells [44]. However, only rAb ON 12-2-46 induces nuclear translocation of nuclear factor kB (NF-kB) p65, which is a marker of cell activation [43]. BMECs activation causes increased secretion of vascular endothelium growth factor (VEGF) and metaloproteinases (MMP)-2/9 which result in a down regulation of claudin 5 and disruption of the BBB. Leakage of the BBB allows entrance of AQP4-IgG to the CNS and its binding to AQP4 in the astrocytic endfeet. Evidences showing the causal role of AQP4-IgG in NMOSD include its nearly absolute specificity for the disease; its correlation with disease activity, higher number of relapses and more severe course as compared with seronegative patients; some distinct demographic and clinical features; increased concentration of AQP4-positive plasmablasts in NMOSD patients, mainly during disease relapses; and decreased serum AQP4-IgG concentration following successful treatments and during disease remission [45–47]. Histopathological features such as a marked loss of astrocytes and accumulation of IgG and IgM around blood vessels, the site of AQP4 expression; spare of myelin and axons in some lesions suggesting that astrocytes (which have a higher expression of AQP4) are the initial cell target in the disease, whereas in more recent lesions there may be preservation of glial fibrillary acidic protein (GFAP), a marker of astrocyte damage, suggesting that AQP4 is the primary target of the immune attack. The initial loss of AQP4 with astrocyte preservation might reflect the internalization of AQP4 of either M1-AQP4 or both isoforms before a complement becomes locally available to mediate a lytic inflammatory process. This would account for the rapid reversal of some MRI abnormalities in the area postrema and some parts of the cerebrum. The disease individual clinical phenotype and severity may be related to the ratio of AQP4-M1 to M23 in the optic nerves, brain, and spinal cord. While CNS regions with a higher proportion of M1 would rapidly internalize, avoiding a cascade of tissue damage, areas richer in AQP4-M23 isoform would be more liable to necrotic lesions and cavitation [44–46].

Additionally, following a decreased serum concentration of AQP4-IgG, the AQP4-M1 isoform is rapidly replaced in the astrocytic membrane. Experimental studies have showed that a passive transfer of AQP4-IgG from NMOSD patients to animals with disrupted BBB by previous experimental autoimmune encephalomyelitis (EAE), or through pretreatment with Freund's adjunct, develop CNS typical NMO histopathological lesions [37,48–51].

2.2. Epidemiology

Some caveats are needed before looking at published data on the epidemiology of NMOSD. First, studies on the frequency and distribution of the disease across the world are still scanty and most of them are based on small cohorts. Additionally, they employed non-standardized methodology and inconsistent inclusion of seronegative patients, and differ regarding used diagnostic criteria and assays for AQP4 antibodies detection. In spite of these limitations, a number of issues related to disease prevalence, ethnicity and geography have been clarified. Studies in different populations and geographic regions show that NMOSD is a rare disorder with worldwide distribution [52]. However, an exception to these studies is the seroprevalence study from Olmsted County, in the United States, and Martinique [53] which showed a 2.5-fold higher prevalence rate of the disease in Martinique (10 per 100,000) than in Olmsted County (3.9 per 100,000), all other studies [52] indicated a fairly uniform prevalence rate below 5 per 100,000 people in different regions and populations (Table 1). Likewise, incidence rates were also homogeneous in different countries, ranging from 0.2 per 1 million per year, in Mexico [54] to 4.0 in Denmark [55]. Although most studies point to incidence rate below 1 per 1 million, a peak incidence rate of 7.3 per 1 million was again found in Martinique [53].

Table 1. Incidence and prevalence of NMOSD across the world.

Authors, Year	Country	Number of Cases	Incidence (95% CI) (per Million per Year)	Prevalence (95% CI) (per 100,000)
Rivera et al., 2008 [54]	Mexico	34	0.20 (0.05–0.35)	1
Cabrera-Gómez et al., 2009 [56]	Cuba	58	0.44 (0.3–0.62)	0.43 (0.29–0.61)
Asgari et al., 2011 [55]	Denmark	42	4 (3.0–5.4)	4.41 (3.1–5.7)
Aboul Enein et al., 2011 [57]	Austria	71	0.54 (0.01–0.03)	0.71 (0.17–0.96)
Cossburn et al., 2012 [58]	UK	14	NA	1.96 (1.22–2.97)
Houzen et al., 2012 [59]	Japan	3	0.8 (0.3–1.6)	0.72 (0.31–1.42)
Jacob et al., 2013 [60]	UK	13	0.8 (0.3–1.6)	0.72 (0.31–1.42)
Etemadifar et al., 2014 [61]	Iran	95	NA	1.95 (1.62–2.23)
Pandit et al., 2014 [62]	India	11	NA	2.6
Kashipazha et al., 2015 [63]	Iran	51	NA	0.8 (0.54–1.06)
Flanagan et al., 2016 [53]	USA	6	0.7 (0.0–2.1)	3.9 (0.8–7.1)
	Martinique	39	7.3 (4.1–10.1)	10.0 (6.8–13.2)
van Pelt et al., 2016 [64]	Netherlands		1.2	NA
Houzen et al., 2017 [65]	Japan	14	NA	4.1 (2.2–6.9)
Hor et al., 2017 [66]	Malaysia	14	NA	1.99 (1.09–3.35)
Bukhari et al., 2017 [67]	ANZ	81	0.37 (0.36–0.38)	0.7 (0.66–0.74)
Sepulveda et al., 2017 [68]	Spain	74	0.63 (0.45–0.8)	0.89 (0.87–0.91)
Holroyd et al., 2018 [69]	United Arab Emirates	10	0.59	0.34

NMOSD: neuromyelitis optica spectrum disorders; NA: not available; ANZ: Australia and New Zealand.

Although NMOSD has been regarded to have a predilection for non-Caucasians, the similarity of prevalence and incidence rates in different geographic regions and distinct ethnicities may suggest that, as in opposition to MS, latitude and genetic factors may not play a key role in NMOSD pathogenesis [70]. This contradicts the ethnicity-specific higher prevalence for blacks in Olmsted County, which was similar to that found in the black population of Martinique [53]. The Australian-New Zealand study also observed higher prevalence rate in people with Asian ancestry than in Caucasians [67].

Ethnicity, however, influences age at onset and phenotype of AQP4 seropositive NMOSD. A recent study comparing the clinical manifestations and outcome of 603 NMOSD patients of three different races (Asians, Caucasians and Afro-Americans/Afro-Europeans) showed that non-white patients are younger at disease onset, and more frequently have brain attacks at onset or during the disease course, as well as more frequent abnormalities on brain MRI. Afro-American and Afro-European patients have more severe attacks at onset than Asians and Caucasians, but the outcome at the last follow-up was similar in the different racial groups [71]. This observed that the similarity of the outcome at the last follow-up for all racial groups is in opposition to previous reports of a more severe outcome of NMOSD in Afro-Caribbean than in Caucasian patients [56,72,73].

Usually, the initial clinical manifestations of NMOSD occur at an age of around 35-45 years (median age at onset is 39), but children and the elderly account for 18% of cases. Women comprise 70% to 90% of all cases, but there is no gender predilection in children [74]. The estimated proportion of familial cases (3%) is greater than expected based on the disease prevalence [75]. In some populations, human leukocyte antigen (HLA) has been reported to be associated with susceptibility to NMOSD, such as HLA-DPB1*0501 allele in Japanese and Chinese populations [76,77] and HLA-DPB1*03 in Caucasian, Afro-Caribbean, and Indian patients [78–81]. These genetic factors may account for the phenotypic variability among racial groups.

2.3. Clinical Manifestations

For a long time, the hallmark of NMOSD had been considered as the preferential involvement of the optic nerves and the spinal cord in absence of brain symptoms. However, following the discovery of NMO-IgG in 2004, a wide variety of brainstem, diencephalic and cerebral signs were described in seropositive patients [34]. In 2015 the International Panel for NMO Diagnosis (IPND) added area postrema, brainstem, diencephalic and cerebral manifestations to optic neuritis and LETM to the revised diagnostic criteria for NMOSD [35]. Table 2 shows the clinical manifestations of NMOSD. Clinical analysis of the largest international cohort of AQP4-seropositive NMOSD so far published [71] shows that the disease was relapsing in 85% of the cases. Myelitis was the initial manifestation in 48%, optic neuritis in 42%, area postrema syndrome in 10%, brainstem/diencephalic/cerebral symptoms in 14%, and simultaneous optic neuritis and myelitis in 4%. During the disease course, 84% of the patients presented myelitis, 63% optic neuritis, 15% APS, 17% brainstem syndrome, 3% diencephalic syndrome and 14% cerebral syndrome. In almost one half of the patients (45%) the inaugural attack was severe (defined as an Expanded Disability Status Scale (EDSS) score at ≥6.0 or visual acuity ≤0.1 in at least one eye at nadir).

Severe transverse myelitis in NMOSD most commonly causes symmetrical motor and sensory loss, mainly of the lower limbs, associated with sphincter disturbances. Hiccups and respiratory failure may result from an extension of cervical lesions to the medulla oblongata. Intractable nausea, vomiting and hiccups indicate involvement of the area postrema. The area postrema is the chemosensitive vomiting center located in the dorsal part of the medulla oblongata. It is highly vascularized, lacks blood brain barrier and has a high AQP-4 expression. Its fenestrated capillaries and loosely apposed astrocytic processes likely facilitate IgG access to the CNS [82]. This increased exposure to AQP4-IgG may explain the frequent occurrence of incoercible nausea/vomiting/hiccups in AQP4-IgG seropositive patients. Cervical lesions with rostral extension to the area postrema as seen on MRI, have been observed in other conditions, such as sarcoidosis, lymphoma, paraneoplastic myelitis, spondylosis and dural arteriovenous fistula. However, area postrema lesions on MRI occurring in association with incoercible nausea, vomiting or hiccups are specific for NMOSD [83].

Table 2. Clinical manifestations of NMOSD according to anatomic involvement *.

Site	Symtoms
Optic nerve/chiasm	Eye pain or headache Blurred vision Disturbance of color vision Amaurosis Optic disc edema Optic atrophy Scotomas and other visual field defects
Spinal cord	Limb weakness Lower limb spasticity Gait abnormalities Sensory disturbances Radicular pain Pruritus Painful tonic spasms Trunk and limb ataxia Sphincter disturbances Respiratory weakness Lhermitte phenomenon
Brainstem	Motor and sensory disturbances Incoercible nausea, vomiting and hiccups Intractable cough Weight loss Anorexia Diplopia/ocular movement disorders Facial dysesthesia and trigeminal neuralgia Dysgeusia Facial paralysis Hearing loss, tinnitus Vertigo Dysarthria/dysphagia Narcolepsy
Diencephalon	Hypophyseal abnormalities Antidiuretic hormone syndrome Pre-syncopal symptoms Disturbances of body temperature Anhydrosis/excessive sweating Hyperphagia Posterior reversible encephalopathy syndrome (PRES)
Cerebrum	Mental confusion Seizures Aphasia Apraxia Cognitive dysfunction Psychiatric symptoms

* Modified from Lana-Peixoto and Callegaro, 2012 [34]. NMOSD: neuromyelitis optica spectrum disorders.

Optic neuritis in NMOSD may differ from isolated idiopathic optic neuritis, and from optic neuritis occurring in MS. In NMOSD, optic neuritis is characterized by more severe visual loss at onset, bilateral involvement of the optic nerves or optic chiasm, relapsing course, poor response to IV corticosteroid pulses, poor recovery with permanent visual deficits, and association with normal brain MRI, or with unspecific lesions on brain MRI. Bitemporal hemianopsia points to the presence of chiasmal involvement, which is more common in AQP4-IgG NMOSD than in MS or anti-MOG syndromes.

Brainstem symptoms occur in about one third of the NMOSD patients and are the inaugural manifestation of the disease in about one half of these cases. The most commonly observed brainstem symptoms are vomiting (33%), hiccups (22%), oculomotor dysfunction (20%), and pruritus (12%), followed by hearing loss, facial palsy, vertigo, and trigeminal neuralgia (about 2% each) [84].

In a study of a multi-racial cohort, associated systemic autoimmune diseases were observed in 30% of the Caucasian, 9% of Asian, and 19% of the Afro-American/Afro-European AQP4-seropositive patients [71]. Serum autoantibodies associated with autoimmune conditions are frequently found in NMOSD patients, even in the absence of clinical manifestations. The most common autoimmune abnormalities associated with NMOSD include those related to thyroid disease, systemic lupus erythematosus, and Sjögren syndrome [46].

2.4. Laboratorial Characteristics

Patients with suspected NMOSD need a careful history and physical examination followed by a comprehensive laboratory work-up to rule out mimickers. Laboratory evaluation should include tests for infectious diseases, sarcoidosis, lymphomas and other tumors, paraneoplastic disorders, metabolic and nutritional disorders as well as a number of other autoimmune conditions. Testing for serum AQP4-IgG and MOG-IgG has diagnostic relevance for all patients with suspected NMOSD. Previously employed techniques for serum detection of AQP4-IgG such as indirect immunofluorescence and enzyme-linked immunosorbent assay (ELISA) proved to have lower sensitivity and specificity than cell-based assays (CBA) (mean sensitivity of indirect immunofluorescence and ELISA were 63% and 64%, respectively). Moreover, ELISA may yield 0.5%–1.2% of false-positive results [85–87]). There is a marked variation in assay sensitivity, which ranges from 48.7% to 76.7%, with the highest sensitivity obtained with CBA [88]. The specificity of the different assays ranged from 86.9% to 100% with the commercial fixed CBA having higher specificity than the live CBA. False negative results are higher during remissions, after plasma exchange, or in use of immunosuppressive drugs [88].

Recommendations for testing for serum AQP4-IgG include: (1) patients with acute transverse myelitis associated with a LETM lesion on spinal MRI, or with myelitis associated with normal brain MRI or without evidences of MS or other causes; (2) patients with optic neuritis with atypical features, such as the occurrence of relapses, bilateral simultaneous involvement of the optic nerves or chiasmal involvement, poor recovery, or optic neuritis associated with a long lesion of the optic nerve; (3) patients with area postrema syndrome; (4) patients with diencephalic symptoms and MRI abnormalities of unknown etiology; and (5) patients with encephalopathy of unknown nature. Testing for AQP4-IgG is not recommended in patients with typical clinical and imaging evidences of MS [14,88].

Cerebrospinal fluid (CSF) analysis usually discloses distinct features from those found in MS. While oligoclonal bands (OCB) restricted to the CSF occur in more than 90% of the MS population [89], they were found in only 18% of a large NMOSD cohort [90]. Interestingly, OCB restricted to the CSF are less frequently observed in Asian than in Caucasian or African-American/African European NMOSD patients [71]. During acute relapses a variable pleocytosis with presence of neutrophils and eosinophils may be observed [46].

2.5. Diagnostic Criteria

Current diagnostic criteria for NMOSD were developed by the IPND in 2015 [35]. The panel took the following decisions: (1) unify NMO and NMOSD under the single term "NMOSD"; (2) define (i) optic neuritis; (ii) acute myelitis; (iii) area postrema syndrome or episode of otherwise unexplained hiccups or nausea and vomiting; (iv) acute brainstem syndrome; (v) symptomatic narcolepsy or acute diencephalic clinical syndrome with NMOSD-typical diencephalic MRI lesions; and (vi) symptomatic cerebral syndrome with NMOSD-typical brain lesions as the six "core clinical characteristics" of NMOSD, according to involvement of anatomic sites; (3) establish diagnostic criteria for both NMOSD with AQP4-IgG and NMOSD without AQP4-IgG (negative serology or not performed test) (Table 3); (4) require additional supportive MRI characteristics to diagnostic criteria for NMOSD without AQP4-IgG or with unknown AQP4-IgG in order to enhancing specificity; (5) recommend the use of CBA for AQP4-IgG detection due to their higher sensitivity and specificity; (6) list some clinical features as well as laboratory and imaging findings that may point to alternative diagnoses, and therefore must be seen as "red flags".

Table 3. International consensus diagnostic criteria for NMOSD *.

1. Diagnostic criteria for NMOSD with AQP4-IgG
1. At least one core clinical characteristic
2. Exclusion of alternative diagnoses
2. Diagnostic criteria for NMOSD without AQP4-IgG or NMOSD with unknown AQP4-IgG status
1. At least two core clinical characteristics meeting all of the following requirements:
a. At least one core clinical characteristic must be optic neuritis, acute myelitis with LETM, or area postrema syndrome
b. Dissemination in space (two or more different core clinical characteristics)
c. Core clinical syndromes must be associated with respective MRI findings:
i. Optic neuritis:
1. Brain MRI is normal or with nonspecific lesions; OR
2. Optic nerve lesion extending over $\frac{1}{2}$ of the optic nerve length; or chiasmal lesion
ii. Acute myelitis: MRI with lesion or spinal atrophy extending over ≥3 contiguous segments
iii. Area postrema syndrome: MRI with dorsal medulla/area postrema lesions
iv. Acute brainstem syndrome: MRI with periependymal brainstem lesions
v. Narcolepsy or acute diencephalic clinical syndrome: MRI with NMOSD-typical diencephalic lesions
2. Exclusion of alternative diagnoses

* Modified from Wingerchuk et al., 2015 [35]. NMOSD: neuromyelitis optica spectrum disorders; AQP4: aquaporin-4; IgG: immunoglobulin G; LETM: longitudinally extensive transverse myelitis lesions.

Table 3 shows the international consensus diagnostic criteria for NMOSD with AQP4-IgG, and the diagnostic criteria for NMOSD without AQP4-IgG or with AQP4-IgG unknown status. For AQP4-IgG seropositive individuals, at least one of six "core clinical characteristics" must be present. For individuals without AQP4-IgG or with unknown AQP4-IgG status, diagnosis of NMOSD requires at least two of the six core clinical characteristics. One of the six core clinical characteristics must be optic neuritis, transverse myelitis or area postrema syndrome, and all of them need additional supportive MRI characteristics.

Clinical signs, CSF, MRI and optic coherence tomography (OCT) findings usually distinguish NMOSD from MS. Most frequently, atypical features for NMOSD ("red flags") point to the diagnosis of MS (Table 4). However, a number of other conditions may mimic NMOSD by involvement of the optic nerves and/or the spinal cord (Table 5) [91].

Table 4. Distinctive characteristics between MS and NMOSD.

Distinctive characteristics of MS
Progressive course
Partial transverse myelitis
Brain MRI features
Perpendicular periventricular lesions (Dawson fingers)
Periventricular lesions in the inferior temporal lobe
Juxtacortical lesions involving subcortical U-fibers
Cortical lesions
More severe brain atrophy
Spinal cord MRI features
Lesions <3 complete vertebral segments
Lesions located predominantly in the peripheral cord
Diffuse, indistinct signal change on T2-weighted sequences
Cerebrospinal fluid analysis
Presence of oligoclonal bands
Optic coherence tomography features
Predominant atrophy of temporal RNFL
Distinctive characteristics of NMOSD
Complete transverse myelitis
Brain MRI features
Multiple patchy enhancement with blurred margin in adjacent regions (cloud-like enhancement)
Large and edematous callosal lesions
Large and confluent white matter lesions (as in PRES)
Predominantly posterior brainstem lesions (around the fourth ventricle lesions and periaqueductal lesions)
Hypothalamic lesions
Extensive optic nerve lesions and chiasmal lesions
Spinal cord MRI features
Longitudinally extensive transverse myelitis lesions ($\geq$3 contiguous segments)
Longitudinally extensive spinal cord atrophy ($\geq$3 contiguous segments)
Centrally-located or holomedullary spinal cord lesions
Cerebrospinal fluid analysis
Moderate or marked pleocytosis
Presence of neutrophils and eosinophils
Optic coherence tomography features
Predominant atrophy of superior and inferior RNFL

MS: multiple sclerosis; NMOSD: neuromyelitis optica spectrum disorders; PRES: posterior reversible encephalopathy syndrome; RNFL: retinal nerve fiber layer.

Table 5. Differential diagnosis of NMOSD.

Multiple Sclerosis
Acute disseminated encephalomyelitis
MOG-related disorders
Sarcoidosis
Lymphoma
Paraneoplastic disease
Central nervous system infections
Syphilis
Tuberculosis
Human T-lymphotropic virus-I (HTLV-I) infection
Herpes virus infection
Dengue-virus infection
Lyme disease
Schistosomiasis
Sjogren syndrome
Systemic lupus erythematosus
Neuro-Behçet's disease
Spinal dural arteriovenous fistula

NMOSD: neuromyelitis optica spectrum disorders.

2.6. Magnetic Resonance Imaging

Magnetic resonance imaging of the brain and spinal cord is an essential tool for the diagnosis and management of demyelinating diseases of the CNS. The correct differentiation of NMOSD and anti-MOG syndromes from MS is important to provide patients with the most appropriate treatment.

Longitudinally extensive transverse myelitis, is the most specific imaging feature of NMOSD (Figure 1a). The length of the lesion has been considered the most distinguishing feature from MS, although long lesions may occur in MS and short lesions in NMOSD. Frequently, LETM lesions exhibit non-homogeneous contrast-enhancing that may persists for months following acute attacks. An extensive centrally-located hypointense signal in T1-sequence denotes cavitation secondary to tissue necrosis (Figure 1b). Cervical lesions may extend rostrally to the medulla oblongata (Figure 1c). Longitudinally extensive cord atrophy results from severe or recurring myelitis (Figure 1d). Short lesions, characterized by extension < three vertebral segments have been reported, predominantly at disease onset in 14% of the patients [92].

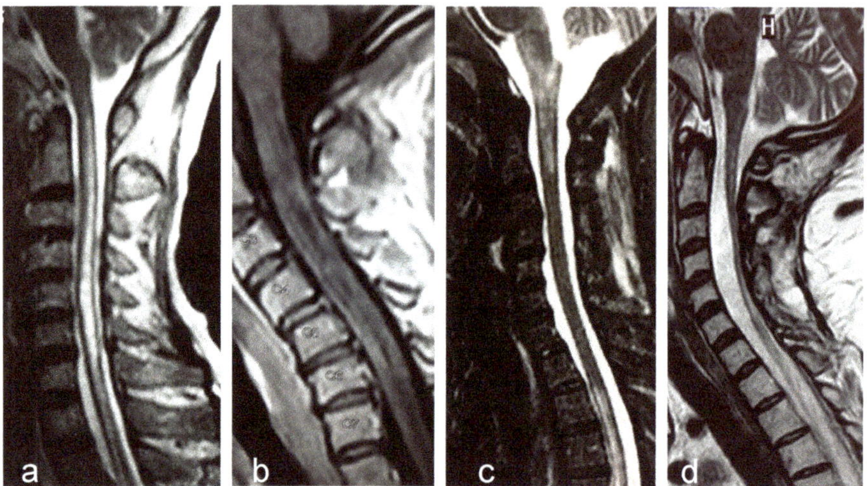

Figure 1. Examples of longitudinally extensive spinal cord lesions detected by MRI in AQP4-seropositive NMOSD patients. (**a**). T2-weighted central longitudinally extensive cervical lesion. (**b**). T1-weighted lesion with gadolinium showing multiple hypointensities (cavitations) throughout the cervical cord. (**c**). T2-weighted cervical lesion extending to brainstem. Another lesion is seen in the upper thoracic levels. (**d**). Longitudinally extensive spinal cord atrophy of the cervical cord.

Optic nerve abnormalities differ between, NMOSD and MS. Thickened, contrast-enhancing and long (≥ one-half the length of the optic nerve) lesions, as well as preference for involvement of the posterior segment of the nerve or chiasm are all in favor of NMOSD (Figure 2).

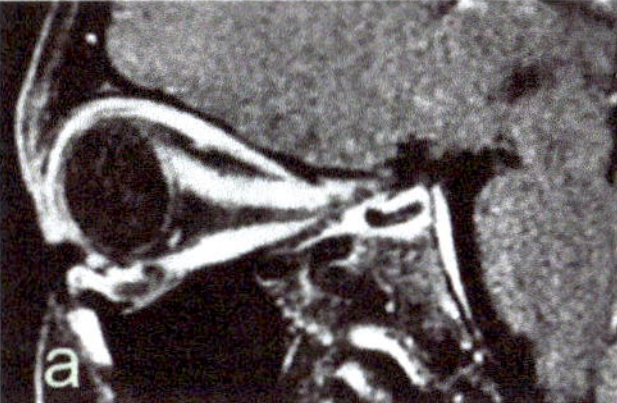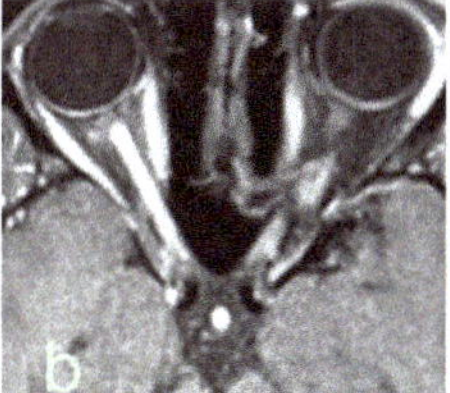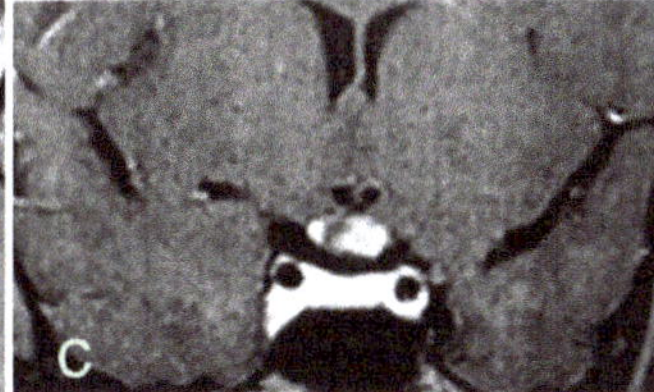

Figure 2. Optic nerve abnormalities on MRI in AQP4-seropositive NMOSD patients. (**a**). Sagittal T1-weighted MRI shows edematous gadolinium-enhancing optic nerve lesion extending from the eye to the intracranial segment. (**b**). Axial T1-weighted extensive gadolinium-enhancing lesion in both optic nerves. (**c**). Coronal T1-weighted MRI shows edematous gadolinium enhancing lesion in the optic chiasm.

Most NMOSD patients have abnormalities on brain MRI [93]. More commonly, brain MRI lesions are unspecific, but they fulfill Barkoff's criteria for MS in up to 42% of patients [93,94]. In a minority of cases, NMOSD typical brain lesions can be identified mainly in AQP4 enriched regions, such as around the lateral, third and fourth ventricles [93]. Brain lesions that favor NMOSD more than MS include peri-ependymal lesions surrounding the ventricles and aqueduct, hemispheric tumefactive lesions, extensive lesions involving corticospinal tracts, and "cloud-like" enhancing lesions [95]. One recent study [96] showed that criteria comprising (1) at least one lesion adjacent to the body of the lateral ventricle and in the inferior temporal lobe; or (2) the presence of an S-shaped U-fiber lesion; or (3) a Dawson's finger type lesion were fulfilled by 90.9% RRMS, 12.9% AQP4-IgG NMOSD, and 4.8% MOG-IgG NMOSD patients.

Adults and children with MOG antibody disease frequently had fluffy brainstem lesions, often located in pons and/or adjacent to fourth ventricle. Children across all conditions showed more frequent bilateral, large, brainstem and deep grey matter lesions. MOG antibody disease spontaneously separated from multiple sclerosis, but overlapped with AQP4 antibody disease. Multiple sclerosis was discriminated from MOG antibody disease and from AQP4 antibody disease with high predictive values, while MOG antibody disease could not be accurately discriminated from AQP4 antibody disease. The best classifiers between MOG antibody disease and multiple sclerosis were similar in adults and children, and included ovoid lesions adjacent to the body of lateral ventricles, Dawson's fingers T1 hypointense lesions (multiple sclerosis), fluffy lesions and three lesions or less (MOG antibody). In the validation cohort patients with antibody-mediated conditions were differentiated from multiple sclerosis with high accuracy [96].

2.7. Treatment

In spite of their clinical similarities, NMOSD and MS have different treatment. It has been shown that most MS disease modifying drugs, including beta-interferons, glatiramer acetate, natalizumab, alemtuzumab, fingolimod and dimethyl-fumarate are not only inefficacious in NMOSD, but may cause disease exacerbation [97].

In NMOSD the outcome of attacks is usually poor. Recent analysis of 871 attacks revealed that complete remission occurred in only 21% of them and 6% of them had no improvement [98]. The sequence of treatments is of fundamental importance to improve the outcome. Medical therapy, therefore, aims both to enfeeble an ongoing inflammatory attack, and avoid future relapses.

2.7.1. Therapy of Acute Relapses

Relapses are usually treated with intravenous pulses of methylprednisolone (one gram/day for five days). In severe NMOSD attacks, or when corticosteroids fail to stabilize progression of symptoms plasma exchange (PLEX) must be added [99]. Apheresis eliminates the pathogenic antibodies, from circulation and has higher therapeutic efficacy than IV corticosteroids. Its early use as first-line therapy following attack is a predictor of better remission.

Post-infusion oral prednisone is usually recommended, mainly when an immunosuppressive agent with delayed onset of action is prescribed as prophylaxis of new events [100]. Azathioprine, mycophenolate mofetil, and rituximab are the most commonly used immunosuppressive treatments for prevention of new attacks of the disease.

2.7.2. Therapy for Relapses Prevention

Table 6 shows the various drugs used for prevention of relapses in NMOSD. Prednisone, azathioprine, mycophenolate mofetil and rituximab are the first-line drugs. The choice of the initial treatment depends on availability, costs, co-morbidities, and disease course. Prednisone is inexpensive and has a rapid-onset therapeutic action, but adverse effects frequently restrain its continuation for a long time.

Table 6. Drugs used in relapse prevention in neuromyelitis optica spectrum disorders.

Drugs	Route	Regimen	Comments
Prednisone	Oral	≥30 mg/d	Keep until until azathioprine or mycophenolate fully effective, then taper over six months
Azathioprine	Oral	2-3 mg/kg/d in 2 doses	First line treatment; latency four to six months; target dose guided by ALC and MCV; monitor liver function
Mycophenolate mofetil	Oral	1500–3000 mg/d in 2 doses	Target dose guided by ALC and blood concentration (1–2 µg/mL)
Rituximab	IV	1000 mg given twice, 14 d apart.Repeat every 6 mo or based on reemergence of CD19 B cells	First-line therapy; CD19 B cells as a marker
Methotrexate	Oral	15–25.0 mg weekly	Supplement with folic acid 1 mg/d, monitor liver function
Ciclosporin A	Oral	2–5 mg/kg/day in 2 doses	Nephrotoxic, target dose guided by blood concentration (70–100 ng/mL)
Tacrolimus	Oral	1–6 mg/day in 2 doses	Nephrotoxic, target dose guided by blood concentration (5–10 ng/mL)
Mitoxantrone	IV	12 mg/m2 every 1–3 months	Cardiac monitoring (LVEF), target dose guided by leukocyte count; total cumulative dose 100 mg/m2
Tocilizumab	IV	8 mg/kg every 4 weeks	8 mg/kg every four weeks; monitoring for infections; CRP no reliable biomarker for infection

ALC = absolute lymphocyte count; MCV = mean corpuscular volume; IV = intravenously; LVEF = left ventricular ejection fraction; CRP = C-reactive protein.

Azathioprine is probably the most commonly used drug in the preventive treatment of attacks in NMOSD. Initially, it should be combined with prednisone for three to six months until its maximal therapeutic effect can be reached. The lymphocyte count should decrease to 600–1000/cubic millimeter and the mean erythrocyte volume should increase five points from baseline. Thiopurine methyltransferase enzyme activity testing, when available is recommended before the administration of the drug to avoid higher risk of adverse effects. Monitoring of blood cell count and liver function tests on a regular basis is mandatory.

Mycophenolate mofetil is recommended as an alternative treatment in patients who develop intolerance or poor response to azathioprine.

Rituximab is a chimeric monoclonal anti-CD20 antibody that produces rapid depletion of circulating CD20 B cells. A number of studies have showed its efficacy and tolerance in the treatment of NMOSD, but some aspects of treatment strategy and long-term safety still remain to be clarified [101].

Monoclonal antibodies will probably play a most important role in treatment of NMOSD in the coming years. Eculizumab and tocilizumab have already shown their efficacy in small groups of patients [102].

Eculizumab is a humanized monoclonal antibody that inhibits the complement protein C5 and blocks terminal complement activation [103]. The complement cascade is a fundamental part in the inflammation process in NMOSD lesions. In spite of eculizumab efficacy in preventing relapses the increased risk of patients developing meningococcal meningitis raises important safety concerns [104].

Tocilizumab is a monoclonal antibody that targets Interleukin-6 (IL-6) receptor and decrease survival of the antibody-producing plasmablasts. Inebelizumab is a humanized anti-CD19 monoclonal antibody that targets B cell lineage. Although there is still no open-label study supporting its use, it is probably more efficacious than rituximab, which targets the more mature CD20. Inebelizumab removes plasmablasts that express CD19, decreasing the production of AQP4-IgG [102].

Satralizumab is an anti-IL-6 receptor monoclonal antibody. A recent communication on results of a phase III study showed that Satralizumab is a promising therapeutic agent by reducing the risk of relapses by 62% in NMOSD patients [105].

Tolerization is a recent therapeutic approach that uses innovative techniques to restore immune tolerance to host antigens and suppress autoimmune diseases [106]. Tolerization techniques include inverse DNA vaccination, T-cell vaccination, peptide-coupling strategies, tolerogenic dendritic cell vaccination, as well as T-cell receptor engineering-, and chimeric antigen receptor-based therapeutics. As AQP-4 is a specific target to NMO-IgG, there is reason for optimism that this new approach might offer marked beneficial to NMOSD patients, avoiding the wide variety of adverse effects of chronic immunosuppressive agents.

3. Anti-Myelin Oligodendrocyte Glycoprotein Syndromes

Myelin oligodendrocyte glycoprotein is a component of myelin expressed exclusively in myelin produced by oligodendrocytes in the CNS, making up less than 0.05% of total myelin proteins. It presents a length of 245 amino acids with a molecular weight of approximately 26–28 kDa [107–109].

The introduction of experimental autoimmune encephalomyelitis (EAE) as an animal model of demyelination raised the interest in the search of anti-MOG antibodies in MS patients. Some investigators reported a prevalence as high as 41% of anti-MOG antibodies serum positivity in MS patients [110]. Others, however, found similar rates of positive MOG-IgG serostatus inpatients with MS, other neurological disorders and healthy controls [111–117]. Recently, the introduction of CBA in substitution to enzyme-linked immunosorbent assays and immunoprecipitation techniques for the detection of MOG-IgG, methods which were not reliable, led to a major change in the understanding of the relationship between MOG-IgG and CNS disorders in humans. Using CBA, a technique that preserve the conformational structure of full-length human MOG, antibodies targeting MOG have been identified in both children and adults with a variety of phenotypes such as ADEM, optic neuritis, transverse myelitis, NMOSD, and brainstem encephalitis [118–122]. Conversely, MOG-IgG has rarely been found in patients with MS phenotype [123,124].

3.1. Pathophysiology

While the role of AQP4-IgG in the pathophysiology of NMOSD has been established by a large number of clinical and experimental evidences the innermost mechanisms underlying the variety of human demyelinating phenotypes in association with anti-MOG antibodies remain to be better clarified.

Anti-MOG antibodies are produced peripherally and usually reach the CNS following a breakdown of the BBB secondary to infections. A history of preceding infectious prodrome is reported in almost 50% of the patients [124]. The absence of restrict oligoclonal bands in the CSF of patients with anti-MOG syndromes supports the notion of its peripheral origin. Circulating lymphocytes may also migrate to CNS with subsequent clonal expansion [125].

Both in vivo and in vitro studies have suggested the presence of complement in mediating demyelination [126,127]. The observation of complement-mediated cytotoxicity from in vitro studies, and the development of a NMOSD-like disorder in animal models are strong evidences in favor of MOG-IgG pathogenicity [18,128,129].

However, in some instances there are reversible alterations to myelin without complement activation or inflammatory cell infiltration [130]. This is in consonance with the better recovery of some patients with anti-MOG syndromes as compared with NMOSD [119,131].

There are few pathological studies on anti-MOG syndromes [7,10]. A brain biopsy from a patient with MOG-antibody-associated encephalomyelitis revealed typical MS-type II histopathological features characterized by deposition of IgG and activated complement at sites of ongoing demyelination. There were well demarcated areas of loss of myelin with relative preservation of axons and astrocytes, numerous lipid-laden macrophages containing myelin debris, and inflammatory infiltrates with predominately perivascular T cells and some perivascular B-cells [7]. However, search for MOG-IgG and a number of other autoantibodies in a series of patients with Type-II MS failed to show any direct relation between type II-MS and MOG-IgG [6]. In contrast with seropositive AQP4-IgG NMOSD, co-existing serum autoantibodies are rare in anti-MOG syndromes. Associated autoimmune disorders are found in over one third of patients with AQP4-IgG seropositive NMOSD, but in only 9% of the anti-MOG syndromes.

3.2. Epidemiology

Major published series show that anti-MOG syndromes have an earlier age at onset, a lower female to male ratio, and a different racial predisposition as compared with seropositive AQP4-IgG NMOSD [96,119,124,132]. In a recent analysis of 50 cases [6], the age at onset ranged from 6 to 70 years (median 31 years) and 64% were females. Caucasians comprised 73% of the 59 patients in Australia/New Zealand series [124].

3.3. Clinical Manifestations

Almost all patients with anti-MOG syndromes present a relapsing course. The proportion of patients with a monophasic disease declines with extension of the follow-up. Relapses occurred in 93% of patients with disease duration ≥8 years [6]. In a study of 276 relapses in 50 patients, optic neuritis occurred in 88%, acute myelitis in 56%, brainstem attacks in 24%, supratentorial encephalitis in 14%, and cerebellitis in 4% of the patients. Bilateral simultaneous optic neuritis occurred in 51% and simultaneous optic neuritis and myelitis in 18 % of the patients [6].

Anti-MOG syndromes have distinct clinical features in children and adults. In children MOG-IgG most frequently expresses clinically as ADEM phenotype, whereas optic neuritis, usually with bilateral involvement, predominates in adults. In a study of 59 patients with relapsing anti-MOG syndromes (33 children and 26 adults) [124] the inaugural symptoms in the pediatric group were ADEM (36%), bilateral optic neuritis (24%), unilateral optic neuritis (15%). In adults, optic neuritis was the presenting symptom in 73% (bilateral optic neuritis 42%; unilateral optic neuritis 31%). Simultaneous involvement of the optic nerves and spinal cord (NMOSD phenotype was the presenting symptom in two children (6%) and five adults (19%). ADEM did not occur in the adult group. Transverse myelitis was less common. Conversely, myelitis occurred at disease presentation in 34% of the patients in another series [6], whereas optic neuritis in 74%, brainstem encephalitis in 8%, cerebral symptoms in 6% and cerebellar symptoms in 2%. At presentation, most patients exhibit either isolated optic neuritis (64%), isolated myelitis (18%), or combined optic neuritis and myelitis (10%). [6]. Optic neuritis is usually severe. Visual acuity ≥20/200 is observed in almost 70% of patients and optic nerve head swelling in the vast majority of the cases [124,132].

Interestingly, 25% to 32% of the patients in both series fulfilled the 2015 International consensus criteria for NMOSD, whereas 15% to 33% of them fulfilled revised McDonald criteria for MS [124,132].

3.4. Anti-MOG Testing

The recently introduced CBA techniques to detect specific autoantibodies that recognize conformational epitopes of membrane proteins, are the currently recommended method for the detection of AQP4-IgG and MOG-IgG. Indications for testing are based on the presence of specific clinical and paraclinical abnormalities that are considered typical for these disorders and atypical for MS. As some patients with MOG-related disorders may test negative for MOG-IgG during disease remission and treatment with immunosuppressive agents, it is recommended that the search for the antibody should be performed during acute relapses.

Many factors influence the sensitivity and specificity for anti-MOG antibody detection and the discrepancies found in early studies are now considered as a result of the use of inappropriate methodology for antibody detection, such as ELISA and immunoblot techniques. Using CBA antibodies targeting MOG have been recently identified in both children and adults with demyelination disorders including acute disseminated encephalomyelitis (ADEM), optic neuritis (ON), transverse myelitis (TM), and AQP4-seronegative NMOSD [124].

3.5. Cerebrospinal Fluid Analysis

Pleocytosis is found in over one half of patients with anti-MOG syndromes. White cell counts $\geq$100 cell/μL have been reported in 28% of cases [132]. Neutrophils may be present in variable proportion. Intrathecal IgG synthesis as measured by the presence of restricted oligoclonal bands in CSF was found in 11% to 13% of patients [124,132].

3.6. MRI Features

Optic neuritis in anti-MOG syndrome exhibits some peculiar features that may distinguish it from optic neuritis in AQP4-IgG NMOSD and MS. Bilateral optic nerve lesions occur more commonly in MOG (and AQP4-IgG) optic neuritis than in MS optic neuritis (Figure 3a). Usually, lesions are longitudinally extensive and tend to locate in the retrobulbar and orbital segments of the optic nerve. Chiasmal involvement is very rare. Perioptic contrast enhancement which may extend to surrounding orbital tissues (Figure 3b) is observed in over one third of patients [132].

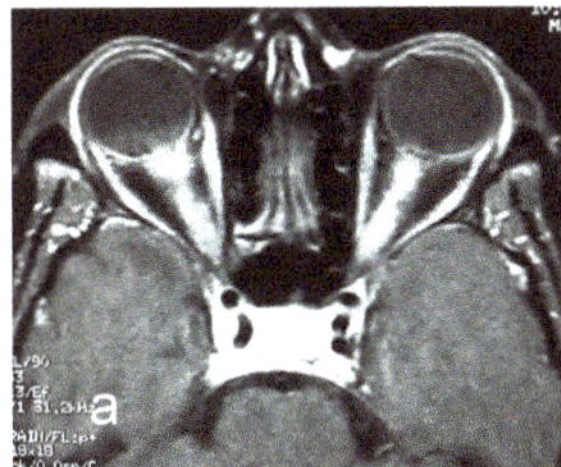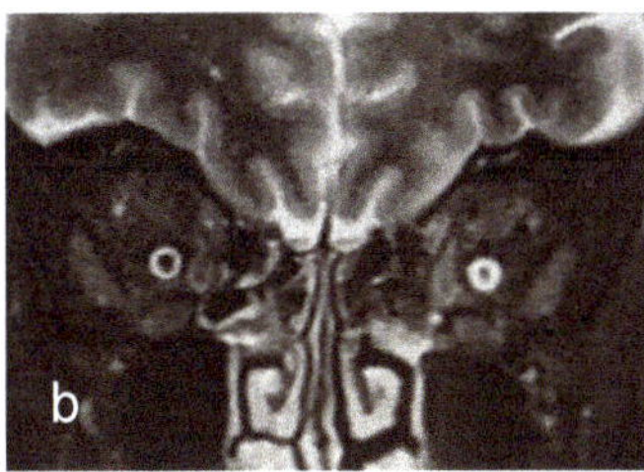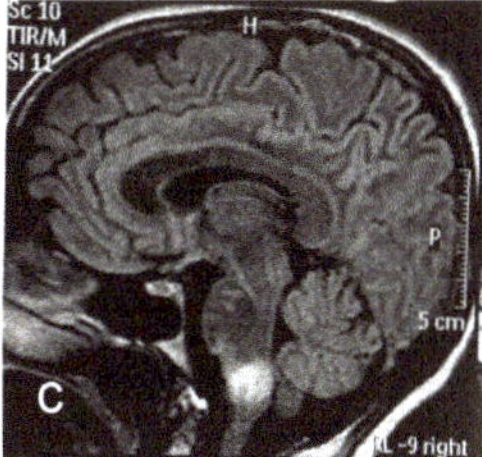

Figure 3. Examples of MRI abnormalities in anti-MOG syndrome. (**a**). Axial T1-weighted MRI reveals longitudinal extensive gadolinium enhancement of both optic nerves. (**b**). Coronal T2-weighted MRI shows hyperintense thickening of perioptic nerve sheath. (**c**). Sagittal T2/FLAIR-weighted image shows large fluffy lesion in the medulla.

Spinal MRI shows in patients with acute myelitis at disease onset LETM lesions in two thirds lesions occur and short lesions (<3 vertebral segments) in one third of patients. Swelling and contrast enhancement of the lesions are frequently observed [131].

Brain MRI is normal in a large majority of anti-MOG NMOSD patients. However, when brain MRI is abnormal, some lesion characteristics may discriminate between anti-MOG NMOSD and MS with high predictive values [96]. Imaging features that are useful to differ between the two conditions are the presence of three lesions or less, and of fluffy brainstem lesions in the pons/or adjacent to fourth ventricle (anti-MOG syndrome) (Figure 3c); and of ovoid lesions adjacent to the body of lateral ventricles, or Dawson's fingers T1 hypointense lesions (MS). On the other hand, brain MRI does not discriminate anti-MOG-NMOSD from AQP4-IgG NMOSD [96].

3.7. Diagnosis

Recently, an international panel of experts [133] formulated the diagnostic criteria for MOG-related disorders in adults. Accordingly, MOG-related disorders should be diagnosed in patients who meet all of the following criteria:

1. Monophasic or relapsing acute ON, myelitis, brainstem encephalitis, or any combination of these symptoms
2. MRI or electrophysiological (visual evoked potentials in patients with isolated ON) findings compatible with CNS demyelination
3. Seropositivity for MOG-IgG as detected by means of a cell-based assay employing full length human MOG as target antigen.

Clinical, laboratory and imaging features that favor the diagnosis of conditions other than MOG-related disorders ("red-flags") include:

a. Chronic progressive course (progressive MS, sarcoidosis and tumors) or acute onset (ischemia);
b. Clinical and paraclinical findings suggesting other conditions such as:

    i.   Tuberculosis, borreliosis, syphilis, Behçet's disease, subacute combined degeneration of the spinal cord, Leber's hereditary optic neuropathy, lymphoma, and paraneoplastic disorders;
    ii. Peripheral demyelination

c. Brain MRI abnormalities such as:

    i.   Lesion adjacent to lateral ventricle associated with inferior temporal lobe lesion, or Dawson's finger-type lesion;
    ii. Increasing number of lesions between relapses.

d. Serum MOG-IgG at low titers.

It is recommended that patients who test positive for MOG-IgG but in whom a "red flag" is suspected undergo retesting, preferably employing a different CBA [133].

3.8. Treatment

Patients with anti-MOG syndrome are usually responsive to steroids, but frequently relapse after prednisone withdrawal or with a rapid taper [134]. More severe attacks or those with suboptimal response to steroid may be treated with plasma exchange or IV immunoglobulin. As relapsing disease is the rule with extended follow-up long-term immunosuppression should follow first-line treatment [132]. Azathioprine, mycophenolate mofetil and rituximab have all been used but studies on their comparative efficacy are still lacking. Multicenter studies are needed to provide physicians with more robust data on the most appropriate way to treat this rare condition.

3.9. Conclusions

The understanding of NMOSD has enormously advanced in the last few years. Pathophysiological and clinical studies have cleared up a number of uncertainties and deeply changed the concept of the disease. Previously considered as a variant of MS, characterized by monophasic course and exclusive involvement of the optic nerves and spinal cord, NMOSD is now recognized as an independent disorder, most frequently with relapsing course and a variety of clinical manifestations. The 2015 diagnostic criteria [35] allows for the identification of NMOSD in both patients with AQP4-IgG seropositivity and without the antibody, or who were not tested. High doses of IV steroids and PLEX are the main therapeutic measures during relapses, whereas immunosupressive drugs and rituximab are most useful to prevent new attacks. Monoclonal antibodies and tolerization are emerging and promising therapeutic approaches. Recently, MOG-IgG was identified in patients with relapsing optic neurits, acute myelitis, NMOSD phenotypes, and brainstem encephalitis, in addition to ADEM. Although these patients are treated with IV corticosteroids and immunosupressive agents, data are too scanty to evaluate the real efficacy of these drugs.

As NMOSD and anti-MOG syndromes are rare conditions, international collaborative efforts are necessary to determine their distribution in different regions and populations, their intimate pathophysiological mechanisms and the most efficacious therapeutic approach, in order to improving patients care.

Funding: This article received no external funding.

Conflicts of Interest: M.L.-P. serves on scientific advisory board for Roche; has received funding for travel and speaker honoraria from Roche, Biogen Idec, Teva, Novartis and Sanofi Genzyme. N.T. declares no conflict of interest.

References

1. Kleiter, I.; Hellwig, K.; Berthele, A.; Kumpfel, T.; Linker, R.A.; Hartung, H.P.; Paul, F.; Aktas, O. Failure of natalizumab to prevent relapses in neuromyelitis optica. *Arch. Neurol.* **2012**, *69*, 239–245. [CrossRef] [PubMed]
2. Min, J.H.; Kim, B.J.; Lee, K.H. Development of extensive brain lesions following fingolimod (fty720) treatment in a patient with neuromyelitis optica spectrum disorder. *Mult. Scler.* **2012**, *18*, 113–115. [CrossRef] [PubMed]
3. Trebst, C.; Jarius, S.; Berthele, A.; Paul, F.; Schippling, S.; Wildemann, B.; Borisow, N.; Kleiter, I.; Aktas, O.; Kumpfel, T. Update on the diagnosis and treatment of neuromyelitis optica: Recommendations of the neuromyelitis optica study group (nemos). *J. Neurol.* **2014**, *261*, 1–16. [CrossRef] [PubMed]
4. van Pelt, E.D.; Wong, Y.Y.; Ketelslegers, I.A.; Hamann, D.; Hintzen, R.Q. Neuromyelitis optica spectrum disorders: Comparison of clinical and magnetic resonance imaging characteristics of aqp4-igg versus mog-igg seropositive cases in the netherlands. *Eur. J. Neurol.* **2016**, *23*, 580–587. [CrossRef] [PubMed]
5. Narayan, R.; Simpson, A.; Fritsche, K.; Salama, S.; Pardo, S.; Mealy, M.; Paul, F.; Levy, M. Mog antibody disease: A review of mog antibody seropositive neuromyelitis optica spectrum disorder. *Mult. Scler. Relat. Disord.* **2018**, *25*, 66–72. [CrossRef] [PubMed]
6. Jarius, S.; Metz, I.; Konig, F.B.; Ruprecht, K.; Reindl, M.; Paul, F.; Bruck, W.; Wildemann, B. Screening for mog-igg and 27 other anti-glial and anti-neuronal autoantibodies in 'pattern ii multiple sclerosis' and brain biopsy findings in a mog-igg-positive case. *Mult. Scler.* **2016**, *22*, 1541–1549. [CrossRef] [PubMed]
7. Spadaro, M.; Gerdes, L.A.; Mayer, M.C.; Ertl-Wagner, B.; Laurent, S.; Krumbholz, M.; Breithaupt, C.; Hogen, T.; Straube, A.; Giese, A.; et al. Histopathology and clinical course of mog-antibody-associated encephalomyelitis. *Ann. Clin. Transl. Neurol.* **2015**, *2*, 295–301. [CrossRef] [PubMed]
8. Misu, T.; Hoftberger, R.; Fujihara, K.; Wimmer, I.; Takai, Y.; Nishiyama, S.; Nakashima, I.; Konno, H.; Bradl, M.; Garzuly, F.; et al. Presence of six different lesion types suggests diverse mechanisms of tissue injury in neuromyelitis optica. *Acta Neuropathol.* **2013**, *125*, 815–827. [CrossRef] [PubMed]
9. Reindl, M.; Rostasy, K. Mog antibody-associated diseases. *Neurol. Neuroimmunol. Neuroinflamm.* **2015**, *2*, e60. [CrossRef]
10. Di Pauli, F.; Hoftberger, R.; Reindl, M.; Beer, R.; Rhomberg, P.; Schanda, K.; Sato, D.; Fujihara, K.; Lassmann, H.; Schmutzhard, E.; et al. Fulminant demyelinating encephalomyelitis: Insights from antibody studies and neuropathology. *Neurol. Neuroimmunol. Neuroinflamm.* **2015**, *2*, e175. [CrossRef]
11. Ramanathan, S.; Dale, R.C.; Brilot, F. Anti-mog antibody: The history, clinical phenotype, and pathogenicity of a serum biomarker for demyelination. *Autoimmun. Rev.* **2016**, *15*, 307–324. [CrossRef] [PubMed]

12. Jarius, S.; Probst, C.; Borowski, K.; Franciotta, D.; Wildemann, B.; Stoecker, W.; Wandinger, K.P. Standardized method for the detection of antibodies to aquaporin-4 based on a highly sensitive immunofluorescence assay employing recombinant target antigen. *J. Neurol. Sci.* **2010**, *291*, 52–56. [CrossRef] [PubMed]

13. Waters, P.J.; McKeon, A.; Leite, M.I.; Rajasekharan, S.; Lennon, V.A.; Villalobos, A.; Palace, J.; Mandrekar, J.N.; Vincent, A.; Bar-Or, A.; et al. Serologic diagnosis of nmo: A multicenter comparison of aquaporin-4-igg assays. *Neurology* **2012**, *78*, 665–671; discussion 669. [CrossRef] [PubMed]

14. Waters, P.J.; Pittock, S.J.; Bennett, J.L.; Jarius, S.; Weinshenker, B.G.; Wingerchuk, D.M. Evaluation of aquaporin-4 antibody assays. *Clin. Exp. Neuroimmunol.* **2014**, *5*, 290–303. [CrossRef] [PubMed]

15. Jarius, S.; Ruprecht, K.; Kleiter, I.; Borisow, N.; Asgari, N.; Pitarokoili, K.; Pache, F.; Stich, O.; Beume, L.A.; Hummert, M.W.; et al. Mog-igg in nmo and related disorders: A multicenter study of 50 patients. Part 1: Frequency, syndrome specificity, influence of disease activity, long-term course, association with aqp4-igg, and origin. *J. Neuroinflamm.* **2016**, *13*, 279. [CrossRef] [PubMed]

16. Ishikawa, N.; Tajima, G.; Hyodo, S.; Takahashi, Y.; Kobayashi, M. Detection of autoantibodies against nmda-type glutamate receptor in a patient with recurrent optic neuritis and transient cerebral lesions. *Neuropediatrics* **2007**, *38*, 257–260. [CrossRef] [PubMed]

17. Kruer, M.C.; Koch, T.K.; Bourdette, D.N.; Chabas, D.; Waubant, E.; Mueller, S.; Moscarello, M.A.; Dalmau, J.; Woltjer, R.L.; Adamus, G. Nmda receptor encephalitis mimicking seronegative neuromyelitis optica. *Neurology* **2010**, *74*, 1473–1475. [CrossRef] [PubMed]

18. Mader, S.; Gredler, V.; Schanda, K.; Rostasy, K.; Dujmovic, I.; Pfaller, K.; Lutterotti, A.; Jarius, S.; Di Pauli, F.; Kuenz, B.; et al. Complement activating antibodies to myelin oligodendrocyte glycoprotein in neuromyelitis optica and related disorders. *J. Neuroinflamm.* **2011**, *8*, 184. [CrossRef] [PubMed]

19. Jarius, S.; Wandinger, K.P.; Borowski, K.; Stoecker, W.; Wildemann, B. Antibodies to cv2/crmp5 in neuromyelitis optica-like disease: Case report and review of the literature. *Clin. Neurol. Neurosurg.* **2012**, *114*, 331–335. [CrossRef] [PubMed]

20. Devic, E. Myelite subaigue compliquee de nevrite optique. *Bull. Med.* **1894**, *8*, 1033.

21. Gault, F. De la neuromyélite optique aiguë. Ph.D. Thesis, Alexandre Rey, imprimeur de la faculté de médecine, Faculté de Medicine et de Pharmacie de Lyon, Lyon, France, 1894.

22. Acchiote, P. Sur un cas de neuromyélite subaiguë ou maladie de devic. *Rev. Neurol.* **1907**, *20*, 775–777.

23. Jarius, S.; Wildemann, B. The case of the marquis de causan (1804): An early account of visual loss associated with spinal cord inflammation. *J. Neurol.* **2012**, *259*, 1354–1357. [CrossRef] [PubMed]

24. Jarius, S.; Wildemann, B. 'Noteomielite' accompanied by acute amaurosis (1844). An early case of neuromyelitis optica. *J. Neurol. Sci.* **2012**, *313*, 182–184. [CrossRef] [PubMed]

25. Jarius, S.; Wildemann, B. An early british case of neuromyelitis optica (1850). *BMJ Clin. Res. Ed.* **2012**, *345*, e6430. [CrossRef] [PubMed]

26. Jarius, S.; Wildemann, B. An early case of neuromyelitis optica: On a forgotten report by jacob lockhart clarke, frs. *Mult. Scler.* **2011**, *17*, 1384–1386. [CrossRef] [PubMed]

27. Allbutt, T.C. On the ophthalmoscopic signs of spinal disease. *Lancet* **1870**, *95*, 76–78. [CrossRef]

28. Erb, W. Ueber das zusammenvorkommen von neuritis optica und myelitis subacuta. *Eur. Arch. Psychiatry Clin. Neurosci.* **1880**, *10*, 146–157. [CrossRef]

29. Seguin, E.C. Art. I.—On the coincidence of optic neuritis and subacute transverse myelitis. *J. Nerv. Ment. Dis.* **1880**, *7*, 177–188. [CrossRef]

30. Marques, A. Da neuromielite ótica: Contribuição clínica e etiológica. *Hospital* **1943**, *24*, 49–63.

31. Lennon, V.A.; Wingerchuk, D.M.; Kryzer, T.J.; Pittock, S.J.; Lucchinetti, C.F.; Fujihara, K.; Nakashima, I.; Weinshenker, B.G. A serum autoantibody marker of neuromyelitis optica: Distinction from multiple sclerosis. *Lancet* **2004**, *364*, 2106–2112. [CrossRef]

32. Lennon, V.A.; Kryzer, T.J.; Pittock, S.J.; Verkman, A.S.; Hinson, S.R. Igg marker of optic-spinal multiple sclerosis binds to the aquaporin-4 water channel. *J. Exp. Med.* **2005**, *202*, 473–477. [CrossRef] [PubMed]

33. Wingerchuk, D.M.; Lennon, V.A.; Lucchinetti, C.F.; Pittock, S.J.; Weinshenker, B.G. The spectrum of neuromyelitis optica. *Lancet Neurol.* **2007**, *6*, 805–815. [CrossRef]

34. Lana-Peixoto, M.A.; Callegaro, D. The expanded spectrum of neuromyelitis optica: Evidences for a new definition. *Arq. Neuro-Psiquiatr.* **2012**, *70*, 807–813. [CrossRef]

35. Wingerchuk, D.M.; Banwell, B.; Bennett, J.L.; Cabre, P.; Carroll, W.; Chitnis, T.; de Seze, J.; Fujihara, K.; Greenberg, B.; Jacob, A.; et al. International consensus diagnostic criteria for neuromyelitis optica spectrum disorders. *Neurology* **2015**, *85*, 177–189. [CrossRef] [PubMed]

36. Jin, B.J.; Rossi, A.; Verkman, A.S. Model of aquaporin-4 supramolecular assembly in orthogonal arrays based on heterotetrameric association of m1-m23 isoforms. *Biophys. J.* **2011**, *100*, 2936–2945. [CrossRef] [PubMed]

37. Papadopoulos, M.C.; Verkman, A.S. Aquaporin 4 and neuromyelitis optica. *Lancet Neurol.* **2012**, *11*, 535–544. [CrossRef]

38. Verkman, A.S.; Anderson, M.O.; Papadopoulos, M.C. Aquaporins: Important but elusive drug targets. *Nat. Rev. Drug Discov.* **2014**, *13*, 259–277. [CrossRef]

39. Saadoun, S.; Waters, P.; Bell, B.A.; Vincent, A.; Verkman, A.S.; Papadopoulos, M.C. Intra-cerebral injection of neuromyelitis optica immunoglobulin g and human complement produces neuromyelitis optica lesions in mice. *Brain J. Neurol.* **2010**, *133*, 349–361. [CrossRef]

40. Lucchinetti, C.F.; Mandler, R.N.; McGavern, D.; Bruck, W.; Gleich, G.; Ransohoff, R.M.; Trebst, C.; Weinshenker, B.; Wingerchuk, D.; Parisi, J.E.; et al. A role for humoral mechanisms in the pathogenesis of devic's neuromyelitis optica. *Brain J. Neurol.* **2002**, *125*, 1450–1461. [CrossRef]

41. Jarius, S.; Franciotta, D.; Paul, F.; Ruprecht, K.; Bergamaschi, R.; Rommer, P.S.; Reuss, R.; Probst, C.; Kristoferitsch, W.; Wandinger, K.P.; et al. Cerebrospinal fluid antibodies to aquaporin-4 in neuromyelitis optica and related disorders: Frequency, origin, and diagnostic relevance. *J. Neuroinflamm.* **2010**, *7*, 52. [CrossRef]

42. Chihara, N.; Aranami, T.; Sato, W.; Miyazaki, Y.; Miyake, S.; Okamoto, T.; Ogawa, M.; Toda, T.; Yamamura, T. Interleukin 6 signaling promotes anti-aquaporin 4 autoantibody production from plasmablasts in neuromyelitis optica. *Proc. Natl. Acad. Sci. USA* **2011**, *108*, 3701–3706. [CrossRef] [PubMed]

43. Shimizu, F.; Schaller, K.L.; Owens, G.P.; Cotleur, A.C.; Kellner, D.; Takeshita, Y.; Obermeier, B.; Kryzer, T.J.; Sano, Y.; Kanda, T.; et al. Glucose-regulated protein 78 autoantibody associates with blood-brain barrier disruption in neuromyelitis optica. *Sci. Transl. Med.* **2017**, *9*, eaai9111. [CrossRef] [PubMed]

44. Shimizu, F.; Nishihara, H.; Kanda, T. Blood-brain barrier dysfunction in immuno-mediated neurological diseases. *Immunol. Med.* **2018**, *41*, 120–128. [CrossRef] [PubMed]

45. Jarius, S.; Wildemann, B.; Paul, F. Neuromyelitis optica: Clinical features, immunopathogenesis and treatment. *Clin. Exp. Immunol.* **2014**, *176*, 149–164. [CrossRef] [PubMed]

46. Weinshenker, B.G.; Wingerchuk, D.M. Neuromyelitis spectrum disorders. *Mayo Clin. Proc.* **2017**, *92*, 663–679. [CrossRef] [PubMed]

47. Hinson, S.R.; Pittock, S.J.; Lucchinetti, C.F.; Roemer, S.F.; Fryer, J.P.; Kryzer, T.J.; Lennon, V.A. Pathogenic potential of igg binding to water channel extracellular domain in neuromyelitis optica. *Neurology* **2007**, *69*, 2221–2231. [CrossRef]

48. Bennett, J.L.; Lam, C.; Kalluri, S.R.; Saikali, P.; Bautista, K.; Dupree, C.; Glogowska, M.; Case, D.; Antel, J.P.; Owens, G.P.; et al. Intrathecal pathogenic anti-aquaporin-4 antibodies in early neuromyelitis optica. *Ann. Neurol.* **2009**, *66*, 617–629. [CrossRef]

49. Bradl, M.; Misu, T.; Takahashi, T.; Watanabe, M.; Mader, S.; Reindl, M.; Adzemovic, M.; Bauer, J.; Berger, T.; Fujihara, K.; et al. Neuromyelitis optica: Pathogenicity of patient immunoglobulin in vivo. *Ann. Neurol.* **2009**, *66*, 630–643. [CrossRef]

50. Kinoshita, M.; Nakatsuji, Y.; Kimura, T.; Moriya, M.; Takata, K.; Okuno, T.; Kumanogoh, A.; Kajiyama, K.; Yoshikawa, H.; Sakoda, S. Neuromyelitis optica: Passive transfer to rats by human immunoglobulin. *Biochem. Biophys. Res. Commun.* **2009**, *386*, 623–627. [CrossRef]

51. Kinoshita, M.; Nakatsuji, Y.; Kimura, T.; Moriya, M.; Takata, K.; Okuno, T.; Kumanogoh, A.; Kajiyama, K.; Yoshikawa, H.; Sakoda, S. Anti-aquaporin-4 antibody induces astrocytic cytotoxicity in the absence of cns antigen-specific t cells. *Biochem. Biophys. Res. Commun.* **2010**, *394*, 205–210. [CrossRef]

52. Etemadifar, M.; Nasr, Z.; Khalili, B.; Taherioun, M.; Vosoughi, R. Epidemiology of neuromyelitis optica in the world: A systematic review and meta-analysis. *Mult. Scler. Int.* **2015**, *2015*, 174720. [CrossRef] [PubMed]

53. Flanagan, E.P.; Cabre, P.; Weinshenker, B.G.; Sauver, J.S.; Jacobson, D.J.; Majed, M.; Lennon, V.A.; Lucchinetti, C.F.; McKeon, A.; Matiello, M.; et al. Epidemiology of aquaporin-4 autoimmunity and neuromyelitis optica spectrum. *Ann. Neurol.* **2016**, *79*, 775–783. [CrossRef] [PubMed]

54. Rivera, J.F.; Kurtzke, J.F.; Booth, V.A.; Corona, T. Characteristics of devic's disease (neuromyelitis optica) in mexico. *J. Neurol.* **2008**, *255*, 710–715. [CrossRef] [PubMed]

55. Asgari, N.; Lillevang, S.T.; Skejoe, H.P.; Falah, M.; Stenager, E.; Kyvik, K.O. A population-based study of neuromyelitis optica in caucasians. *Neurology* **2011**, *76*, 1589–1595. [CrossRef] [PubMed]

56. Cabrera-Gomez, J.A.; Kurtzke, J.F.; Gonzalez-Quevedo, A.; Lara-Rodriguez, R. An epidemiological study of neuromyelitis optica in cuba. *J. Neurol.* **2009**, *256*, 35–44. [CrossRef] [PubMed]

57. Aboul-Enein, F.; Seifert-Held, T.; Mader, S.; Kuenz, B.; Lutterotti, A.; Rauschka, H.; Rommer, P.; Leutmezer, F.; Vass, K.; Flamm-Horak, A.; et al. Neuromyelitis optica in austria in 2011: To bridge the gap between neuroepidemiological research and practice in a study population of 8.4 million people. *PLoS ONE* **2013**, *8*, e79649. [CrossRef] [PubMed]

58. Cossburn, M.; Tackley, G.; Baker, K.; Ingram, G.; Burtonwood, M.; Malik, G.; Pickersgill, T.; te Water Naude, J.; Robertson, N. The prevalence of neuromyelitis optica in south east wales. *Eur. J. Neurol.* **2012**, *19*, 655–659. [CrossRef] [PubMed]

59. Houzen, H.; Niino, M.; Hirotani, M.; Fukazawa, T.; Kikuchi, S.; Tanaka, K.; Sasaki, H. Increased prevalence, incidence, and female predominance of multiple sclerosis in northern japan. *J. Neurol. Sci.* **2012**, *323*, 117–122. [CrossRef] [PubMed]

60. Jacob, A.; Panicker, J.; Lythgoe, D.; Elsone, L.; Mutch, K.; Wilson, M.; Das, K.; Boggild, M. The epidemiology of neuromyelitis optica amongst adults in the merseyside county of united kingdom. *J. Neurol.* **2013**, *260*, 2134–2137. [CrossRef] [PubMed]

61. Etemadifar, M.; Dashti, M.; Vosoughi, R.; Abtahi, S.H.; Ramagopalan, S.V.; Nasr, Z. An epidemiological study of neuromyelitis optica in isfahan. *Mult. Scler.* **2014**, *20*, 1920–1922. [CrossRef] [PubMed]

62. Pandit, L.; Kundapur, R. Prevalence and patterns of demyelinating central nervous system disorders in urban mangalore, south india. *Mult. Scler.* **2014**, *20*, 1651–1653. [CrossRef] [PubMed]

63. Kashipazha, D.; Mohammadianinejad, S.E.; Majdinasab, N.; Azizi, M.; Jafari, M. A descriptive study of prevalence, clinical features and other findings of neuromyelitis optica and neuromyelitis optica spectrum disorder in khuzestan province, iran. *Iran. J. Neurol.* **2015**, *14*, 204–210. [PubMed]

64. Danielle van Pelt, E.; Wong, Y.Y.M.; Ketelslegers, I.A.; Siepman, D.A.; Hamann, D.; Hintzen, R.Q. Incidence of aqp4-igg seropositive neuromyelitis optica spectrum disorders in the netherlands: About one in a million. *Mult. Scler. J. Exp. Transl. Clin.* **2016**, *2*, 2055217315625652. [CrossRef] [PubMed]

65. Houzen, H.; Kondo, K.; Niino, M.; Horiuchi, K.; Takahashi, T.; Nakashima, I.; Tanaka, K. Prevalence and clinical features of neuromyelitis optica spectrum disorders in northern japan. *Neurology* **2017**, *89*, 1995–2001. [CrossRef] [PubMed]

66. Hor, J.Y.; Lim, T.T.; Chia, Y.K.; Ching, Y.M.; Cheah, C.F.; Tan, K.; Chow, H.B.; Arip, M.; Eow, G.B.; Easaw, P.E.S.; et al. Prevalence of neuromyelitis optica spectrum disorder in the multi-ethnic penang island, malaysia, and a review of worldwide prevalence. *Mult. Scler. Relat. Disord.* **2018**, *19*, 20–24. [CrossRef] [PubMed]

67. Bukhari, W.; Prain, K.M.; Waters, P.; Woodhall, M.; O'Gorman, C.M.; Clarke, L.; Silvestrini, R.A.; Bundell, C.S.; Abernethy, D.; Bhuta, S.; et al. Incidence and prevalence of nmosd in australia and new zealand. *J. Neurol. Neurosurg. Psychiatry* **2017**, *88*, 632–638. [CrossRef] [PubMed]

68. Sepulveda, M.; Aldea, M.; Escudero, D.; Llufriu, S.; Arrambide, G.; Otero-Romero, S.; Sastre-Garriga, J.; Romero-Pinel, L.; Martinez-Yelamos, S.; Sola-Valls, N.; et al. Epidemiology of nmosd in catalonia: Influence of the new 2015 criteria in incidence and prevalence estimates. *Mult. Scler.* **2017**, *24*, 1843–1851. [CrossRef] [PubMed]

69. Holroyd, K.B.; Aziz, F.; Szolics, M.; Alsaadi, T.; Levy, M.; Schiess, N. Prevalence and characteristics of transverse myelitis and neuromyelitis optica spectrum disorders in the united arab emirates: A multicenter, retrospective study. *Clin. Exp. Neuroimmunol.* **2018**, *9*, 155–161. [CrossRef]

70. Mori, M.; Kuwabara, S.; Paul, F. Worldwide prevalence of neuromyelitis optica spectrum disorders. *J. Neurol. Neurosurg. Psychiatry* **2018**, *89*, 555–556. [CrossRef]

71. Kim, S.H.; Mealy, M.A.; Levy, M.; Schmidt, F.; Ruprecht, K.; Paul, F.; Ringelstein, M.; Aktas, O.; Hartung, H.P.; Asgari, N.; et al. Racial differences in neuromyelitis optica spectrum disorder. *Neurology* **2018**, *91*, e2089–e2099. [CrossRef]

72. Kitley, J.; Leite, M.I.; Nakashima, I.; Waters, P.; McNeillis, B.; Brown, R.; Takai, Y.; Takahashi, T.; Misu, T.; Elsone, L.; et al. Prognostic factors and disease course in aquaporin-4 antibody-positive patients with neuromyelitis optica spectrum disorder from the united kingdom and japan. *Brain J. Neurol.* **2012**, *135*, 1834–1849. [CrossRef] [PubMed]

73. Sepulveda, M.; Armangue, T.; Sola-Valls, N.; Arrambide, G.; Meca-Lallana, J.E.; Oreja-Guevara, C.; Mendibe, M.; Alvarez de Arcaya, A.; Aladro, Y.; Casanova, B.; et al. Neuromyelitis optica spectrum disorders: Comparison according to the phenotype and serostatus. *Neurol. Neuroimmunol. Neuroinflamm.* **2016**, *3*, e225. [CrossRef] [PubMed]

74. McKeon, A.; Lennon, V.A.; Lotze, T.; Tenenbaum, S.; Ness, J.M.; Rensel, M.; Kuntz, N.L.; Fryer, J.P.; Homburger, H.; Hunter, J.; et al. Cns aquaporin-4 autoimmunity in children. *Neurology* **2008**, *71*, 93–100. [CrossRef] [PubMed]

75. Matiello, M.; Kim, H.J.; Kim, W.; Brum, D.G.; Barreira, A.A.; Kingsbury, D.J.; Plant, G.T.; Adoni, T.; Weinshenker, B.G. Familial neuromyelitis optica. *Neurology* **2010**, *75*, 310–315. [CrossRef] [PubMed]

76. Matsushita, T.; Matsuoka, T.; Isobe, N.; Kawano, Y.; Minohara, M.; Shi, N.; Nishimura, Y.; Ochi, H.; Kira, J. Association of the hla-dpb1*0501 allele with anti-aquaporin-4 antibody positivity in japanese patients with idiopathic central nervous system demyelinating disorders. *Tissue Antigens* **2009**, *73*, 171–176. [CrossRef] [PubMed]

77. Wang, H.; Dai, Y.; Qiu, W.; Zhong, X.; Wu, A.; Wang, Y.; Lu, Z.; Bao, J.; Hu, X. Hla-dpb1 0501 is associated with susceptibility to anti-aquaporin-4 antibodies positive neuromyelitis optica in southern han chinese. *J. Neuroimmunol.* **2011**, *233*, 181–184. [CrossRef] [PubMed]

78. Blanco, Y.; Ercilla-Gonzalez, G.; Llufriu, S.; Casanova-Estruch, B.; Magraner, M.J.; Ramio-Torrenta, L.; Mendibe-Bilbao, M.M.; Ucles-Sanchez, A.J.; Casado-Chocan, J.L.; Lopez de Munain, A.; et al. hla-drb1 typing in caucasians patients with neuromyelitis optica. *Rev. De Neurol.* **2011**, *53*, 146–152.

79. Pandit, L.; Malli, C.; D'Cunha, A.; Mustafa, S. Human leukocyte antigen association with neuromyelitis optica in a south indian population. *Mult. Scler.* **2015**, *21*, 1217–1218. [CrossRef]

80. Deschamps, R.; Paturel, L.; Jeannin, S.; Chausson, N.; Olindo, S.; Bera, O.; Bellance, R.; Smadja, D.; Cesaire, D.; Cabre, P. Different hla class ii (drb1 and dqb1) alleles determine either susceptibility or resistance to nmo and multiple sclerosis among the french afro-caribbean population. *Mult. Scler.* **2011**, *17*, 24–31. [CrossRef]

81. Zephir, H.; Fajardy, I.; Outteryck, O.; Blanc, F.; Roger, N.; Fleury, M.; Rudolf, G.; Marignier, R.; Vukusic, S.; Confavreux, C.; et al. Is neuromyelitis optica associated with human leukocyte antigen? *Mult. Scler.* **2009**, *15*, 571–579. [CrossRef]

82. Popescu, B.F.; Lennon, V.A.; Parisi, J.E.; Howe, C.L.; Weigand, S.D.; Cabrera-Gomez, J.A.; Newell, K.; Mandler, R.N.; Pittock, S.J.; Weinshenker, B.G.; et al. Neuromyelitis optica unique area postrema lesions: Nausea, vomiting, and pathogenic implications. *Neurology* **2011**, *76*, 1229–1237. [CrossRef] [PubMed]

83. Dubey, D.; Pittock, S.J.; Krecke, K.N.; Flanagan, E.P. Association of extension of cervical cord lesion and area postrema syndrome with neuromyelitis optica spectrum disorder. *JAMA Neurol.* **2017**, *74*, 359–361. [CrossRef] [PubMed]

84. Kremer, L.; Mealy, M.; Jacob, A.; Nakashima, I.; Cabre, P.; Bigi, S.; Paul, F.; Jarius, S.; Aktas, O.; Elsone, L.; et al. Brainstem manifestations in neuromyelitis optica: A multicenter study of 258 patients. *Mult. Scler.* **2014**, *20*, 843–847. [CrossRef] [PubMed]

85. Jarius, S.; Wildemann, B. Aquaporin-4 antibodies (nmo-igg) as a serological marker of neuromyelitis optica: A critical review of the literature. *Brain Pathol.* **2013**, *23*, 661–683. [CrossRef] [PubMed]

86. Marignier, R.; Bernard-Valnet, R.; Giraudon, P.; Collongues, N.; Papeix, C.; Zephir, H.; Cavillon, G.; Rogemond, V.; Casey, R.; Frangoulis, B.; et al. Aquaporin-4 antibody-negative neuromyelitis optica: Distinct assay sensitivity-dependent entity. *Neurology* **2013**, *80*, 2194–2200. [CrossRef] [PubMed]

87. Pittock, S.J.; Lennon, V.A.; Bakshi, N.; Shen, L.; McKeon, A.; Quach, H.; Briggs, F.B.; Bernstein, A.L.; Schaefer, C.A.; Barcellos, L.F. Seroprevalence of aquaporin-4-igg in a northern california population representative cohort of multiple sclerosis. *JAMA Neurol.* **2014**, *71*, 1433–1436. [CrossRef] [PubMed]

88. Waters, P.; Reindl, M.; Saiz, A.; Schanda, K.; Tuller, F.; Kral, V.; Nytrova, P.; Sobek, O.; Nielsen, H.H.; Barington, T.; et al. Multicentre comparison of a diagnostic assay: Aquaporin-4 antibodies in neuromyelitis optica. *J. Neurol. Neurosurg. Psychiatry* **2016**, *87*, 1005–1015. [CrossRef] [PubMed]

89. Andersson, M.; Alvarez-Cermeno, J.; Bernardi, G.; Cogato, I.; Fredman, P.; Frederiksen, J.; Fredrikson, S.; Gallo, P.; Grimaldi, L.M.; Gronning, M.; et al. Cerebrospinal fluid in the diagnosis of multiple sclerosis: A consensus report. *J. Neurol. Neurosurg. Psychiatry* **1994**, *57*, 897–902. [CrossRef]

90. Jarius, S.; Ruprecht, K.; Wildemann, B.; Kuempfel, T.; Ringelstein, M.; Geis, C.; Kleiter, I.; Kleinschnitz, C.; Berthele, A.; Brettschneider, J.; et al. Contrasting disease patterns in seropositive and seronegative neuromyelitis optica: A multicentre study of 175 patients. *J. Neuroinflamm.* **2012**, *9*, 14. [CrossRef]

91. Kim, S.M.; Kim, S.J.; Lee, H.J.; Kuroda, H.; Palace, J.; Fujihara, K. Differential diagnosis of neuromyelitis optica spectrum disorders. *Ther. Adv. Neurol. Disord.* **2017**, *10*, 265–289. [CrossRef]

92. Flanagan, E.P.; Weinshenker, B.G.; Krecke, K.N.; Lennon, V.A.; Lucchinetti, C.F.; McKeon, A.; Wingerchuk, D.M.; Shuster, E.A.; Jiao, Y.; Horta, E.S.; et al. Short myelitis lesions in aquaporin-4-igg-positive neuromyelitis optica spectrum disorders. *JAMA Neurol.* **2015**, *72*, 81–87. [CrossRef] [PubMed]

93. Pittock, S.J.; Weinshenker, B.G.; Lucchinetti, C.F.; Wingerchuk, D.M.; Corboy, J.R.; Lennon, V.A. Neuromyelitis optica brain lesions localized at sites of high aquaporin 4 expression. *Arch. Neurol.* **2006**, *63*, 964–968. [CrossRef] [PubMed]

94. Matthews, L.; Marasco, R.; Jenkinson, M.; Kuker, W.; Luppe, S.; Leite, M.I.; Giorgio, A.; De Stefano, N.; Robertson, N.; Johansen-Berg, H.; et al. Distinction of seropositive nmo spectrum disorder and ms brain lesion distribution. *Neurology* **2013**, *80*, 1330–1337. [CrossRef] [PubMed]

95. Kim, H.J.; Paul, F.; Lana-Peixoto, M.A.; Tenembaum, S.; Asgari, N.; Palace, J.; Klawiter, E.C.; Sato, D.K.; de Seze, J.; Wuerfel, J.; et al. Mri characteristics of neuromyelitis optica spectrum disorder: An international update. *Neurology* **2015**, *84*, 1165–1173. [CrossRef] [PubMed]

96. Jurynczyk, M.; Tackley, G.; Kong, Y.; Geraldes, R.; Matthews, L.; Woodhall, M.; Waters, P.; Kuker, W.; Craner, M.; Weir, A.; et al. Brain lesion distribution criteria distinguish ms from aqp4-antibody nmosd and mog-antibody disease. *J. Neurol. Neurosurg. Psychiatry* **2017**, *88*, 132–136. [CrossRef]

97. Kira, J.I. Unexpected exacerbations following initiation of disease-modifying drugs in neuromyelitis optica spectrum disorder: Which factor is responsible, anti-aquaporin 4 antibodies, b cells, th1 cells, th2 cells, th17 cells, or others? *Mult. Scler.* **2017**, *23*, 1300–1302. [CrossRef] [PubMed]

98. Kleiter, I.; Gahlen, A.; Borisow, N.; Fischer, K.; Wernecke, K.D.; Wegner, B.; Hellwig, K.; Pache, F.; Ruprecht, K.; Havla, J.; et al. Neuromyelitis optica: Evaluation of 871 attacks and 1,153 treatment courses. *Ann. Neurol.* **2016**, *79*, 206–216. [CrossRef] [PubMed]

99. Weinshenker, B.G. What is the optimal sequence of rescue treatments for attacks of neuromyelitis optica spectrum disorder? *Ann. Neurol.* **2016**, *79*, 204–205. [CrossRef]

100. Wingerchuk, D.M.; Weinshenker, B.G. Neuromyelitis optica. *Curr. Treat. Options Neurol.* **2008**, *10*, 55–66. [CrossRef]

101. Kim, S.H.; Hyun, J.W.; Kim, H.J. Individualized b cell-targeting therapy for neuromyelitis optica spectrum disorder. *Neurochem. Int.* **2018**, in press. [CrossRef]

102. Paul, F.; Murphy, O.; Pardo, S.; Levy, M. Investigational drugs in development to prevent neuromyelitis optica relapses. *Expert Opin. Investig. Drugs* **2018**, *27*, 265–271. [CrossRef] [PubMed]

103. Kelly, R.J.; Hochsmann, B.; Szer, J.; Kulasekararaj, A.; de Guibert, S.; Roth, A.; Weitz, I.C.; Armstrong, E.; Risitano, A.M.; Patriquin, C.J.; et al. Eculizumab in pregnant patients with paroxysmal nocturnal hemoglobinuria. *N. Engl. J. Med.* **2015**, *373*, 1032–1039. [CrossRef] [PubMed]

104. McNamara, L.A.; Topaz, N.; Wang, X.; Hariri, S.; Fox, L.; MacNeil, J.R. High risk for invasive meningococcal disease among patients receiving eculizumab (soliris) despite receipt of meningococcal vaccine. *Am. J. Transplant. Off. J. Am. Soc. Transplant. Am. Soc. Transpl. Surg.* **2017**, *17*, 2481–2484. [CrossRef]

105. Traboulsee, A.; Greenberg, B.; Bennett, J.L.; Szczechowiski, L.; Fox, E.; Shkrobot, S.; Yamamura, T.; Terada, Y.; Kawata, Y.; Melia, A.; et al. A double-blind placebo-controlled study of satralizumab (sa 237), a recycling anti-il-6 receptor monoclonal antibody, as monotherapy for patients witn neuromyelitis optica spectrum disorder (nmosd). In Proceedings of the ECTRIMS, Berlin, Germany, 10–12 Octorber 2018. Poster 1278.

106. Steinman, L.; Bar-Or, A.; Behne, J.M.; Benitez-Ribas, D.; Chin, P.S.; Clare-Salzler, M.; Healey, D.; Kim, J.I.; Kranz, D.M.; Lutterotti, A.; et al. Restoring immune tolerance in neuromyelitis optica: Part i. *Neurol. Neuroimmunol. Neuroinflamm.* **2016**, *3*, e276. [CrossRef] [PubMed]

107. Brunner, C.; Lassmann, H.; Waehneldt, T.V.; Matthieu, J.M.; Linington, C. Differential ultrastructural localization of myelin basic protein, myelin/oligodendroglial glycoprotein, and 2′,3′-cyclic nucleotide 3′-phosphodiesterase in the cns of adult rats. *J. Neurochem.* **1989**, *52*, 296–304. [CrossRef]

108. Pham-Dinh, D.; Mattei, M.G.; Nussbaum, J.L.; Roussel, G.; Pontarotti, P.; Roeckel, N.; Mather, I.H.; Artzt, K.; Lindahl, K.F.; Dautigny, A. Myelin/oligodendrocyte glycoprotein is a member of a subset of the immunoglobulin superfamily encoded within the major histocompatibility complex. *Proc. Natl. Acad. Sci. USA* **1993**, *90*, 7990–7994. [CrossRef] [PubMed]

109. Gardinier, M.V.; Amiguet, P.; Linington, C.; Matthieu, J.M. Myelin/oligodendrocyte glycoprotein is a unique member of the immunoglobulin superfamily. *J. Neurosci. Res.* **1992**, *33*, 177–187. [CrossRef] [PubMed]

110. Berger, T.; Rubner, P.; Schautzer, F.; Egg, R.; Ulmer, H.; Mayringer, I.; Dilitz, E.; Deisenhammer, F.; Reindl, M. Antimyelin antibodies as a predictor of clinically definite multiple sclerosis after a first demyelinating event. *N. Engl. J. Med.* **2003**, *349*, 139–145. [CrossRef] [PubMed]

111. Reindl, M.; Linington, C.; Brehm, U.; Egg, R.; Dilitz, E.; Deisenhammer, F.; Poewe, W.; Berger, T. Antibodies against the myelin oligodendrocyte glycoprotein and the myelin basic protein in multiple sclerosis and other neurological diseases: A comparative study. *Brain J. Neurol.* **1999**, *122 Pt 11*, 2047–2056. [CrossRef]

112. Karni, A.; Bakimer-Kleiner, R.; Abramsky, O.; Ben-Nun, A. Elevated levels of antibody to myelin oligodendrocyte glycoprotein is not specific for patients with multiple sclerosis. *Arch. Neurol.* **1999**, *56*, 311–315. [CrossRef]

113. Markovic, M.; Trajkovic, V.; Drulovic, J.; Mesaros, S.; Stojsavljevic, N.; Dujmovic, I.; Mostarica Stojkovic, M. Antibodies against myelin oligodendrocyte glycoprotein in the cerebrospinal fluid of multiple sclerosis patients. *J. Neurol. Sci.* **2003**, *211*, 67–73. [CrossRef]

114. Gaertner, S.; de Graaf, K.L.; Greve, B.; Weissert, R. Antibodies against glycosylated native mog are elevated in patients with multiple sclerosis. *Neurology* **2004**, *63*, 2381–2383. [CrossRef] [PubMed]

115. Lindert, R.B.; Haase, C.G.; Brehm, U.; Linington, C.; Wekerle, H.; Hohlfeld, R. Multiple sclerosis: B- and t-cell responses to the extracellular domain of the myelin oligodendrocyte glycoprotein. *Brain J. Neurol.* **1999**, *122 Pt 11*, 2089–2100. [CrossRef]

116. Egg, R.; Reindl, M.; Deisenhammer, F.; Linington, C.; Berger, T. Anti-mog and anti-mbp antibody subclasses in multiple sclerosis. *Mult. Scler.* **2001**, *7*, 285–289. [CrossRef] [PubMed]

117. Kuhle, J.; Lindberg, R.L.; Regeniter, A.; Mehling, M.; Hoffmann, F.; Reindl, M.; Berger, T.; Radue, E.W.; Leppert, D.; Kappos, L. Antimyelin antibodies in clinically isolated syndromes correlate with inflammation in mri and csf. *J. Neurol.* **2007**, *254*, 160–168. [CrossRef] [PubMed]

118. Brilot, F.; Dale, R.C.; Selter, R.C.; Grummel, V.; Kalluri, S.R.; Aslam, M.; Busch, V.; Zhou, D.; Cepok, S.; Hemmer, B. Antibodies to native myelin oligodendrocyte glycoprotein in children with inflammatory demyelinating central nervous system disease. *Ann. Neurol.* **2009**, *66*, 833–842. [CrossRef] [PubMed]

119. Kitley, J.; Waters, P.; Woodhall, M.; Leite, M.I.; Murchison, A.; George, J.; Kuker, W.; Chandratre, S.; Vincent, A.; Palace, J. Neuromyelitis optica spectrum disorders with aquaporin-4 and myelin-oligodendrocyte glycoprotein antibodies: A comparative study. *JAMA Neurol.* **2014**, *71*, 276–283. [CrossRef] [PubMed]

120. Ramanathan, S.; Reddel, S.W.; Henderson, A.; Parratt, J.D.; Barnett, M.; Gatt, P.N.; Merheb, V.; Kumaran, R.Y.; Pathmanandavel, K.; Sinmaz, N.; et al. Antibodies to myelin oligodendrocyte glycoprotein in bilateral and recurrent optic neuritis. *Neurol. Neuroimmunol. Neuroinflamm.* **2014**, *1*, e40. [CrossRef]

121. Hoftberger, R.; Sepulveda, M.; Armangue, T.; Blanco, Y.; Rostasy, K.; Calvo, A.C.; Olascoaga, J.; Ramio-Torrenta, L.; Reindl, M.; Benito-Leon, J.; et al. Antibodies to mog and aqp4 in adults with neuromyelitis optica and suspected limited forms of the disease. *Mult. Scler.* **2015**, *21*, 866–874. [CrossRef]

122. Jarius, S.; Kleiter, I.; Ruprecht, K.; Asgari, N.; Pitarokoili, K.; Borisow, N.; Hummert, M.W.; Trebst, C.; Pache, F.; Winkelmann, A.; et al. Mog-igg in nmo and related disorders: A multicenter study of 50 patients. Part 3: Brainstem involvement—Frequency, presentation and outcome. *J. Neuroinflamm.* **2016**, *13*, 281. [CrossRef]

123. Spadaro, M.; Gerdes, L.A.; Krumbholz, M.; Ertl-Wagner, B.; Thaler, F.S.; Schuh, E.; Metz, I.; Blaschek, A.; Dick, A.; Bruck, W.; et al. Autoantibodies to mog in a distinct subgroup of adult multiple sclerosis. *Neurol. Neuroimmunol. Neuroinflamm.* **2016**, *3*, e257. [CrossRef] [PubMed]

124. Ramanathan, S.; Mohammad, S.; Tantsis, E.; Nguyen, T.K.; Merheb, V.; Fung, V.S.C.; White, O.B.; Broadley, S.; Lechner-Scott, J.; Vucic, S.; et al. Clinical course, therapeutic responses and outcomes in relapsing mog antibody-associated demyelination. *J. Neurol. Neurosurg. Psychiatry* **2018**, *89*, 127–137. [CrossRef] [PubMed]

125. Reindl, M.; Di Pauli, F.; Rostasy, K.; Berger, T. The spectrum of mog autoantibody-associated demyelinating diseases. *Nat. Rev. Neurol.* **2013**, *9*, 455–461. [CrossRef] [PubMed]

126. Kerlero de Rosbo, N.; Honegger, P.; Lassmann, H.; Matthieu, J.M. Demyelination induced in aggregating brain cell cultures by a monoclonal antibody against myelin/oligodendrocyte glycoprotein. *J. Neurochem.* **1990**, *55*, 583–587. [CrossRef] [PubMed]

127. Piddlesden, S.J.; Lassmann, H.; Zimprich, F.; Morgan, B.P.; Linington, C. The demyelinating potential of antibodies to myelin oligodendrocyte glycoprotein is related to their ability to fix complement. *Am. J. Pathol.* **1993**, *143*, 555–564. [CrossRef]

128. Bettelli, E.; Baeten, D.; Jager, A.; Sobel, R.A.; Kuchroo, V.K. Myelin oligodendrocyte glycoprotein-specific t and b cells cooperate to induce a devic-like disease in mice. *J. Clin. Investig.* **2006**, *116*, 2393–2402. [CrossRef] [PubMed]

129. Krishnamoorthy, G.; Lassmann, H.; Wekerle, H.; Holz, A. Spontaneous opticospinal encephalomyelitis in a double-transgenic mouse model of autoimmune t cell/b cell cooperation. *J. Clin. Investig.* **2006**, *116*, 2385–2392. [CrossRef]

130. Saadoun, S.; Waters, P.; Owens, G.P.; Bennett, J.L.; Vincent, A.; Papadopoulos, M.C. Neuromyelitis optica mog-igg causes reversible lesions in mouse brain. *Acta Neuropathol. Commun.* **2014**, *2*, 35. [CrossRef]

131. Sato, D.K.; Callegaro, D.; Lana-Peixoto, M.A.; Waters, P.J.; de Haidar Jorge, F.M.; Takahashi, T.; Nakashima, I.; Apostolos-Pereira, S.L.; Talim, N.; Simm, R.F.; et al. Distinction between mog antibody-positive and aqp4 antibody-positive nmo spectrum disorders. *Neurology* **2014**, *82*, 474–481. [CrossRef]

132. Jarius, S.; Ruprecht, K.; Kleiter, I.; Borisow, N.; Asgari, N.; Pitarokoili, K.; Pache, F.; Stich, O.; Beume, L.A.; Hummert, M.W.; et al. Mog-igg in nmo and related disorders: A multicenter study of 50 patients. Part 2: Epidemiology, clinical presentation, radiological and laboratory features, treatment responses, and long-term outcome. *J. Neuroinflamm.* **2016**, *13*, 280. [CrossRef]

133. Jarius, S.; Paul, F.; Aktas, O.; Asgari, N.; Dale, R.C.; de Seze, J.; Franciotta, D.; Fujihara, K.; Jacob, A.; Kim, H.J.; et al. Mog encephalomyelitis: International recommendations on diagnosis and antibody testing. *J. Neuroinflamm.* **2018**, *15*, 134. [CrossRef] [PubMed]

134. Chalmoukou, K.; Alexopoulos, H.; Akrivou, S.; Stathopoulos, P.; Reindl, M.; Dalakas, M.C. Anti-mog antibodies are frequently associated with steroid-sensitive recurrent optic neuritis. *Neurol. Neuroimmunol. Neuroinflamm.* **2015**, *2*, e131. [CrossRef] [PubMed]

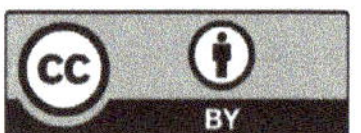

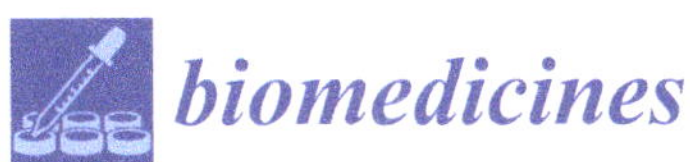

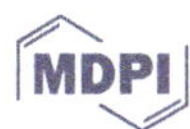

Review

Women's Health: Contemporary Management of MS in Pregnancy and Post-Partum

Kelly Tisovic and Lilyana Amezcua *

Department of Neurology, Keck School of Medicine, University of Southern California, Los Angeles, CA 90033, USA; tisovic@usc.edu
* Correspondence: lamezcua@usc.edu; Tel.: +1-323-442-7589

Received: 12 March 2019; Accepted: 18 April 2019; Published: 19 April 2019

Abstract: Multiple sclerosis (MS) primarily affects women in childbearing age and is associated with an increased risk of adverse post-partum outcomes. Relapses and now fetal exposure to disease modifying treatments in the early phase of pregnancy and thereafter are of concern. Safe and effective contraception is required for women who wish to delay or avoid pregnancy while on disease-modifying treatments. Counseling and planning is essential to assess the risk of both fetal and maternal complications, particularly now in the era of highly efficient and riskier therapies. The purpose of this review is to provide a practical framework using the available data surrounding pregnancy in MS with the goal of optimizing outcomes during this phase in MS.

Keywords: multiple sclerosis; pregnancy; post-partum; treatment

---

1. Introduction

Multiple sclerosis (MS) is an autoimmune disease of the central nervous system (CNS) characterized by inflammation and demyelination with almost 1 million affected in the US [1]. The disease predominantly affects females and often starts in childbearing age [1], making this period a particularly important stage for treatment decisions. Evidence supporting a reduction of disease activity during pregnancy [2] is likely contributing to the recent observation that more women with MS are considering pregnancy [3]. Because most disease-modifying treatments (DMT) are contraindicated during pregnancy, understanding the risk behind discontinuation and early pregnancy exposure is important. In the current era, a neurologist can now be faced with concerns relating to pregnancy, including contraception, fertility, relapses during pregnancy and post-partum, and breastfeeding.

The purpose of this paper is to provide a practical clinical framework to assist physicians in the treatment of women with MS surrounding pregnancy by reviewing the most recent data surrounding pre-conception care, pregnancy and the post-partum phase in MS with the goal of facilitating informed decisions.

2. Methods

We performed a literature search in Pubmed using the search term "multiple sclerosis," with additional search terms of "pregnancy," "breastfeeding," "contraception," "fertility," "disease modifying therapy," "pregnancy outcomes," "guidelines," and "counseling" in the last 10 years. The studies felt to be most relevant for clinical practice were selected for inclusion in this review.

3. Pre-Pregnancy

3.1. Family Planning and Counseling

The rates of pregnancies in MS patients has increased in the US from 2006 to 2014, from 7.91% to 9.47%, while the rate of women without MS decreased from 8.83% to 7.75% over this time [3]. Because there is a high rate of unintentional pregnancies [4] and safety concerns surrounding certain MS DMTs in pregnancy [5], counseling should be performed for all women with MS of reproductive age. In addition, the neurologist should be aware of other related issues such as contraception, fertility, and the low risk of transmission of MS to offspring (2–3% if one parent is affected and about 20% if both parents are affected) [5]. Once a patient has decided to become pregnant, a number of steps can be taken in an effort to achieve optimal outcomes. These are described below, and are outlined in Figure 1.

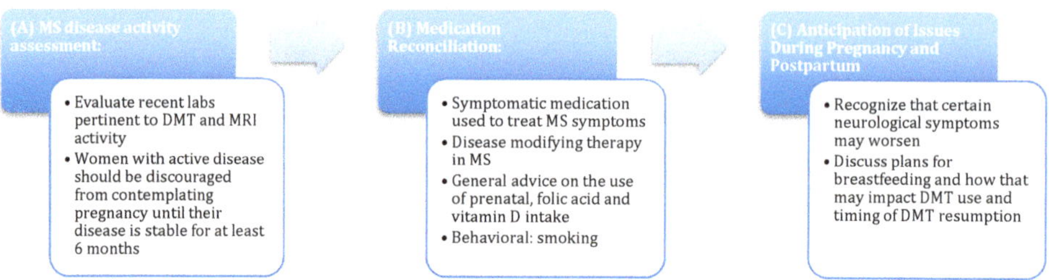

Figure 1. Pre-pregnancy care. (**A**) Multiple sclerosis (MS) disease activity assessment, (**B**) medication reconciliation, (**C**) anticipation of issues during pregnancy and post-partum.

3.1.1. MS Disease Activity Assessment

The current MS disease activity should be evaluated. Appropriate laboratory analysis and MRIs should be included in this assessment. For those with active MS disease activity, postponing attempted conception until disease is stable for at least six months is recommended.

3.1.2. Medication Reconciliation

The current symptomatic MS medications a patient is taking and their safety in pregnancy should be evaluated. This should be performed with the assistance of a patient's obstetrician-gynecologist whenever possible. Current DMT use should be discussed in regards to safety and optimal discontinuation timing, which is typically 5 maximal half lives of the DMT, but this time frame may vary in specific circumstances [6]. Standard prenatal medications including prenatal vitamins and folic acid supplementation is advised [6]. Optimal Vitamin D supplementation is important to maintain throughout pregnancy, as an increased risk of MS was seen in offspring of women with low gestational Vitamin D (25(OH)D) levels of less than 30nmol/L in a Finnish study [7]. Smoking cessation is recommended for all patients, given its impact on both MS disease activity and on pregnancy [6].

3.1.3. Anticipation of Issues Encountered during Pregnancy and Post-partum

Physicians should discuss the potential for MS symptoms to worsen or for new MS symptoms to appear, especially during the less-protective phases of pregnancy and especially in patients with highly active disease or on DMTs with risk for rebound activity. Plans regarding breastfeeding should also be discussed pre-conception, as this will affect the timing of DMT resumption.

3.2. Oral Contraceptives and Multiple Sclerosis (MS) Disease Activity

Estrogen has known anti-inflammatory properties and has shown to be neuroprotective in preclinical studies [8]. The reduction in disease activity observed during pregnancy is thought to be related to high levels of estriol, especially in the third trimester [9]. In experimental autoimmune encephalomyelitis (EAE) models, administration of estriol improved EAE, which correlated with a decrease in the number of CNS inflammatory cells [8]. However, retrospective and prospective studies have reported mixed results regarding oral contraceptive (OC) use and MS risk [10–12] and have reported a positive influence on relapse rates [13]. While Hellwig et al. found that OC use was associated with a slightly increased risk of MS/clinically isolated syndrome (CIS) (adjusted odds ratio

(OR) = 1.52, 95% CI = 1.21–1.91; $p < 0.001$ [12], the risk did not change with duration of OC use, suggesting non-causal association. Other studies have supported a positive effect. Rejali et al. found a statistically significant relationship between history of OC use (OR = 0.492, p = 0.002) and MS risk and in the duration of OC use (OR = 0.881, p = 0.008) and MS risk [11]. Holmqvist et al. found the mean age of MS onset was significantly higher in patients with OC use prior to MS onset than those without OC use (26 years old vs. 19 years old, $p < 0.001$). Additionally, age of MS onset increased with increasing time of OC use prior to MS onset [10]. Bove et al. evaluated effects of past-, current- or never-OC use in women with new onset relapsing remitting multiple sclerosis (RRMS) or CIS started on a first-line injectable disease-modifying therapy and found that past OC users had a statistically significant lower annualized relapse rate (ARR) compared to never OC users (Relative Risk (RR) = 0.64, p = 0.031) and that current OC users had a non-statistically significant lower ARR compared to never OC users (RR = 0.97, p = 0.91) [13].

The anti-inflammatory effects of estradiol in combination with injectable MS therapies have been demonstrated in preliminary studies [9,14]. Pozzilli et al. combined low-dose and high-dose oral contraceptives with interferon beta and evaluated disease activity via cumulative number of combined unique active (CUA) lesions on magnetic resonance imagining (MRI) at 96 weeks. There was a 26.5% (p = 0.04) reduction in CUA lesions in the high dose OC group compared to interferon beta alone and a non-significant reduction in the low dose OC group compared to interferon beta alone [14]. Voskuhl et al. published a randomized, double-blind, placebo controlled phase 2 trial to assess the safety and efficacy of estriol and progesterone in combination to glatiramer acetate versus glatiramer acetate alone using a primary endpoint of annualized confirmed relapse rate at 24 months, and using a significance level of p = 0.01. Confirmed relapse rate was 0.25 (95% CI 0.17–0.37) relapses per year in the estriol treated group compared to 0.37 (95% CI 0.25–0.53) relapses per year in the placebo group with an adjusted rate ratio of 0.63 (95% CI 0.37–1.05, p = 0.077) [9]. Larger studies with longer treatment times are needed to better evaluate the effect of OC treatment and to help better stratify the risk-benefit of long term estrogen use.

Clinical considerations: reliable contraception is recommended for patients taking DMT. DMT-specific recommendations for contraceptive use are included in Table 1 [15–20], if provided specifically in the prescribing recommendations. Beyond the need for pregnancy protection while using DMT, oral contraceptive use is considered safe in MS [13], and potential additional benefits on disease activity may be seen with oral contraceptive use in combination with platform injectable therapy [9,14].

Table 1. Summary of prescribing contraception recommendations for MS disease-modifying treatments (DMTs).

Disease Modifying Treatment (DMT)	Prescribing Contraception Recommendations *
Interferon beta	N/A
Glatiramer acetate	N/A
Fingolimod	Effective contraception during treatment and two months following therapy [15]
Dimethyl fumarate	N/A
Teriflunomide	Effective contraception during treatment and until plasma concentrations of teriflunomide are less than 0.02 mg/L [16]

Table 1. *Cont.*

Disease Modifying Treatment (DMT)	Prescribing Contraception Recommendations *
Natalizumab	N/A
Alemtuzumab	Effective contraceptive measures during treatment and for 4 months following that course of treatment [17]
Ocrelizumab	Effective contraception during therapy and for 6 months after the last infusion [18]
Mitoxantrone	Women should not become pregnant during therapy [19]
Cyclophosphamide **	Effective contraception during therapy and for up to 1 year after completion of treatment [20]

* Contraception recommendations included if provided in the prescribing label. ** Not Food and Drug Administration (FDA) approved for use in MS.

3.3. Fertility

3.3.1. Effects of MS on Fertility

There are multiple observational studies supporting the argument that fertility may be influenced by MS [21–25]. An Italian study found that women with MS are more frequently childless compared to the general population, with reported rates of 22% vs. 13%, respectively [21]. However, it is unclear if childlessness is due to behavioral factors such as disability, fear or beliefs about caring for a newborn child or transmitting MS to her offspring, or actually a disease-related pathology [26]. Another important factor impacting fertility in MS patients includes sexual dysfunction, which is very common, reported in 30–70% of MS patients [26] and is beyond the scope of this paper.

Reassuringly, an observational study in a French cohort evaluated fecundity, defined as the time to become pregnant, in MS patients both before and after MS onset [22]. No differences in the time to conception prior to or after MS disease onset were found (on average <1 year). However, despite their normal fecundity, the mean number of children per women with MS was less than in the general French population (1.37 versus 1.99, respectively) [22]. It is important to note that infertility in Western populations is not uncommon, estimated at 10–20%, and because MS occurs at a fertile age, it is possible that infertility is not actually MS mediated [27]. Nevertheless, assisted reproductive techniques (ART) have been reported to be more common in women with MS [23].

Other studies have focused on evaluating hormonal differences, where higher levels of prolactin, luteinizing hormone (LH), and follicle-stimulating hormone (FSH) and lower levels of estrogen have been reported among MS women [24]. Elevated FSH in the early follicular phase is an indicator of low ovarian reserve [25]. Another marker of low ovarian reserve, Anti-Mullerian hormone (AMH), has been found to be decreased in reproductive-aged women with other autoimmune diseases and does not fluctuate with menstrual cycles as FSH and LH levels do. To better understand ovarian reserve in women with MS, serum AMH levels were examined in 76 RRMS patients and in 58 healthy controls and found serum AMH levels to be significantly lower in patients with RRMS than in healthy controls, and a higher proportion of RRMS patients showed very low AMH levels [25]. However, in a follow up study, no significant differences in AMH levels were found [28] indicating that larger studies are needed to better understand if lower ovarian reserve is found in reproductive-aged women with MS. Thus, the ability to conceive may be influenced by various factors which makes fertility a concern for many women affected with MS.

If a woman with MS does suffer from infertility, ART should be considered with caution. Gonadotropin-releasing hormone (GnRH) agonists and antagonists are used to suppress the influence of the hypothalamic-pituitary gland axis, preventing an LH surge and thus spontaneous ovulation. Subsequent ovarian hyperstimulation is accomplished by administration of gonadotropins. Following stimulation, controlled ovulation is accomplished by human choriongonadotropin (hCG), and administration of progesterone to support the luteal phase. Fertilization is completed by intrauterine insemination, in vitro fertilization, or intracytoplasmatic sperm injection [27].

There are no randomized control trials to evaluate the safety or changes in relapse rate in MS patients who are treated with ART. Despite the clinical improvements seen with the use of GnRH agonists in EAE models [29], their use in humans with MS have shown opposite effects [27]. ART therapy in MS patients may cause increased disease activity, and patients who plan to pursue these therapies should be counseled about this risk sufficiently. Hellwig et al. published a review of five small studies evaluating ART use in MS patients using various reproductive techniques. This collection of studies demonstrated an increase in relapse rate following unsuccessful ART and increased MRI activity. Downregulation of pituitary GnRH receptors via GnRH agonists might account for this increased relapse rate. Additional theories behind worsening MS activity following ART include discontinuation of DMT, stress related to infertility, rapidly changing hormone levels inducing pro-inflammatory changes, and ART-mediated increases in immune cell movement across the blood-brain-barrier via induction of interleukin-8 (IL-8), vascular endothelial growth factor (VEGF), and CXC chemokine ligand 12 (CXCL-12) [27].

3.3.2. Effects of Disease-Modifying Treatments (DMTs) on Fertility

In evaluating the potential influence of DMT use on fertility, information on humans is currently scarce. Table 2 summarizes reported effects of DMTs on fertility with special concerns to the following DMTs: interferon beta [30], natalizumab [31], alemtuzumab [17], mitoxantrone [31], and cyclophosphamide [31]. An additional concern exists for autologous stem cell transplant in combination with high-dose chemotherapy, which is an experimental MS treatment and may decrease fertility [32].

Table 2. Summary of reported MS DMT effects on fertility.

DMT	Fertility
Interferon beta	Reduced fertility in animals; no information in humans [30]
Glatiramer acetate	No effects
Fingolimod	No effects
Dimethyl Fumarate	No effects
Teriflunomide	No effects
Natalizumab	Reduced fertility in animals; no information in humans [31]
Alemtuzumab	Reduced fertility in animals; no information in humans [17]
Ocrelizumab	No effects
Mitoxantrone	Amenorrhea and transient azoospermia have been reported [31]
Cyclophosphamide *	Amenorrhea and transient azoospermia have been reported [31]

* Not FDA approved for the treatment of MS.

Clinical considerations: because it is prudent to optimize a patient's chance of conception off of DMT, strategies such as substituting barrier methods for OC, waiting for ovulation cycles to resume prior to discontinuing DMT, and referrals for evaluation of fertility if pregnancy does not result after 6 months of attempt should be considered [6].

4. Pregnancy

4.1. Pregnancy and the Risk of MS

There are multiple studies supporting the argument that pregnancy can be protective. Both a reduction in MS risk [10,11,33–35] and a delay in MS onset [10] has been reported. For example, Runmarker et al. found a higher risk of MS in nulliparous women compared to parous women, suggesting that pregnancy can be protective. This risk appeared to increase with older age [35]. Magyari et al. reported a 46% reduced risk of MS in Danish women during the five years following childbirth [33], while Ponsonby et al. found that a higher parity and a higher number of offspring was associated with reduced risk of a first clinical demyelinating event, and that each pregnancy conferred a decreased risk [34]. Similarly, in a case-controlled study, Rejali et al. found a significant relationship between the number of pregnancies and reduced risk of MS (OR = 0.586, 95% CI = 0.461–0.745), suggesting that higher parity also influences MS risk [11]. Holmqvist et al. found that pregnancy significantly delayed the mean age at MS onset in women who had given birth prior to disease onset. This increase in age was seen for each child born to a woman prior to MS onset, suggesting a protective effect of each pregnancy [10] which could be related to long-term epigenetic effects [36].

4.2. Pregnancy and Risk of Disease Activity

During pregnancy, the female's immune system is reported to be more immunotolerant due to a shift in the ratio of T helper 1 and 2 cells, mediated by high levels of estrogens, especially estradiol, in addition to other important hormones including progesterone and androgens [6,10]. Some of these changes support the clinical observation of decrease relapses during pregnancy and likely also support the return of disease activity observed in months post-partum.

One of the pivotal studies to support this was reported in 1998, where Confravreux et al. prospectively reported on the natural history of MS in pregnancy. A reduction in ARR during pregnancy of 70%, especially during the third trimester, compared with the year prior to pregnancy was reported and was followed by an increase in ARR during three months post-partum. The relapse rate subsequently returned to the pre-partum relapse rate [37]. Contrary to Poser's report [38], there was no negative effect of pregnancy on disability progression [37]. In 2004, a two-year post-partum follow up by Vukusic et al. noted that the risk of post-partum relapse was correlated to the number of relapses in the year prior to pregnancy, in the number of relapses during pregnancy, and in those with a higher Expanded Disability Status Scale (EDSS) at baseline [39]. Other studies [40,41] published worldwide have found similar trends in the pattern of relapse occurrence during pregnancy and post-partum which supports that the observations are more likely to be return of activity.

Clinical considerations: because there is the theoretical risk for relapses to occur in the early phases of pregnancy, it is important to provide a recommendation in the clinical setting concerning treatment. This risk of early relapses has become more apparent in patients who are becoming pregnant while on fingolimod and natalizumab.

Previous studies have reported on treatment effects with interferon beta or glatiramer acetate on relapse rates but little information is available concerning second-line therapies that are only more recently available and are not typically used during pregnancy due to safety concerns [42]. There is data to support the argument that the older treatments, such as glatiramer acetate or interferon beta had no effect [43]. There have been reports of rebound with newer and higher efficacy DMT with discontinuation of therapy prior to or during pregnancy [42]. A cross-sectional study of 99 pregnancies with nearly 90% of women treated with DMTs during the year prior to pregnancy showed a higher relapse occurrence during pregnancy than previously reported [42]. A four-fold increase in relapses during pregnancy occurred, mostly during the first and third trimesters. Relapses were primarily seen in patients treated with natalizumab and fingolimod before pregnancy. Longer DMT washout periods before pregnancy resulted in a higher probability of relapse (OR 3.9, 95% CI 1.4–10.6, p = 0.008), and were seen in patients previously treated with natalizumab and fingolimod who relapsed during the first trimester of pregnancy [42].

It is important to recognize that there are certain DMT's that can place a woman at risk for relapse prior to or during pregnancy. Discontinuing fingolimod has been reported to increase risk of rebound disease and a suggested washout of 2 months is recommended [15]. Women taking fingolimod should be counseled regarding the risk of rebound activity, and switching to a safer medication such as glatiramer acetate or interferon beta should be considered, based on newer data from postmarking studies [42,44–46]. Patients taking natalizumab may also be at increased risk of rebound disease activity and switching to glatiramer acetate or interferon beta may be similarly considered [42,46]. For women on natalizumab with highly active disease, Thone et al. [45] recommends a consideration of either shortening the washout period, continuing natalizumab until conception, or continuing natalizumab during pregnancy with extended interval dosing every 6 weeks through gestation week 30, with a pediatric check upon delivery for hematologic abnormalities. This should be done on a case-by-case basis and after a discussion about the risks with each patient [45]. Continuation of natalizumab during the entire pregnancy has also been suggested in those patients with high disease activity who are at high risk of rebound [47]. However, a full discussion between patient and physician needs to occur highlighting the potential risk of fetal hematologic abnormalities reported with natalizumab use [46,47]. If exposed, we recommend that women be under the care of a high-risk obstetrician and consider delivering in a hospital where a pediatrician is accessible to assess the newborn for potential complications [47]. Other considerations for these patients include discontinuation of DMT followed by empiric treatment with prophylactic monthly high-dose corticosteroids during attempted conception after a negative pregnancy test [6], switching treatment to alemtuzumab and waiting 4 months before attempted conception [17], or switching treatment to B-cell therapy and waiting 6 months before attempted conception [18]. These studies are part of the recommendations found in the joint European Committee of Treatment and Research in Multiple Sclerosis (ECTRIMS) and European Academy of Neurology (EAN) guidelines for treatment of women with MS who wish to become pregnant [48] (Table 3).

Table 3. European Committee of Treatment and Research in Multiple Sclerosis (ECTRIMS)/European Academy of Neurology (EAN) Guidelines for management of DMT in women with MS in pregnancy.

Only Glatiramer Acetate 20 mg/mL is Approved for Use during Pregnancy (Consensus) [48].
For women who are at risk of disease reactivation and planning pregnancy:
○ Consider switching the glatiramer acetate or interferon beta until conception is confirmed (weak) [48].   ○ For specific cases in women with active disease, consider continuing treatment throughout pregnancy (weak) [48].
Delaying pregnancy is advised for women with persistent, highly active disease.
○ Women who become pregnant unintentionally or despite recommendation, treatment with natalizumab during pregnancy can be considered after counseling about the potential consequences (weak) [48].   ○ For planned pregnancies with very active disease, alemtuzumab can be considered, but treatment must be followed by 4 months of effective contraception (weak) [48].

Relapses during pregnancy should have clinical and radiologic assessments when indicated. A brain MRI without contrast does not appear to be harmful to the fetus [49]. Treatment with prednisone, prednisolone, or methylprednisolone can be used to shorten symptom duration, as these medications are metabolized by the placenta by about 90% [50]. However, their use in the first trimester of pregnancy is considered teratogenic and an increased risk of cleft lip or palate has been reported [51].

4.3. Maternal and Delivery Complications

The effect of MS on pregnancy outcomes in the US and throughout the world has been previously described, with conflicting results [40,41,52–55]. A meta-analysis cited a relatively higher prevalence of abortions, cesarean sections, prematurity, and low birth weight in women with MS. However, due to the high heterogeneity between the studies, they felt the effects of regional, legal, and cultural differences could have hyper-inflated the abortion and cesarean section rates [40]. Studies using claims databases have mixed reports. A higher risk of both antenatal [53] or post-partum [52] hospitalization of mothers with MS were reported in two studies, whereas other studies found no increased risk [3,54,55]. Reports of maternal infections such as urinary tract infections (UTI) [54] and sexually transmitted diseases (STD) [3], cesarean section rates [53,54] and induction of labor [54] were increased in women with MS compared to controls. Risk of premature labor [3] and preterm delivery [55] have also been reported.

The conflicting evidence regarding pregnancy outcomes in women with MS may stem from ascertainment bias and other confounding variables. Both older age and an increased prevalence of co-morbidities in women with MS can independently affect pregnancy outcomes. There are several potential issues with using claims based databases, where coding and billing might simply reflect increased health care use in MS patients due to increased caution by their providers [41], where different databases capture differing MS subpopulations based on the health insurance included in that database, where reliance on hospital discharge summaries for identification of MS patients may not capture all patients if they are asymptomatic at the time of delivery and no code for MS is entered, and where a lack of vital background information including MS disease duration, disability, prior IV corticosteroid use during pregnancy, other medications used during pregnancy, and prior pregnancy outcomes limit interpretation of the results [3,52–55].

There is still much to be learned about MS and whether it is associated with adverse pregnancy outcomes. Well-designed analyses not reliant on recall, standardized and more detailed data collection, and increased participation in pregnancy registries are all vital to our future knowledge [3].

4.4. Fetal and Neonatal Complications

A majority of reported data regarding fetal and neonatal outcomes in women with MS has been reassuring [40,52–55]. Rates of malformations and neonatal deaths have been reported as low as 1.13–6.25%, which is similar to US reported rates [40,56]. Several US claims based studies have evaluated the rate of fetal malformations in newborns born to mothers with and without MS, and most [52–55], but not all [3], have not demonstrated an increased risk. Houtchens et al. alone found that a higher proportion of patients with MS than without MS had claims for acquired fetal damage (27.8% vs. 23.5% $p = 0.002$) and congenital fetal malformations (13.2% vs. 10.3% $p = 0.004$) [3]. Importantly, in this study, both MS and control groups had a higher rate of labor and delivery complications than reported in the general population [56]. Additional considerations include the fact that MS patients were older, were more likely to have other chronic medications conditions, and due to the study design, other pertinent health and pregnancy information was not available. Thus, independent predictors of adverse pregnancy outcomes were present, but were not able to be appropriately interpreted, again highlighting the need for additional information which could not be ascertained from the data [3,56].

Clinical considerations: none of the current US Food and Drug Administration (FDA) approved DMTs used to treat MS are specifically approved for women who are trying to conceive, who are currently pregnant, or who are breastfeeding. There are variations in DMT washout prior to pregnancy [15–19,57,58] which are summarized in Table 4 along with their associated FDA pregnancy categorization [46,59]. The recommendations differ in other countries from those in the US, especially for glatiramer acetate [48].

Table 4. FDA pregnancy categories and recommended washout periods for MS DMTs.

DMT	FDA Pregnancy Category	Recommended Washout Period
Interferon beta	Category C [46]	0–1 Menstrual cycles [57,58]
Glatiramer acetate	Category B [46]	0–1 Menstrual cycles [57,58]
Fingolimod	Category C [46]	2 Menstrual cycles [15]
Dimethyl Fumarate	Category C [46]	0–1 Menstrual cycles [57,58]
Teriflunomide	Category X [46]	Either: (1) Wait 24 Menstrual cycles, OR (2) Perform accelerated elimination until plasma concentration <0.02 mg/dL [16]

Table 4. *Cont.*

DMT	FDA Pregnancy Category	Recommended Washout Period
Natalizumab *	Category C [46]	1–3 Menstrual cycles [58]
Alemtuzumab	Category C [46]	4 Menstrual cycles [17]
Ocrelizumab	N/A	6 Menstrual cycles [18]
Mitoxantrone	Category D [46]	6 Menstrual cycles [19]

* Natalizumab: Case by case decision should be made in females with highly active disease or with history of severe natalizumab withdrawal relapse after full discussion of the risks and benefits with the patient.

A summary of prescribing recommendations in pregnancy can be found in the labels of MS DMTs, including a summary of their safety, lactation warnings, and contraception guidelines. Most FDA approved MS DMTs have established pregnancy registries, and providers should encourage patients with DMT exposures during pregnancy to enroll. Interestingly, a recent retrospective study using an international MS pregnancy database found an increasing percentage of MS patients becoming pregnant on DMTs, rising from 27% in 2006 to 62% in 2016, with a median exposure duration of one month. The proportion of pre-term births or miscarriages compared to the unexposed pregnancies were no different [60]. Updated information on the safety of DMT use during pregnancy based from the FDA label, registry data and other sources may be found in the Supplementary Materials, Table S1 [15–19,30,31,46,57,61–78].

5. Post-Partum

5.1. Post-Partum and the Risk of Disease Activity

Several studies have down that the post-partum period is a time of risk for increased disease activity [37,41,42]. In a cross-sectional study of 512 patients, Poser et al. found that women at six months post-partum were at increased risk of developing MS, disability progression, and of experiencing a higher number of relapses compared with during pregnancy [38]. Pregnancy may also increase the risk of conversion from radiologically isolated syndrome (RIS) to CIS [79]. In a small French cohort of 60 women with RIS, those who became pregnant developed a first neurologic event earlier or had more active MRI lesions than those who did not become pregnant [79]. Due to its small sample size and the rarity of RIS, larger studies are needed to better understand the influence of pregnancy on the risk of conversion from RIS to CIS.

As none of the current DMTs are FDA-approved for use during breastfeeding, it is important to discuss the appropriate time to resume DMT. To balance the risk of relapse to the mother with the benefit of breastfeeding to the baby in considering resuming DMT, the physician must consider a patient's likelihood to experience post-partum disease activity. Research supports that there is a relationship between post-partum relapse rates and prior disease activity the year before pregnancy [39]. The highest predictor of post-partum relapse was a higher annualized relapse rate in the 2 years prior to pregnancy [80]. For women at increased risk of relapse, a discussion regarding benefits of resuming DMT versus the risks of relapse with breastfeeding should occur. Women who chose to forego breastfeeding to resume DMT or who simply do not wish to breastfeed should resume DMT in 7–10 days post-partum [45].

5.2. Breastfeeding and Disease Activity

Breastfeeding has numerous health benefits to both the mother and infant. Exclusive breastfeeding for six months should be encouraged if possible, as recommended by the World Health Organization [81]. The reported effects of breastfeeding on post-partum relapse rate in MS have varied [6,37,82–84] and generally the patient is advised to make an informed decision.

Several prospective studies have found a benefit with breastfeeding and in particular exclusive breastfeeding on post-partum relapse rates [37,82,83] (Table 5). Exclusive breastfeeding is thought to provoke lactational amenorrhea and ovarian suppression, which may be important in the pathophysiology behind the observed benefit in MS [85]. In a small prospective study, women who exclusively breastfed were five times less likely to experience a relapse in the year following pregnancy compared to those who did not and exclusive breastfeeding was associated with protracted lactational amenorrhea. This study was limited by its small size, but showed a consistent benefit of exclusive breastfeeding when women with more highly active disease, a source of possible confounding, were excluded from analysis [82]. A meta-analysis of the effects of breastfeeding on relapse rate reported that women who breastfed were half as likely to have a post-partum relapse than women who did not [84]. Limitations included high heterogeneity between studies, exclusivity of breastfeeding was not always defined or was simplistically defined, and recall bias in the included retrospective studies. A larger prospective study was conducted using the German MS and Pregnancy Registry that enrolled pregnant MS women based on their intention to exclusively or non-exclusively breastfeed. A lower risk of relapse in the six months post-partum was seen in women who chose to breastfeed exclusively compared to those who did not, and compared to those who resumed DMT within 30 days [83].

Table 5. Annualized relapse rates (ARR) in breastfeeding.

Study	Breastfeeding	ARR Pre-Pregnancy	ARR During Pregnancy	ARR Post Partum
Confavreux et al. [37]	Yes	0.6	0.3	1–3 months: 1.2 4–6 months: 0.9
	No	0.8	0.5	1–3 months: 1.3 4–6 months: 1.0
Hellwig et al. [83]	Exclusive	N/A	0.22	0.48
	Non-Exclusive	N/A	0.36	0.77
Langer-Gould et al. [82]	Exclusive	0.57	0.19	0.36
	Non-Exclusive	0.83	0.18	0.87

A recent study examined the effects of breastfeeding on the risk of MS in the nursing mother. The authors hypothesized that breast-feeding leads to anovulation, which confers decreased MS risk. Interestingly, in this matched case-control study, a cumulative duration of breastfeeding for ≥ 15 months was associated with a reduced risk of developing MS (adjusted OR 0.47, 95% CI 0.28–0.77; $p = 0.003$) compared to <4 months of breastfeeding, concluding that longer breastfeeding confers protection of developing MS to the nursing mother. Interestingly, the authors did not find an association between ovulatory years and MS risk. Limitations of this study included recall bias, the lack of hypothesized association of ovulatory years with MS risk, and lack of information as to why women chose not to breastfeed [86]. The effect of breastfeeding on MS risk requires further evaluation.

Clinical considerations: when resuming DMT, it is important to consider that the patients with more highly active disease pre-pregnancy and/or during pregnancy are more likely to chose not to breastfeed and to resume DMT post-partum and thus confound the above results [6], although the authors did account for this as best they could [82,83]. A larger, prospective study evaluating the effects of exclusive breastfeeding on post-partum relapse is needed. At the least, breastfeeding appears to be safe in women with MS, and exclusive breastfeeding may be beneficial until food supplementation is introduced into the infant's diet. For women who wish to breastfeed, the data support greater benefit from exclusive and without supplementation.

In patients who wish to breastfeed but are at a high risk of post-partum relapse, a protective strategy is using monthly corticosteroids [87]. Although only about 10% of an infant's endogenous corticosteroid production is ingested from breast milk, the long-term risks are unknown. Thus, a four-hour period of delayed breastfeeding, or "pumping and dumping," is recommended [88]. For monitoring purposes, routine screening MRI with gadolinium after delivery, again followed by delayed breastfeeding for 24 h, in breastfeeding mothers is recommended to help identify subclinical MS activity, and those who may need DMT earlier than anticipated [6].

5.3. Newborn Care

Women with MS are faced with balancing their own needs with those of their newborn child during the post-partum period. Sleep management, rehabilitation (often in the form of pelvic floor exercises), and resumption of DMT are important maternal considerations. Family or paid assistance should be encouraged. Women should also be screened for post-partum depression due to its high overall prevalence in the population, with the strongest risk factor of having baseline depression [5].

6. Conclusions

Women with MS are becoming pregnant with increasing rates, while newer and more effective DMTs are used to treat MS patients. Knowledge about safe and effective DMT use and the pattern of disease activity around pregnancy is vital. Decisions regarding breastfeeding and DMT resumption post-partum are shared between patient and physician, but with appropriate discussion about risks and benefits. Special consideration should be taken with women who have highly active disease, or who take medications that might cause rebound disease activity. Generally speaking, women should feel reassured and confident about the management of their MS in the reproductive years.

Supplementary Materials: The following are available online at http://www.mdpi.com/2227-9059/7/2/32/s1: Table S1: Updated information on the safety of DMT use during pregnancy.

Funding: This research received no external funding.

Acknowledgments: Tisovic's Multiple Sclerosis Clinical Care Physician Fellowship is funded by the National Multiple Sclerosis Society.

Conflicts of Interest: Amezcua has received personal compensation for consulting, serving on a scientific advisory board, or other activities with Genzyme and Serono. She has clinical trial research funding from Medday.

References

1. Wallin, M.T.; Culpepper, W.J.; Campbell, J.D.; Nelson, L.M.; Langer-Gould, A.; Marrie, R.A.; Cutter, G.R.; Kaye, W.E.; Wagner, L.; Tremlett, H.; et al. The prevalence of MS in the United States: A population-based estimate using health claims data. *Neurology* **2019**, *92*, e1029–e1040. [CrossRef] [PubMed]
2. D'Hooghe, M.B.; Nagels, G.; Bissay, V.; De Keyser, J. Modifiable factors influencing relapses and disability in multiple sclerosis. *Mult. Scler.* **2010**, *16*, 773–785. [CrossRef]
3. Houtchens, M.K.; Edwards, N.C.; Schneider, G.; Stern, K.; Phillips, A.L. Pregnancy rates and outcomes in women with and without MS in the United States. *Neurology* **2018**, *91*, e1559–e1569. [CrossRef] [PubMed]
4. Finer, L.B.; Zolna, M.R. Unintended pregnancy in the United States: Incidence and disparities, 2006. *Contraception* **2011**, *84*, 478–485. [CrossRef]
5. Bove, R.; Alwan, S.; Friedman, J.M.; Hellwig, K.; Houtchens, M.; Koren, G.; Lu, E.; McElrath, T.F.; Smyth, P.; Tremlett, H.; et al. Management of multiple sclerosis during pregnancy and the reproductive years: A systematic review. *Obstet. Gynecol.* **2014**, *124*, 1157–1168. [CrossRef]
6. Rankin, K.; Bove, R. Caring for Women with Multiple Sclerosis Across the Lifespan. *Curr. Neurol. Neurosci. Rep.* **2018**, *18*, 36. [CrossRef] [PubMed]
7. Munger, K.L.; Aivo, J.; Hongell, K.; Soilu-Hanninen, M.; Surcel, H.M.; Ascherio, A. Vitamin D Status During Pregnancy and Risk of Multiple Sclerosis in Offspring of Women in the Finnish Maternity Cohort. *JAMA Neurol.* **2016**, *73*, 515–519. [CrossRef]
8. Spence, R.D.; Voskuhl, R.R. Neuroprotective effects of estrogens and androgens in CNS inflammation and neurodegeneration. *Front. Neuroendocrinol.* **2012**, *33*, 105–115. [CrossRef]
9. Voskuhl, R.R.; Wang, H.; Wu, T.C.; Sicotte, N.L.; Nakamura, K.; Kurth, F.; Itoh, N.; Bardens, J.; Bernard, J.T.; Corboy, J.R.; et al. Estriol combined with glatiramer acetate for women with relapsing-remitting multiple sclerosis: A randomised, placebo-controlled, phase 2 trial. *Lancet Neurol.* **2016**, *15*, 35–46. [CrossRef]

10. Holmqvist, P.; Hammar, M.; Landtblom, A.M.; Brynhildsen, J. Age at onset of multiple sclerosis is correlated to use of combined oral contraceptives and childbirth before diagnosis. *Fertil. Steril.* **2010**, *94*, 2835–2837. [CrossRef] [PubMed]

11. Rejali, M.; Hosseini, S.M.; Kazemi Tabaee, M.S.; Etemadifar, M. Assessing the Risk Factors for Multiple Sclerosis in Women of Reproductive Age Suffering the Disease in Isfahan Province. *Int. J. Prev. Med.* **2016**, *7*, 58. [CrossRef] [PubMed]

12. Hellwig, K.; Chen, L.H.; Stancyzk, F.Z.; Langer-Gould, A.M. Oral Contraceptives and Multiple Sclerosis/Clinically Isolated Syndrome Susceptibility. *PLoS ONE* **2016**, *11*, e0149094. [CrossRef]

13. Bove, R.; Rankin, K.; Chua, A.S.; Saraceno, T.; Sattarnezhad, N.; Greeke, E.; Stuart, F.; LaRussa, A.; Glanz, B.I.; Chitnis, T. Oral contraceptives and MS disease activity in a contemporary real-world cohort. *Mult. Scler.* **2018**, *24*, 227–230. [CrossRef] [PubMed]

14. Pozzilli, C.; De Giglio, L.; Barletta, V.T.; Marinelli, F.; Angelis, F.D.; Gallo, V.; Pagano, V.A.; Marini, S.; Piattella, M.C.; Tomassini, V.; et al. Oral contraceptives combined with interferon beta in multiple sclerosis. *Neurol. Neuroimmunol. Neuroinflamm.* **2015**, *2*, e120. [CrossRef] [PubMed]

15. Gilenya (Fingolimod) Capsules, for Oral Use. Highlights of Prescribing Information. Available online: https://www.pharma.us.novartis.com/sites/www.pharma.us.novartis.com/files/gilenya.pdf (accessed on 29 January 2019).

16. Aubagio (Teriflunomide) Tablets, for Oral Use. Highlights of Prescribing Information. Available online: http://products.sanofi.us/aubagio/aubagio.pdf (accessed on 28 January 2019).

17. Lemtrada (Alemtuzumab) Injection, for Intravenous Use. Highlights of Prescribing Information. Available online: http://products.sanofi.us/lemtrada/lemtrada.pdf?s_mcid=ps-LP-google-BRsitelink-pi (accessed on 28 January 2019).

18. Ocrevus (Ocrelizumab) Injection, for Intravenous Use. Highlights of Prescribing Information. Available online: https://www.gene.com/download/pdf/ocrevus_prescribing.pdf (accessed on 29 January 2019).

19. Novantrone, Mitoxantrone for Injection Concentrate. Available online: https://www.accessdata.fda.gov/drugsatfda_docs/label/2009/019297s030s031lbl.pdf (accessed on 29 January 2019).

20. yclophosphamide Injection, for Intravenous Use. Cyclophosphamide Tablets, for Oral Use. Highlights of prescribing information. Available online: https://www.accessdata.fda.gov/drugsatfda_docs/label/2013/012141s090,012142s112lbl.pdf (accessed on 29 January 2019).

21. Ferraro, D.; Simone, A.M.; Adani, G.; Vitetta, F.; Mauri, C.; Strumia, S.; Senesi, C.; Curti, E.; Baldi, E.; Santangelo, M.; et al. Definitive childlessness in women with multiple sclerosis: A multicenter study. *Neurol Sci* **2017**, *38*, 1453–1459. [CrossRef]

22. Roux, T.; Courtillot, C.; Debs, R.; Touraine, P.; Lubetzki, C.; Papeix, C. Fecundity in women with multiple sclerosis: An observational mono-centric study. *J. Neurol* **2015**, *262*, 957–960. [CrossRef] [PubMed]

23. Jalkanen, A.; Alanen, A.; Airas, L. Pregnancy outcome in women with multiple sclerosis: Results from a prospective nationwide study in Finland. *Mult. Scler.* **2010**, *16*, 950–955. [CrossRef]

24. Grinsted, L.; Heltberg, A.; Hagen, C.; Djursing, H. Serum sex hormone and gonadotropin concentrations in premenopausal women with multiple sclerosis. *J. Intern. Med.* **1989**, *226*, 241–244. [CrossRef]

25. Thone, J.; Kollar, S.; Nousome, D.; Ellrichmann, G.; Kleiter, I.; Gold, R.; Hellwig, K. Serum anti-Mullerian hormone levels in reproductive-age women with relapsing-remitting multiple sclerosis. *Mult. Scler.* **2015**, *21*, 41–47. [CrossRef]

26. Cavalla, P.; Rovei, V.; Masera, S.; Vercellino, M.; Massobrio, M.; Mutani, R.; Revelli, A. Fertility in patients with multiple sclerosis: Current knowledge and future perspectives. *Neurol. Sci.* **2006**, *27*, 231–239. [CrossRef]

27. Hellwig, K.; Correale, J. Artificial reproductive techniques in multiple sclerosis. *Clin. Immunol.* **2013**, *149*, 219–224. [CrossRef]

28. Sepulveda, M.; Ros, C.; Martinez-Lapiscina, E.H.; Sola-Valls, N.; Hervas, M.; Llufriu, S.; La Puma, D.; Casals, E.; Blanco, Y.; Villoslada, P.; et al. Pituitary-ovary axis and ovarian reserve in fertile women with multiple sclerosis: A pilot study. *Mult. Scler.* **2016**, *22*, 564–568. [CrossRef] [PubMed]

29. Guzman-Soto, I.; Salinas, E.; Hernandez-Jasso, I.; Quintanar, J.L. Leuprolide acetate, a GnRH agonist, improves experimental autoimmune encephalomyelitis: A possible therapy for multiple sclerosis. *Neurochem. Res.* **2012**, *37*, 2190–2197. [CrossRef] [PubMed]

30. AVONEX (Interferon beta-1a) Intramuscular Injection. Highlights of Prescribing Information. Available online: https://www.avonex.com/content/dam/commercial/multiple-sclerosis/avonex/pat/en_us/pdf/Avonex_US_Prescribing_Information.pdf (accessed on 29 January 2019).

31. Amato, M.P.; Portaccio, E. Fertility, pregnancy and childbirth in patients with multiple sclerosis: Impact of disease-modifying drugs. *CNS Drugs* **2015**, *29*, 207–220. [CrossRef] [PubMed]

32. Holmoy, T.; Torkildsen, O. Family planning, pregnancy and breastfeeding in multiple sclerosis. *Tidsskr. Nor. Laegeforen* **2016**, *136*, 1726–1729. [CrossRef]

33. Magyari, M. Role of socio-economic and reproductive factors in the risk of multiple sclerosis. *Acta Neurol. Scand.* **2015**, *132*, 20–23. [CrossRef]

34. Ponsonby, A.L.; Lucas, R.M.; van der Mei, I.A.; Dear, K.; Valery, P.C.; Pender, M.P.; Taylor, B.V.; Kilpatrick, T.J.; Coulthard, A.; Chapman, C.; et al. Offspring number, pregnancy, and risk of a first clinical demyelinating event: The AusImmune Study. *Neurology* **2012**, *78*, 867–874. [CrossRef]

35. Runmarker, B.; Andersen, O. Pregnancy is associated with a lower risk of onset and a better prognosis in multiple sclerosis. *Brain* **1995**, *118 Pt 1*, 253–261. [CrossRef]

36. Mehta, D.; Wani, S.; Wallace, L.; Henders, A.K.; Wray, N.R.; McCombe, P.A. Cumulative influence of parity-related genomic changes in multiple sclerosis. *J. Neuroimmunol* **2019**, *328*, 38–49. [CrossRef]

37. Confavreux, C.; Hutchinson, M.; Hours, M.M.; Cortinovis-Tourniaire, P.; Moreau, T. Rate of pregnancy-related relapse in multiple sclerosis. Pregnancy in Multiple Sclerosis Group. *N. Engl. J. Med.* **1998**, *339*, 285–291. [CrossRef]

38. Poser, S.; Poser, W. Multiple sclerosis and gestation. *Neurology* **1983**, *33*, 1422–1427. [CrossRef]

39. Vukusic, S.; Hutchinson, M.; Hours, M.; Moreau, T.; Cortinovis-Tourniaire, P.; Adeleine, P.; Confavreux, C. Pregnancy and multiple sclerosis (the PRIMS study): Clinical predictors of post-partum relapse. *Brain* **2004**, *127*, 1353–1360. [CrossRef]

40. Finkelsztejn, A.; Brooks, J.B.; Paschoal, F.M., Jr.; Fragoso, Y.D. What can we really tell women with multiple sclerosis regarding pregnancy? A systematic review and meta-analysis of the literature. *BJOG* **2011**, *118*, 790–797. [CrossRef]

41. Houtchens, M.K.; Edwards, N.C.; Phillips, A.L. Relapses and disease-modifying drug treatment in pregnancy and live birth in US women with MS. *Neurology* **2018**, *91*, e1570–e1578. [CrossRef]

42. Alroughani, R.; Alowayesh, M.S.; Ahmed, S.F.; Behbehani, R.; Al-Hashel, J. Relapse occurrence in women with multiple sclerosis during pregnancy in the new treatment era. *Neurology* **2018**, *90*, e840–e846. [CrossRef]

43. Fragoso, Y.D.; Boggild, M.; Macias-Islas, M.A.; Carra, A.; Schaerer, K.D.; Aguayo, A.; de Almeida, S.M.; Alvarenga, M.P.; Alvarenga, R.M.; Alves-Leon, S.V.; et al. The effects of long-term exposure to disease-modifying drugs during pregnancy in multiple sclerosis. *Clin. Neurol. Neurosurg.* **2013**, *115*, 154–159. [CrossRef]

44. Vukusic, S.; Marignier, R. Multiple sclerosis and pregnancy in the 'treatment era'. *Nat. Rev. Neurol.* **2015**, *11*, 280–289. [CrossRef]

45. Thone, J.; Thiel, S.; Gold, R.; Hellwig, K. Treatment of multiple sclerosis during pregnancy - safety considerations. *Expert Opin. Drug Saf.* **2017**, *16*, 523–534. [CrossRef] [PubMed]

46. Vaughn, C.; Bushra, A.; Kolb, C.; Weinstock-Guttman, B. An Update on the Use of Disease-Modifying Therapy in Pregnant Patients with Multiple Sclerosis. *CNS Drugs* **2018**, *32*, 161–178. [CrossRef] [PubMed]

47. Haghikia, A.; Langer-Gould, A.; Rellensmann, G.; Schneider, H.; Tenenbaum, T.; Elias-Hamp, B.; Menck, S.; Zimmermann, J.; Herbstritt, S.; Marziniak, M.; et al. Natalizumab use during the third trimester of pregnancy. *JAMA Neurol.* **2014**, *71*, 891–895. [CrossRef] [PubMed]

48. Montalban, X.; Gold, R.; Thompson, A.J.; Otero-Romero, S.; Amato, M.P.; Chandraratna, D.; Clanet, M.; Comi, G.; Derfuss, T.; Fazekas, F.; et al. ECTRIMS/EAN guideline on the pharmacological treatment of people with multiple sclerosis. *Eur. J. Neurol.* **2018**, *25*, 215–237. [CrossRef] [PubMed]

49. Kanal, E.; Barkovich, A.J.; Bell, C.; Borgstede, J.P.; Bradley, W.G., Jr.; Froelich, J.W.; Gimbel, J.R.; Gosbee, J.W.; Kuhni-Kaminski, E.; Larson, P.A.; et al. ACR guidance document on MR safe practices: 2013. *J. Magn. Reson. Imaging* **2013**, *37*, 501–530. [CrossRef] [PubMed]

50. Elliott, A.B.; Chakravarty, E.F. Immunosuppressive medications during pregnancy and lactation in women with autoimmune diseases. *Womens Health (Lond.)* **2010**, *6*, 431–442. [CrossRef]

51. Xiao, W.L.; Liu, X.Y.; Liu, Y.S.; Zhang, D.Z.; Xue, L.F. The relationship between maternal corticosteroid use and orofacial clefts-a meta-analysis. *Reprod. Toxicol.* **2017**, *69*, 99–105. [CrossRef]

52. Mueller, B.A.; Zhang, J.; Critchlow, C.W. Birth outcomes and need for hospitalization after delivery among women with multiple sclerosis. *Am. J. Obst. Gynecol.* **2002**, *186*, 446–452. [CrossRef]

53. Kelly, V.M.; Nelson, L.M.; Chakravarty, E.F. Obstetric outcomes in women with multiple sclerosis and epilepsy. *Neurology* **2009**, *73*, 1831–1836. [CrossRef] [PubMed]

54. Fong, A.; Chau, C.T.; Quant, C.; Duffy, J.; Pan, D.; Ogunyemi, D.A. Multiple sclerosis in pregnancy: Prevalence, sociodemographic features, and obstetrical outcomes. *J. Matern Fetal. Neonatal. Med.* **2018**, *31*, 382–387. [CrossRef] [PubMed]

55. MacDonald, S.C.; McElrath, T.F.; Hernandez-Diaz, S. Pregnancy Outcomes in Women With Multiple Sclerosis. *Am. J. Epidemiol.* **2019**, *188*, 57–66. [CrossRef] [PubMed]

56. Update on overall prevalence of major birth defects—Atlanta, Georgia, 1978–2005. *MMWR Morb. Mortal. Wkly. Rep.* **2008**, *57*, 1–5.

57. Voskuhl, R.; Momtazee, C. Pregnancy: Effect on Multiple Sclerosis, Treatment Considerations, and Breastfeeding. *Neurotherapeutics* **2017**, *14*, 974–984. [CrossRef]

58. Coyle, P.K. Multiple sclerosis and pregnancy prescriptions. *Expert Opin. Drug Saf.* **2014**, *13*, 1565–1568. [CrossRef] [PubMed]

59. Brucker, M.C.; King, T.L. The 2015 US Food and Drug Administration Pregnancy and Lactation Labeling Rule. *J. Midwifery Womens Health* **2017**, *62*, 308–316. [CrossRef]

60. Nguyen, A.L.; Havrdova, E.K.; Horakova, D.; Izquierdo, G.; Kalincik, T.; van der Walt, A.; Terzi, M.; Alroughani, R.; Duquette, P.; Girard, M.; et al. Incidence of pregnancy and disease-modifying therapy exposure trends in women with multiple sclerosis: A contemporary cohort study. *Mult. Scler. Relat. Disord.* **2019**, *28*, 235–243. [CrossRef]

61. Thiel, S.; Langer-Gould, A.; Rockhoff, M.; Haghikia, A.; Queisser-Wahrendorf, A.; Gold, R.; Hellwig, K. Interferon-beta exposure during first trimester is safe in women with multiple sclerosis-A prospective cohort study from the German Multiple Sclerosis and Pregnancy Registry. *Mult. Scler.* **2016**, *22*, 801–809. [CrossRef]

62. Coyle, P.K.; Sinclair, S.M.; Scheuerle, A.E.; Thorp, J.M., Jr.; Albano, J.D.; Rametta, M.J. Final results from the Betaseron (interferon beta-1b) Pregnancy Registry: A prospective observational study of birth defects and pregnancy-related adverse events. *BMJ Open* **2014**, *4*, e004536. [CrossRef]

63. Glatiramer Acetate (Glatiramer Acetate Injection) for Subcutaneous Use. Highlights of Prescribing Information. Available online: https://www.copaxone.com/Resources/pdfs/PrescribingInformation.pdf (accessed on 29 January 2019).

64. Herbstritt, S.; Langer-Gould, A.; Rockhoff, M.; Haghikia, A.; Queisser-Wahrendorf, A.; Gold, R.; Hellwig, K. Glatiramer acetate during early pregnancy: A prospective cohort study. *Mult. Scler.* **2016**, *22*, 810–816. [CrossRef]

65. Sandberg-Wollheim, M.; Neudorfer, O.; Grinspan, A.; Weinstock-Guttman, B.; Haas, J.; Izquierdo, G.; Riley, C.; Ross, A.P.; Baruch, P.; Drillman, T.; et al. Pregnancy Outcomes from the Branded Glatiramer Acetate Pregnancy Database. *Int. J. MS Care* **2018**, *20*, 9–14. [CrossRef] [PubMed]

66. Geissbuhler, Y.; Vile, J.; Koren, G.; Guennec, M.; Butzkueven, H.; Tilson, H.; MacDonald, T.M.; Hellwig, K. Evaluation of pregnancy outcomes in patients with multiple sclerosis after fingolimod exposure. *Ther. Adv. Neurol. Disord.* **2018**, *11*, 1756286418804760. [CrossRef] [PubMed]

67. Tecfidera (Dimethyl Fumarate) Delayed-Release Capsules, for Oral Use. Highlights of Prescribing Information. Available online: https://www.tecfidera.com/content/dam/commercial/multiple-sclerosis/tecfidera/pat/en_us/pdf/full-prescribing-info.pdf (accessed on 28 January 2019).

68. Kieseier, B.C.; Benamor, M. Pregnancy outcomes following maternal and paternal exposure to teriflunomide during treatment for relapsing-remitting multiple sclerosis. *Neurol. Ther.* **2014**, *3*, 133–138. [CrossRef] [PubMed]

69. Tysabri (Natalizumab) Injection, for Intravenous Use. Highlights of Prescribing Information. Available online: https://www.tysabri.com/content/dam/commercial/multiple-sclerosis/tysabri/pat/en_us/pdfs/tysabri_prescribing_information.pdf (accessed on 29 January 2019).

70. Ebrahimi, N.; Herbstritt, S.; Gold, R.; Amezcua, L.; Koren, G.; Hellwig, K. Pregnancy and fetal outcomes following natalizumab exposure in pregnancy. A prospective, controlled observational study. *Mult. Scler.* **2015**, *21*, 198–205. [CrossRef]

71. Friend, S.; Richman, S.; Bloomgren, G.; Cristiano, L.M.; Wenten, M. Evaluation of pregnancy outcomes from the Tysabri(R) (natalizumab) pregnancy exposure registry: A global, observational, follow-up study. *BMC Neurol.* **2016**, *16*, 150. [CrossRef] [PubMed]

72. Alroughani, R.; Altintas, A.; Al Jumah, M.; Sahraian, M.; Alsharoqi, I.; AlTahan, A.; Daif, A.; Dahdaleh, M.; Deleu, D.; Fernandez, O.; et al. Pregnancy and the Use of Disease-Modifying Therapies in Patients with Multiple Sclerosis: Benefits versus Risks. *Mult. Scler. Int.* **2016**, *2016*, 1034912. [CrossRef] [PubMed]

73. De Santis, M.; Straface, G.; Cavaliere, A.F.; Rosati, P.; Batocchi, A.P.; Caruso, A. The first case of mitoxantrone exposure in early pregnancy. *Neurotoxicology* **2007**, *28*, 696–697. [CrossRef] [PubMed]

74. Baumgartner, A.K.; Oberhoffer, R.; Jacobs, V.R.; Ostermayer, E.; Menzel, H.; Voigt, M.; Schneider, K.T.; Pildner von Steinburg, S. Reversible foetal cerebral ventriculomegaly and cardiomyopathy under chemotherapy for maternal AML. *Onkologie* **2009**, *32*, 40–43. [CrossRef] [PubMed]

75. Hellwig, K.; Schimrigk, S.; Chan, A.; Epplen, J.; Gold, R. A newborn with Pierre Robin sequence after preconceptional mitoxantrone exposure of a female with multiple sclerosis. *J. Neurol. Sci.* **2011**, *307*, 164–165. [CrossRef] [PubMed]

76. Rituxan (Rituximab) Injection, for Intravenous Use. Highlights of Prescribing Information. Available online: https://www.gene.com/download/pdf/rituxan_prescribing.pdf (accessed on 29 January 2019).

77. Chakravarty, E.F.; Murray, E.R.; Kelman, A.; Farmer, P. Pregnancy outcomes after maternal exposure to rituximab. *Blood* **2011**, *117*, 1499–1506. [CrossRef]

78. Das, G.; Damotte, V.; Gelfand, J.M.; Bevan, C.; Cree, B.A.C.; Do, L.; Green, A.J.; Hauser, S.L.; Bove, R. Rituximab before and during pregnancy: A systematic review, and a case series in MS and NMOSD. *Neurol. Neuroimmunol. Neuroinflamm.* **2018**, *5*, e453. [CrossRef] [PubMed]

79. Lebrun, C.; Le Page, E.; Kantarci, O.; Siva, A.; Pelletier, D.; Okuda, D.T. Impact of pregnancy on conversion to clinically isolated syndrome in a radiologically isolated syndrome cohort. *Mult. Scler.* **2012**, *18*, 1297–1302. [CrossRef]

80. Hughes, S.E.; Spelman, T.; Gray, O.M.; Boz, C.; Trojano, M.; Lugaresi, A.; Izquierdo, G.; Duquette, P.; Girard, M.; Grand'Maison, F.; et al. Predictors and dynamics of postpartum relapses in women with multiple sclerosis. *Mult. Scler.* **2014**, *20*, 739–746. [CrossRef] [PubMed]

81. Section on Breastfeeding. Breastfeeding and the use of human milk. *Pediatrics* **2012**, *129*, e827–e841. [CrossRef] [PubMed]

82. Langer-Gould, A.; Huang, S.M.; Gupta, R.; Leimpeter, A.D.; Greenwood, E.; Albers, K.B.; Van Den Eeden, S.K.; Nelson, L.M. Exclusive breastfeeding and the risk of postpartum relapses in women with multiple sclerosis. *Arch. Neurol.* **2009**, *66*, 958–963. [CrossRef] [PubMed]

83. Hellwig, K.; Rockhoff, M.; Herbstritt, S.; Borisow, N.; Haghikia, A.; Elias-Hamp, B.; Menck, S.; Gold, R.; Langer-Gould, A. Exclusive Breastfeeding and the Effect on Postpartum Multiple Sclerosis Relapses. *JAMA Neurol.* **2015**, *72*, 1132–1138. [CrossRef]

84. Pakpoor, J.; Disanto, G.; Lacey, M.V.; Hellwig, K.; Giovannoni, G.; Ramagopalan, S.V. Breastfeeding and multiple sclerosis relapses: A meta-analysis. *J. Neurol.* **2012**, *259*, 2246–2248. [CrossRef]

85. Howie, P.W.; McNeilly, A.S.; Houston, M.J.; Cook, A.; Boyle, H. Fertility after childbirth: Infant feeding patterns, basal PRL levels and post-partum ovulation. *Clin. Endocrinol (Oxf.)* **1982**, *17*, 315–322. [CrossRef] [PubMed]

86. Langer-Gould, A.; Smith, J.B.; Hellwig, K.; Gonzales, E.; Haraszti, S.; Koebnick, C.; Xiang, A. Breastfeeding, ovulatory years, and risk of multiple sclerosis. *Neurology* **2017**, *89*, 563–569. [CrossRef] [PubMed]

87. de Seze, J.; Chapelotte, M.; Delalande, S.; Ferriby, D.; Stojkovic, T.; Vermersch, P. Intravenous corticosteroids in the postpartum period for reduction of acute exacerbations in multiple sclerosis. *Mult Scler* **2004**, *10*, 596–597. [CrossRef] [PubMed]

88. Ost, L.; Wettrell, G.; Bjorkhem, I.; Rane, A. Prednisolone excretion in human milk. *J. Pediatr.* **1985**, *106*, 1008–1011. [CrossRef]

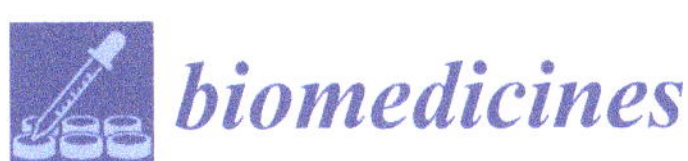 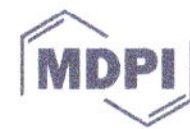

Review

Assessment and Impact of Cognitive Impairment in Multiple Sclerosis: An Overview

Miguel Ángel Macías Islas [1],* and Ethel Ciampi [2]

[1] Department of Neurosciences, CUCS. University of Guadalajara and Mexico, Guadalajara 44160, Mexico

[2] Neurology, Pontificia Universidad Católica de Chile, Neurology, Hospital Dr. Sótero del Río, Santiago 8320000, Chile; ethelciampi@gmail.com

* Correspondence: miguelangelmacias@hotmail.com; Tel.: +52-(33)-3124-0294

Received: 11 January 2019; Accepted: 14 March 2019; Published: 19 March 2019

Abstract: Cognitive impairment affects 40–60% of patients with multiple sclerosis. It may be present early in the course of the disease and has an impact on a patient's employability, social interactions, and quality of life. In the last three decades, an increasing interest in diagnosis and management of cognitive impairment has arisen. Neuropsychological assessment and neuroimaging studies focusing on cognitive impairment are now being incorporated as primary outcomes in clinical trials. However, there are still key uncertainties concerning the underlying mechanisms of damage, neural basis, sensitivity and validity of neuropsychological tests, and efficacy of pharmacological and non-pharmacological interventions. The present article aimed to present an overview of the assessment, neural correlates, and impact of cognitive impairment in multiple sclerosis.

Keywords: multiple sclerosis; demyelinating diseases; cognitive impairment; cognitive dysfunction

---

1. Introduction

Multiple sclerosis (MS) is a chronic inflammatory demyelinating disease of the central nervous system (CNS). Typically, the disease affects the brain, spinal cord, and optic nerves, with acute inflammation as seen during MS relapses, and variable degrees of chronic inflammation and neurodegenerative processes within the white and gray matter, associated with progressive accumulation of disability. In about 85% of the patients, MS begins as a relapsing-remitting course and secondarily evolves to a progressive stage (secondary-progressive MS) in about 15–30% of patients [1,2]. From the onset, about 15% of the patients will develop a primary progressive course [3].

Most people experience their first symptoms of MS between the ages of 20 and 40. The clinical heterogeneity of MS, as well as the findings of different pathological patterns, suggests that MS may be a spectrum of diseases representing different processes [4–7]. MS can be clinically categorized in different phenotypes, including clinically isolated syndrome (CIS), relapsing/remitting (RRMS), primary progressive and secondary progressive MS (SPMS), and can be subclassified according to its clinical and radiological activity [8]. These phenotypes are related to potentially different pathophysiological disease mechanisms, including acute/chronic inflammation, axonal/neuronal loss and gliosis, and variable degrees of tissue repair, as well as plasticity and clinical recovery, mainly related to each individual [7], although these differences have yet to be demonstrated at the molecular level [2].

Clinical symptoms of MS may include motor dysfunction (pyramidal); tremor, dysmetria, or ataxia (cerebellar); diplopia or nystagmus (brainstem); numbness (sensory); urinary/bowel hesitancy, incontinence, or retention; disturbances in vision and cognitive impairment. The latter functional systems can be measured with the Expanded Disability Status Scale (EDSS), which range from 0 (normal neurological examination), to 10 (death due to MS) [9], and although it is the most widely used disability score worldwide, cognitive impairment related to the disease seems fairly underrepresented, even when cognitive and neuropsychiatric symptoms are a major cause of disability, loss of employment, and poor quality of life of patients and their families [10].

Although more than a century ago J.M. Charcot described "marked enfeeblement of the memory" with "conceptions that are formed slowly" in persons with "sclérose en plaques" [11], this elegant clinical observation was almost forgotten for more than a hundred years as a remarkable symptom of what is now known as MS. In 1991, S. Rao brought renewed attention to cognitive impairment in MS patients [12]. Since then, it has been a topic of clinical and basic research, trying to reveal the precise mechanisms behind its presentation, in order to develop effective treatments that include cognitive impairment as an outcome in clinical trials, many of them with unsatisfactory results [13].

The following manuscript is not a systematic review about the topic, but an overview that aims to raise awareness on the cognitive deficits in MS, including the most affected cognitive domains and related neuropsychological batteries for their assessment, their neural correlates with an emphasis on neuroimaging, and a potential therapeutic approach as well as future perspectives.

2. Cognitive Impairment in Multiple Sclerosis

Cognition represents the function of several neural pathways involved in the processing of information in the brain, including several correlated and interdependent cognitive domains such as executive function, perceptual-motor function, language, learning and memory, complex attention, and social cognition, as defined by the Diagnostic and Statistical Manual of Mental Disorders 5th edition (DSM-5) [14]. Impairment of individual domains may cause dysfunction of the global cognitive performance [15].

Although impairment in cognitive function occurs in different neurologic diseases, the clinical syndromes, the degree of dysfunction, and related disability, depend on the involvement of different brain structures (cortical or subcortical), the extent of neural damage or number of affected domains, and the patient's previous cognitive reserve and performance. In MS, as a heterogeneous disease, all of the aforementioned characteristics makes it even more difficult to study cognition as a single manifestation of the disease [16,17].

Despite advances in knowledge about the neural basis of cognitive function in MS, there are still key uncertainties concerning what it is called 'normal cognition', and consequently with the assessment of cognitive dysfunction, typically defined as a performance below a chosen threshold in a number of cognitive domains, assessed in a specific neuropsychological test (e.g., 1.5–2 standard deviations below normal of a Z-score of one or more cognitive domains). In these batteries, results are commonly expressed as "intact/preserved" or "impaired" [18], and prevalent studies usually differ in cognitive impairment definitions.

Almost thirty years ago, in a population-based study performed by S. Rao et al., a 45% frequency of cognitive impairment in MS was found [12]. Other epidemiological studies reported frequencies of cognitive impairment in patients with MS between 40–70% in North America and Europe [19]. Frequencies of 40–60% have been reported in Latin America [20]. Even though a variety of different methodological approaches and neuropsychological batteries have been used, results are very similar across all reported populations.

MS is commonly diagnosed during a patient's most productive life period, and employment years and cognitive impairment supposes a severe impact over a patient's behavior, social functioning, adaptative strategies, and profound functional limitations affecting the activities of daily living and employment [10,21]. A large cross-sectional study carried out in nine European countries showed that only 35.8% of MS patients were employed. Low mood and cognitive impairment affecting domains like memory, attention, and slowed information processing speed were reported as frequent determinants of work-related difficulties, but only working memory impairment was responsible for higher unemployment rates [22]. Employment provides higher quality of life, independence, social participation, personal and professional reaffirmation, monetary income, health insurance, financial support for medication, and in some countries access to work benefits and social security [23], so cognition should be a priority in an era with highly active treatments reducing relapses and new lesions, and even new horizons in preventing accumulation of physical disability with new disease modifying treatments available [2].

A review by Shiavolin et al. concluded that difficulties that people with MS can experience with employment are always secondary outcomes of research, and it is quite difficult to address which factors contribute to reduced work participation. In their review, fatigue, mobility reduction, and cognitive impairment were reported as the main drivers of unemployment, and unemployment was related with worse quality of life scores [21].

In the same line, social cognition has gained relevance as a non-traditional cognitive domain present in MS since early stages of the disease, a domain that has been related to the capability for developing deep social interactions [24]. Recent evidence has shown 20% of social cognition impairment among patients, with a similar distribution for different phenotypes [25], and social cognition deficits show a significant correlation with the performance in other cognitive domains as working memory, processing speed, and executive functions [26–28] and exhibit behavioral impact affecting moral evaluation of other individuals' actions [29].

Finally, cognitive impairment not only affects patients, but also affects their relationship with their families and is a frequent complaint of higher burden for caregivers [21]. Mickens et al. studied the mediational effect on the relationships between MS impairments (neurological, cognitive, behavioral, emotional, and functional), unmet family needs (household information, financial, social, support, and health), and caregiver mental health (satisfaction with life, anxiety, burden, and depression) using a structural equation model. They suggested that intervention research on MS caregivers in Latin America may consider focusing on caregiver mental health problems by addressing unmet family needs and teaching caregivers' ways to manage the impairments of the individual with MS [30].

3. Cognitive Domains

All cognitive domains may be affected in MS, but the most affected ones are episodic memory and information processing speed [17,31]. Working memory, executive function, verbal fluency, and attention have also been widely described [12,32,33], with a recent interest in social cognition impairment [24,34]. Although clinical phenotypes may differ in the prevalence or severity of cognitive impairment, main determinants are physical disability as measured by EDSS, and patients' age [35]. Other individual characteristics such as gender, genetic factors, and cognitive reserve may also play a relevant role [36]. For a summary of the most frequent cognitive domains affected in MS see Table 1.

Table 1. Frequency of cognitive impairment in patients with multiple sclerosis (MS) by cognitive domain.

Cognitive Domain	Frequency
Learning Memory	**40–65%**
Visual Episodic Memory	20–75%
Verbal Episodic Memory	15–80%
Complex Attention	**5–25%**
Information processing Speed	15–50%
Executive Function	**15–25%**
Working Memory	15–60%
Inhibitory control	15–30%
Language	**20–58%**
Verbal Fluency	15–25%
Social Cognition	**20–40%**

MS: Multiple sclerosis. Adapted from Rao et al. 1991 [12], Benedict et al. 2006 [32], Chiaravaloti et al. 2008 [17], Dulau 2017 [25], Cotter et al. 2018 [34], Ciampi et al. 2018 [37], Ntoskou et al. 2018 [38].

3.1. Learning Memory

Long-term memory refers to the ability to learn new information and to recall that information at a later time point [39]. It is the most consistently affected cognitive domain in MS patients. Impaired learning of new information seems to be the primary problem [36], but the encoding, storing, and retrieval from long-term storage processes of memory seems to be affected in MS patients, so there is still controversy about which of these components of memory is the most influential factor for explaining memory deficits [40]. Other factors, such as slow processing speed, susceptibility to interference, executive disfunction, and perceptual deficits can also determine poor learning abilities [41].

3.2. Complex Attention—Information Processing

Complex attention domain involves sustained attention, divided attention, selective attention, and processing speed [42]. MS patients usually present with deficits in information processing efficiency, which refers to the ability to maintain and manipulate information in the brain for a short time period (working memory–executive function) [43] and to the speed with which one can process that information (processing speed–complex attention) [44]. It represents a key cognitive deficit in MS patients and might contribute to the presence of impairment in other cognitive domains [45,46].

3.3. Executive Function

Executive function is a complex domain which involves goal-directed behavior to adapt individuals to changes and demands of the environment, including planning, decision-making, working memory, responding to feedback, inhibition, and flexibility [42], and is affected in around 20% of MS patients. Some studies claim the difficulty to differentiate executive impairment from information processing, due to most of the tests used to evaluate executive function imply integrity of information processing and are affected by emotional affections such as depression. Leavitt et al. [47] studied executive functions and speed tasks (trail making test and Wisconsin card sorting test) in MS patients versus healthy controls. They found that MS patients score worse than controls, but differences decreased when corrected for information processing. They concluded that slow information processing accounts for executive function deficits in MS patients. The difficulty in assessing a specific domain, such as executive function, may be extrapolated to all other domains, as cognitive abilities are assessed individually in optimal environments, but patients usually struggle with managing multiple goals simultaneously [18].

3.4. Language

The language domain includes tasks such as object naming, word finding, fluency, grammar and syntax, and receptive language [42]. In MS, language deficits have been less studied than episodic memories or information processing speed. While some articles show intact functionality [48], more recent studies report frequencies of language impairment between 20% and 58% in RRMS or SPMS, respectively [38]. The most affected tasks seem to be phonological and semantic fluency, although verbal fluency tests are directly influenced by executive functions, thus many of the deficits have been considered as due to a dysfunctional executive syndrome [39].

3.5. Social Cognition

Social cognition, including social perception, empathy and theory of the mind, focuses on how people process, store, and apply information about other people and social situations, guiding social interactions [24]. Therefore, it is the sum of these processes that allow subjects of the same species to interact and exchange social codes to obtain information about another's behavior, and about the environment [49]. Its recent inclusion within the six main cognitive domains of the DSM-5, and its association with quality of life and employment, have raised awareness among MS researchers in the last years [34].

Social perception has been defined as the ability to perceive information about the mental state of other subjects based on behavioral signals [50]. Empathy refers to the generation of an emotional response in the observer to situations affecting other subjects (e.g., same or different emotion), and it is an essential component of human emotional experience and social interaction, because when an observed mental state is understood, and affective responses are generated, prosocial and cooperative behaviors can exist [51,52]. Theory of the mind is the ability to represent the psychological perspective of interacting subjects, requiring an internal theorization about their thoughts and beliefs, emotions, affective states, and feelings [53].

Recent studies have shown 20–40% of social cognition impairment in MS patients, with similar distribution across phenotypes, greater impact in theory of the mind tasks, as well as in the recognition of certain negative facial emotion expressions [25,34]. It also seems that social cognition interacts with other cognitive domains, although a distinct patter of association with an exclusive domain (e.g., executive functions) has not been demonstrated [34,37].

4. Neuropsychological Assessment

Cognitive function assessment in MS patients should become a part of everyday clinical practice and as a constant outcome in clinical trials. Ideally, every patient with a diagnosis of MS should undergo a complete neuropsychological assessment and routinely repeat a standardized and validated battery to detect clinically meaningful changes, as well as start a timely and effective treatment, similar to what the Magnetic Resonance Imaging in MS (MAGNIMS) group has proposed for the MRI protocols in the diagnosis and monitoring of the disease [54,55]. Nonetheless, this desire from the cognitive research community has many obstacles, including key knowledge gaps and methodological limitations related to the understanding and measurement of cognitive deficits, neuroimaging of neural bases and correlations of deficits, as well as the development of effective treatments [18].

Mini-Mental State Examination by Folstein in 1975, which was used for dementia, is not sensitive to MS cognitive disorders [56]. The three most frequently used neurocognitive batteries in MS are: (1) The Brief Repeatable Battery of Neuropsychological tests (BRB-N), also known as Rao's battery [57], (2) the minimal assessment of cognitive function in MS (MACFIMS) introduced by Benedict et al. [32], and (3) the Brief International Cognitive Assessment for Multiple Sclerosis (BICAMS), a shorter version that was developed in 2012 by an expert team, and is recommended for small centers with one or few staff members who may not have neuropsychological training [58]. All these screening batteries allow to establish the presence or absence of cognitive dysfunction and the specific domains affected. All of them have similarities and differences but share the fact that they are sensitive, specific, and cover the most frequently affected cognitive domains, and are also reasonably brief.

It is important to note that BICAMS should not be used within one month of recovery from relapse or within one month of steroid therapy, and the recommended order of administration is first the Symbol Digit Modalities Test (SDMT), then the California Verbal Learning Test (CVLT-II T1-5), and then the Brief Visuospatial Memory Test Revised (BVMT-R T1-3). In most clinical situations, yearly or bi-annual BICAMS evaluations will be appropriate.

Emphasis in testing MS cognitive impairment must be focused on the assessment of the most frequently affected domains, learning/memory, and information processing speed. In this context, experts are encouraging the MS multidisciplinary team (e.g., neurologists, nurses, psychologists, speech therapists, etc.) to be trained to use short MS cognitive assessment batteries, such as the BICAMS [12]. The subtests that compose the structure of domain specific evaluation of these batteries are shown in Table 2.

Table 2. Comparison of the three most used neuropsychological batteries in MS.

Cognitive Domain	BRB-N	MACFIMS	BICAMS
Auditory processing speed and working memory	PASAT	PASAT	-
Visual processing speed and working memory	SDMT	SDMT	SDMT
Auditory or verbal episodic memory	SRT	CVLT-II	CVLT-II
Visual or spatial episodic memory	10/36 Spatial Recall Test	BVMT-R	BVMT-R
Expressive language	COWAT	COWAT	-
Spatial processing	-	JLO	-
Executive function	-	DKEFS sorting	-

MS: Multiple sclerosis, BRB-N: Brief Repeatable Battery of Neuropsychological tests, MACFIMS: Minimal assessment of cognitive function in MS, BICAMS: Brief International Cognitive Assessment for Multiple Sclerosis, PASAT: Paced Auditory Serial Addition, SDMT: Symbol Digit Modalities Test, SRT: Selective Reminding Test, CVLT-II: California Verbal Learning Test, BVMT-R: Brief Visuospatial Memory Test Revised, COWAT: Controlled Oral Word Association Test, JLO: Judgement of Line Orientation test, DKEFS: Delis-Kaplan Executive Function System.

For the purpose of this review, we will describe the components of the BICAMS battery, due to its extensive use and validation in many countries, as well as the PASAT as being included as the cognitive test in MSFC, as well as a brief summary of social cognition tasks.

4.1. Information Processing Speed: Symbol Digit Modalities Test (SDMT)

When SDMT was first published in 1982, there were precedents of similar formats since 1927 and was adopted by the United States Army to assess precisely the speed of substitution of symbols by digits. SDMT has been used in almost every MS cognitive assessment battery and found to be exceptionally reliable and sensitive to assess information processing speed. The test consists of single digits paired with abstract symbols, with rows of the nine symbols arranged pseudo-randomly. The patient must say (or write) the number that corresponds with each symbol. The SDMT can be completed within 5 min, including instructions, practice, and testing. The SDMT has a reported sensitivity of 82% and a specificity of 60% [59]. It is the most sensitive task in MS, with good to excellent reliability, well tolerated by patients, has uniformity across languages, with no floor or ceiling effects, and a preliminary clinically meaningful change of 3–4 points [59], so it is recommended for clinical practice and research [18].

4.2. Episodic Verbal Memory: California Learning Verbal Test (CVLT)

This comprises of a 16-item word list, with four items belonging to each of the four categories, arranged randomly. The list is read aloud five times in the same order to the patient, at a slightly slower rate than one item per second. Patients are required to recall as many items as possible, in any order, after each reading. The CVLT-II T1-5 [60] can be completed in 5–10 min. It is recommended for clinical use, and it has high sensitivity with good age and sex adjusted normative data [18].

4.3. Episodic Visuospatial Memory: Brief Visuospatial Memory Test Revised (BVMT-R)

The BVMT-R T1-3 requires the patient to inspect a 2 × 3 stimulus array of abstract geometric figures. There are three learning trials of 10 s. The array is removed, and the patient is required to draw the array from memory, with the correct shapes in the correct position. It is also recommended for clinical and research use and has high sensitivity, it is time efficient, and is well tolerated by patients. Its main disadvantage is for patients with severe motor impairment [18].

4.4. Working Memory: Paced Auditory Serial Addition Test (PASAT-3")

The PASAT is a measure of cognitive function that specifically assesses auditory information processing speed and flexibility, as well as calculation ability [61]. Stimulus presentation rates were adapted for use with MS patients by Rao and colleagues in 1989, and the measure has been widely used in MS studies since then. Single digits are presented either every 3" (or every 2" for the optional PASAT-2", which could be a more accurate assessment of information processing speed) and the patient must add each new digit to the one immediately prior to it. The test score is the number of correct sums given (out of 60 possible sums) in each trial. To minimize familiarity with stimulus items in clinical trials and other serial studies, two alternate forms have been developed; the order of these should be counterbalanced across testing sessions [62,63]. Although it has been widely used in clinical research and clinical trials, and it has been included within the MSFC, there are several disadvantages to this test including a limited reliability due to practice effects, susceptibility to ceiling effect, poor tolerability due to a patient's math ability, and test-related anxiety. Therefore, it is not recommended for cognitive monitoring in clinical practice, nor for clinical trials designed with multiple administrations, but it is better used as a putative cognitive processing task to compare results across previous studies [18].

4.5. Social Cognition

The assessment of social cognition in MS include a myriad of tests used in other neurological disorders, for example the Face and Emotion Recognition (e.g., Ekman faces [64]) for social perception, Faux Pas, or Reading the Mind in the Eyes tests for theory of the mind tasks, or compound batteries previously used in other neurological disorders such as in frontotemporal dementia (e.g., Social Emotion Assessment [65,66]). For example, the mini-Social and Emotional Assessment test (mini-SEA) includes the Faux Pas and the Face Emotion Recognition. The Faux Pas is comprised by ten narrative vignettes or short stories in which a character inadvertently hurts or offends another, using Theory of the Mind tasks to infer another's mental state, making attributions to their knowledge, beliefs, and emotions. Half of the vignette test is control stories and the other half includes a principal character who inadvertently hurts or offends another, the 'victim of the Faux Pas'. The subject is expected to recognize the situations in which a Faux Pas is committed, why the leading character did it (cognitive theory of mind, he did not mean it), and how the victim of the Faux Pas must have felt (affective theory of mind, we expect him to recognize that the victim must have had a negative emotion). The Face Emotion Recognition consists of 35 pictures for face affect recognition of basic emotions among a list presented at the bottom of the screen including happiness, sadness, anger, surprise, fear, disgust, and neutral [66].

There is still the need for a consensus statement from expert groups to select those tests with best sensitivity, specificity, and reliability in MS.

5. Neural Basis of Cognitive Impairment in MS

Underlying neural mechanisms of cognitive damage can be related to the inflammatory and neurodegenerative changes in the MS brain, including grey and white matter structures, both globally and regionally, structurally, and functionally [67]. Although one can appreciate some of these changes at a single-subject level (Figure 1), routine measurements (e.g., brain atrophy) are still not suggested to be used in clinical practice, mainly due to biological changes (e.g., dehydration, pseudo atrophy, etc.), that can exceed the accuracy threshold of current brain analysis software [55]. On the other hand, a myriad of group-analysis studies have been published trying to unveil the neural basis of cognitive impairment in MS. Differences in the results obtained by various studies may represent biased sample selection and differences between the image technology and software utilized in reported studies. Nonetheless, in vivo studies of neural correlations may contribute to early diagnosis, monitoring, and treatment of cognitive impairment in MS.

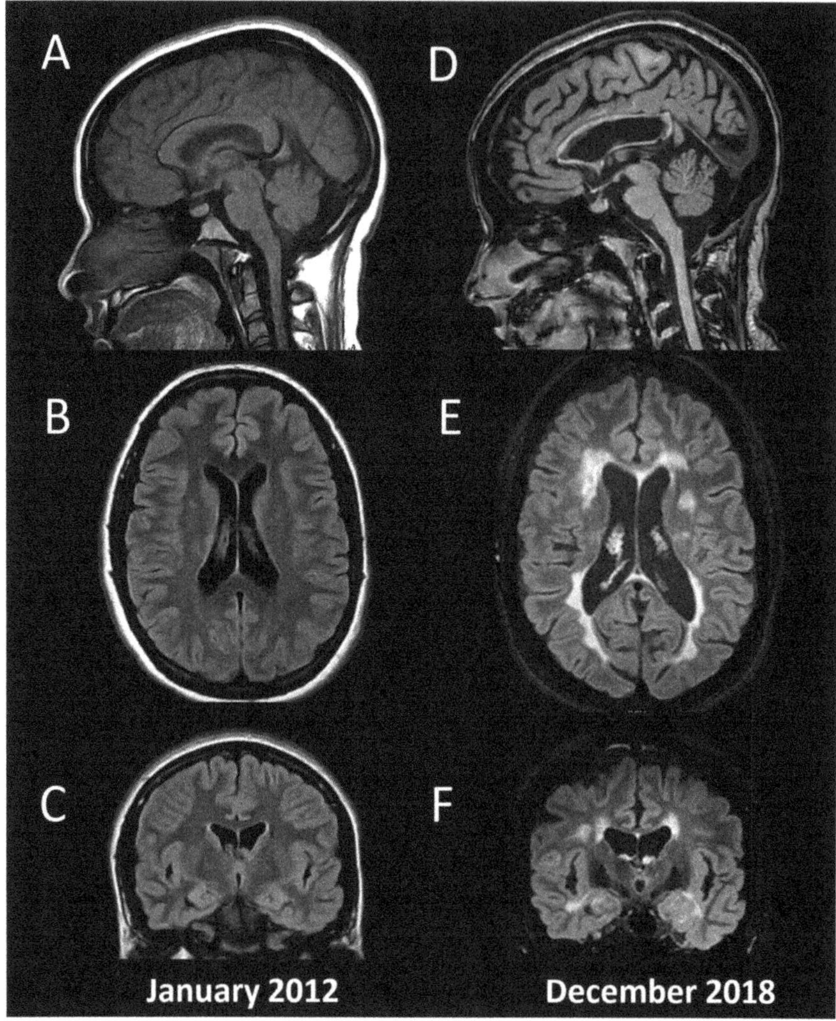

Figure 1. Conventional MRI in a patient with multiple sclerosis and cognitive impairment. Baseline MRI (**A**: Sagittal T1, **B**: Axial FLAIR, **C**: Coronal FLAIR) from a 15-year-old female with fulminant MS (Marburg variant, EDSS 8.0). After initial aggressive treatment in 2012, including myeloablation with cyclophosphamide, the patient remained asymptomatic without disease modifying treatment, until a second supratentorial motor relapse in 2015, confirming her MS diagnosis and beginning fingolimod. Since then, no relapses or new T2/enhancing lesions have appeared, and she had an EDSS 1.0 by the time of the second MRI in 2018 (**D**: Sagittal T1, **E**: Axial FLAIR, **F**: Coronal FLAIR). Her Mini-Mental State Examination was 30 (normal), Beck Depression Inventory 4 (without depression), and her fatigue severity score was 4 (significative fatigue). She had below normal performance ($\leq$1.5 standard deviation) in verbal and visual episodic memory, and in information processing speed tests, with the diagnosis of cognitive impairment according to the MACFIMS battery. Note the widespread brain volume loss including cortical grey matter, ventricular width, and corpus callosum atrophy. The patient gave her written informed consent to present this data.

Structural imaging comprise of measurements of brain volume loss (atrophy), which can include global measurements, such as cross-sectional or longitudinal volumetric or 3D whole brain volume loss using semi-automated software (e.g., brain parenchymal fraction (BPF) [68], structural image evaluation using normalization of atrophy SIENAX—SIENA [69,70]), regional measurements of different tissues (e.g., grey matter or white matter volume, also measured by SIENAX), or specific grey or white matter structures (e.g., using voxel-based morphometry or Free Surfer for regional tissue volume loss or cortical thickness, respectively [71]), as well as manual/linear or 2D assessments such as the Corpus Callosum Index [72–74], or the third ventricle width, the frontal horn width, and the intercaudate distance [75].

From a functional point of view, although positron emission tomography (PET) and single photon emission computed tomography (SPECT) have shown correlations between cerebral blood flow and oxygen use with cognitive impairment in MS patients [76,77], functional MRI (fMRI) has gained its place among cognitive researchers in assessing the neural correlates of disability in MS, with an special emphasis on early changes, with a potential role for treatment monitoring (e.g., during cognitive rehabilitation) [78].

Also, recent interest has developed in the study of water diffusivity in normal-appearing white matter (regions of the white matter where no lesion is seen in conventional MRI studies), using diffusion tensor imaging (DTI), that can be related both with structural and functional disconnection between different regions of the brain [79]. Other non-conventional and advanced MRI techniques are also in study, including magnetization transfer imaging (MTI), proton MR spectroscopy (^{1}H-MRS), and iron imaging [80].

Cognitive impairment has been associated with linear measure changes [75], the extent of white matter lesions and lesion load [29,33,37], focal cortical lesions [81], whole brain atrophy [82], diffuse cortical atrophy [81,83,84], regional grey matter structures such as thalamus, caudate, putamen, hippocampus, and amygdala, cerebellum and corpus callosum [67,85], as well as with widespread subtle pathological changes in normal-appearing white matter [83,86], among others.

Neuroanatomical correlates of memory deficits seem to differ across disease stages [87]. Early brain volume loss is a very precise predictor for the presence of cognitive impairment years later [82,83], and although hippocampal atrophy was not significantly seen in patients with CIS suggestive of MS compared with healthy controls in a study using DTI, hippocampal fractional anisotropy was significantly decreased in CIS patients, and mean diffusivity was correlated with verbal episodic memory performance [88]. An interesting study showed that a predictive model of cognitive performance in MS should include bilateral posterior cingulate cortex and bilateral temporal pole cortical thickness, overall white matter lesion load, normal-appearing white matter integrity, and age, reaffirming the multifactorial etiology of MS cognitive impairment [84].

Episodic memory has been correlated with total grey matter and regional cortical structures (e.g., left precuneus [89]); visuospatial memory has been associated with brain MRI total lesion area, T1 lesion, and FLAIR lesion volume, BPF, third ventricular width, and right superior frontal atrophy, among others [90,91]; verbal episodic memory has been associated with total and regional hippocampal atrophy, total lesion load and BPF [90–93]; information processing speed has been correlated with thalamus, whole grey matter atrophy, and third ventricle width [94], cerebellum atrophy [95,96], as well as with less white matter integrity, and increases in functional connectivity [79]; executive disfunction has been associated with frontal lobe structural and functional damage [97,98] and with dorsolateral prefrontal, orbitofrontal, anterior cingulate, and insular areas [99], as well as with thalamic structural and functional changes [100]; PASAT-3″ scores have been correlated with cortical and subcortical structures such as bilateral precuneus, posterior cingulate, caudate putamen, and cerebellum [101], and acute changes in PASAT score with no physical changes (EDSS) have been associated with presence of acute gadolinium enhancing lesions [102], with similar results observe with transient SDMT changes [103], proposing that patients could also experience "cognitive relapses".

Concerning social cognition, when assessing regional gray matter atrophy in a cohort of progressive MS patients with social cognitive impairment, significant loss was seen within bilateral cortical regions of orbitofrontal, insula and cerebellum, and right regions of fusiform gyrus, and precuneus [37], while functional MRI studies have shown increased activation in the posterior cingulate cortex and precuneus for the identification of anger and disgust faces, and greater activity in the occipital fusiform gyri, the anterior cingulate, and the inferior frontal cortex for the recognition of neutral faces [104]. Also, increased lesion volume has been correlated with lower success in face emotion recognition [105]. When assessing theory of the mind tasks, it seems that a disconnection syndrome, caused by white matter lesions, could also be one of the possible mechanisms underlying this specific impairment [105–109].

Other regions of interest associated with cognitive performance in multiple cognitive domains include the thalamus, as a relay station or cortico-subcortical and cortico-cortical networks [85] (e.g., global cognitive disfunction, information processing speed, attention, verbal memory, spatial memory, verbal fluency, executive function) [91,110–112]; the cerebellum, as a historically understudied region for cognitive performance (attention, working memory, information processing speed, etc.) [37,95,96]; and the corpus callosum, the main white matter tract of the brain (e.g., information processing speed, working memory, verbal fluency, etc.) [73,74].

Finally, we would like to highlight advances of fMRI and cognitive research in MS [78], although there has been some controversies about the real meaning of fMRI results, it seems that early changes can be seen, even in cognitively preserved patients, including higher recruitment of non-related areas, such as supplementary motor cortex during working memory tasks [113] or by changes in activity properties of regions highly related to cognitive functions, as centrality measures of the default mode network [114], changes that may be used as a biomarker for neurocognitive rehabilitation [115] especially, resting state fMRI [116–118].

6. Treatment of Cognitive Impairment in MS

6.1. Pharmacological Interventions

6.1.1. MS Disease Modifying Therapies

MS specific disease modifying therapies such as the injectables interferon beta, glatiramer acetate; oral agents such as fingolimod, teriflunomide, or dimethyl fumarate; and monoclonal antibodies such as natalizumab, alemtuzumab, and ocrelizumab, have shown significant benefits in reducing the annualized relapse rate and MRI activity (new T2 or gadolinium enhancing lesions), with a more discrete efficacy over reducing disability progression or the brain atrophy rate [2]. However, their specific impact on cognitive impairment remains unclear, mainly because most phase III clinical trials established cognitive impairment as a secondary or tertiary outcome measure. Comparative efficacy on cognitive outcomes across trials is even more difficult, because of the different neuropsychological batteries used, the varied methods for evaluation and outcome analysis, and the differences between populations included in the trials.

Pivotal interferons and glatiramer acetate clinical trials did not include cognitive evaluation as primary endpoints. Intramuscular interferon beta 1a versus placebo included neuropsychological evaluation as a secondary outcome measure and showed 52.7% improvement compared with 29% in the placebo group [119], including processing speed and episodic memory outcomes. In the COGIMUS (Cognitive Impairment in Multiple Sclerosis) study, subcutaneous interferon 1a protected RRMS patients from general cognitive decline when reevaluated at 3 [120] and 5 years [121] after therapy onset. Regarding interferon beta 1b, Pishkin reported only improvement of delayed visual reproduction performance [122], and the Betaferon/Betaseron in Newly Emerging Multiple Sclerosis for Initial Treatment (BENEFIT) trial revealed that in patients with CIS interferon beta 1b had beneficial effects on working memory, and the effects remained over 8 years [123]. Glatiramer Acetate trials, while included BRB-N evaluation, did not show significant differences versus placebo [62].

The GOLDEN Study using once-daily oral fingolimod was compared with interferon beta 1b using a trial design that included cognitive impairment as the primary outcome. This study showed improvement in cognitive function (BRB-N and DKEFS) in both treatment arms, favoring fingolimod on MRI parameters [69], although some baseline imbalances may have favored the interferon beta 1b arm, according to the authors. In a patient-reported outcomes study, evaluating global satisfaction in switching treatment from several disease modifying drugs to teriflunomide and using SDMT to measure cognitive impairment, results showed that patients and physicians reported stability of cognition in a 48-week period [124].

Natalizumab pivotal studies showed that it can reduce the risk of progressive working memory impairment by 43% compared with placebo [125]. In a long-term observational study by Jacques et al., natalizumab was reported to preserve cognition over 7 years of continuous therapy using a computed test and the SDMT. No patient showed evidence of sustained cognitive deterioration over a 24-month period [126]. In a study including 21 patients during a 15-month follow-up period, alemtuzumab showed stable cognitive function using an extensive neuropsychological battery [127]. Ocrelizumab has shown improvement in MS Functional Composite score (a composite measure of walking speed, upper-limb movements, and cognition assessed by PASAT) compared with interferon beta 1a [128].

6.1.2. Cognitive Impairment-Specific Treatment

The use of acetylcholinesterase inhibitors (AChEI) in multiple sclerosis patients remains controversial. Few studies in a small number of MS patient populations reported contradictory results. While Krupp in 2004 reported the positive impact of donepezil in verbal learning and memory in a cohort of 69 patients [129], the same investigator reported no significant effect in 2011, which included 120 MS patients [130]. It is important to stress that long term treatments with AChEI compels one to be aware of the side effects. Regarding memantine, similar contradictory findings were reported in a small number of studies prevailing negative outcomes for this drug [131].

Amphetamines significantly improved visuospatial memory and verbal memory [132], fampridine has shown to be able to improve cognitive fatigue, alertness, psychomotor speed, and verbal fluency [133,134], while no benefit on learning were found using modafinil [135].

6.2. Non-Pharmacological Interventions

6.2.1. Neuropsychological Rehabilitation

Only recently, neuropsychological rehabilitation has been established as a useful therapeutic tool. Multidisciplinary and cognitive-behavioral interventions, computer-assisted training and combinations of the above, have been showing consistently better results [13,136], especially when tailored to individual needs. Evidence-based conclusions have only recently become stronger in regards to which interventions may have real benefits for MS patients. In a recent review article and meta-analysis including literature from 2007 to 2016, only one intervention received support for a practice standard in verbal learning and memory (modified Story Memory Technique—mSMT [137]), two computer programs received support as a practice guideline for attention and multicognitive domains (Attention Process Training—APT [138] and RehaCom [139]), and several studies provided support for the practice option in attention, learning, and memory [140].

6.2.2. Exercise

To date, numerous publications have shown the positive impact of physical exercise on different clinical parameters, but evidence remains to be demonstrated, as clinical trials have shown equivocal results [141,142]. A systematic review by Sandroff et al. showed that a few comparable studies did not yield a significant positive impact of physical exercise on cognitive impairment outcomes [143]. Another systematic review of the impact of yoga also failed to show the effect of this discipline in cognitive impairment [144]. This maybe the result of collectively insufficient well–designed research, and again, the fact that cognitive impairment is maintained as a secondary outcome. The cognitive effects of physical exercise in MS is gaining hype among cognitive researchers, as one relevant intervention both in preventing and improving cognitive outcomes, although clear results, as well as doses and regimens (e.g., aerobic versus weight training), are still missing [13].

7. Conclusions

In the last three decades, increasing knowledge in the field of cognitive impairment in MS has arisen. From defining the most sensitive neuropsychological tests and compound batteries for clinical practice and research, to better understanding the neural correlates in specific populations with assistance from conventional-structural and non-conventional/functional neuroimaging, better and more effective treatment, rehabilitation, and prevention strategies are being proposed.

Cognitive function assessment should be included in the standard clinical evaluation and clinical trials involving MS patients, and treatment strategies should be implemented as supported by current evidence. Limitations are still present, especially due to the validation and standardization of both diagnostic and therapeutic tools.

Due to the devastating impact over the working status, social interaction, and self-care of MS patients, improvement in all the aforementioned areas, as well as education to patients, families, and the community should be stated as a priority, and an unmet need.

Funding: This research received no external funding.

Conflicts of Interest: The authors declare no conflict of interest.

References

1. Cree, B.A.; Gourraud, P.A.; Oksenberg, J.R.; Bevan, C.; Crabtree-Hartman, E.; Gelfand, J.M.; Goodin, D.S.; Graves, J.; Green, A.J.; Mowry, E.; et al. Long-term evolution of multiple sclerosis disability in the treatment era. *Ann. Neurol.* **2016**, *80*, 499–510. [PubMed]
2. Thompson, A.J.; Baranzini, S.E.; Geurts, J.; Hemmer, B.; Ciccarelli, O. Multiple sclerosis. *Lancet* **2018**, *391*, 1622–1636. [CrossRef]
3. Miller, D.H.; Leary, S.M. Primary-progressive multiple sclerosis. *Lancet Neurol.* **2007**, *6*, 903–912. [CrossRef]
4. Kakalacheva, K.; L€unemann, J.D. Enviromental triggers of multiple sclerosis. *FEBS Lett.* **2011**, *585*, 3724–3729. [CrossRef] [PubMed]
5. Chitnis, T. Role of puberty in multiple sclerosis risk and course. *Clin. Immunol.* **2013**, *149*, 192–200. [CrossRef]
6. Franciotta, D.; Salvetti, M.; Lolli, F.; Serafini, B.; Aloisi, F. B cells and multiple sclerosis. *Lancet Neurol.* **2008**, *7*, 852–858. [CrossRef]
7. Fletcher, J.M.; Lalor, S.J.; Sweeney, C.M.; Tubridy, N.; Mills, K.H.G.; Lalor, S. T cells in multiple sclerosis and experimental autoimmune encephalomyelitis. *Clin. Exp. Immunol.* **2010**, *162*, 1–11. [CrossRef]
8. Lublin, F.D.; Reingold, S.C.; Cohen, J.A.; Cutter, G.R.; Sørensen, P.S.; Thompson, A.J.; Wolinsky, J.S.; Balcer, L.J.; Banwell, B.; Barkhof, F.; et al. Defining the clinical course of multiple sclerosis: The 2013 revisions. *Neurology* **2014**, *83*, 278–286. [CrossRef]
9. Kurtzke, J.F. Rating neurologic impairment in multiple sclerosis: An expanded disability status scale (EDSS). *Neurology* **1983**, *33*, 1444–1452. [CrossRef]
10. Clemens, L.; Langdon, D. How does cognition relate to employment in multiple sclerosis? A systematic review. *Mult. Scler. Relat. Disord.* **2018**, *26*, 183–191. [CrossRef]
11. Murray, J. Terminology and disease description. In *Multiple Sclerosis the History of a Disease*; DEMOS Medical: New York, NY, USA, 2005; Volume 2, pp. 21–26.
12. Rao, S.; Leo, G.; Bernardin, I.; Unverzagt, F. Cognitive dysfunction in multiple sclerosis: Frequency, patterns, and predictions. *Neurology* **1991**, *41*, 94–97. [CrossRef]
13. Sokolov, A.A.; Grivaz, P.; Bove, R. Cognitive Deficits in Multiple Sclerosis: Recent Advances in Treatment and Neurorehabilitation. *Curr. Treat. Options Neurol.* **2018**, *20*, 53. [CrossRef] [PubMed]
14. American Psychiatric Association. *Diagnostic and Statistical Manual of Mental Disorders*, 5th ed.; American Psychiatric Publishing: Arlington, VA, USA, 2013; pp. 5–25, ISBN 978-0-89042-555-8.

15. Wooddruff, B.K. Disorders of cognition. *Semin. Neurol.* **2011**, *31*, 18–28. [CrossRef] [PubMed]

16. Amato, P.; Langdon, D.; Montalvan, X.; Benedict, R.; DeLuca, J.; Krupp, L.B.; Thompson, A.J.; Comi, G. Treatment of cognitive impairment in multiple sclerosis: Position paper. *J. Neurol.* **2013**, *260*, 1452–1468. [CrossRef] [PubMed]

17. Chiaravaloti, N.D.; DeLuca, J. Cognitive impairment in multiple sclerosis. *Lancet* **2008**, *7*, 1139–1151. [CrossRef]

18. Sumowski, J.F.; Benedict, R.; Enzinger, C.; Filippi, M.; Geurts, J.J.; Hamalainen, P.; Hulst, H.; Inglese, M.; Leavitt, V.M.; Rocca, M.A.; et al. Cognition in multiple sclerosis, State of the field and priorities for the future. *Neurology* **2018**, *90*, 278–288. [CrossRef] [PubMed]

19. DiGiuseppe, G.; Blair, M.; Morrow, S.A. Prevalence of cognitive impairment in newly diagnosed relapsing-remitting multiple sclerosis. *Int. J. MS Care* **2018**, *20*, 153–157. [CrossRef]

20. Vanotti, S.; Caceres, F.J. Cognitive and neuropsychiatric disorders among MS patients from Latin America. *MSJ Exp. Trans. Clin.* **2017**, *3*. [CrossRef]

21. Schiavolin, S.; Leonardi, M.; Giovannetti, A.M.; Antozzi, C.; Brambilla, L.; Confalonieri, P.; Mantegazza, R.; Raggi, A. Factors related to difficulties with employment in patients with multiple sclerosis: A review of 2002–2011 literature. *Int. J. Rehabil. Res.* **2013**, *36*, 105–111. [CrossRef]

22. Raggi, A.; Covelli, V.; Schiavolin, S.; Scaratti, C.; Leonardi, M.; Willems, M. Work-related problems in multiple sclerosis: A literature review on its associates and determinants. *Disabil. Rehabil.* **2016**, *38*, 936–944. [CrossRef]

23. Yamout, B.; Issa, Z.; Herlopian, A.; El Bejjani, M.; Khalifa, A.; Ghadieh, A.S.; Habib, R.H. Predictors of quality of life among multiple sclerosis patients: A comprehensive analysis. *Eur. J. Neurol.* **2013**, *20*, 756–764. [CrossRef] [PubMed]

24. Labbé, T.; Ciampi, E.; Carcamo Rodríguez, C. Social cognition: Concepts, neural basis and its role in multiple sclerosis. *Neurol. Clin. Neurosci.* **2018**, *6*, 3–8. [CrossRef]

25. Dulau, C.; Deloire, M.; Diaz, H.; El Bejjani, M.; Khalifa, A.; Ghadieh, A.S.; Habib, R.H. Social cognition according to cognitive impairment in different clinical phenotypes of multiple sclerosis. *J. Neurol.* **2017**, *264*, 740–748. [CrossRef] [PubMed]

26. Raimo, S.; Trojano, L.; Pappacena, S.; Alaia, R.; Spitaleri, D.; Grossi, D.; Santangelo, G. Neuropsychological Correlates of Theory of Mind Deficits in Patients with Multiple Sclerosis. *Neuropsychology* **2017**. [CrossRef] [PubMed]

27. Carotenuto, A.; Arcara, G.; Orefice, G.; Cerillo, I.; Giannino, V.; Rasulo, M.; Iodice, R.; Bambini, V. Communication in Multiple Sclerosis: Pragmatic Deficit and its Relation with Cognition and Social Cognition. *Arch. Clin. Neuropsychol.* **2017**, *33*, 194–205. [CrossRef] [PubMed]

28. Henry, A.; Tourbah, A.; Chaunu, M.P.; Bakchine, S.; Montreuil, M. Social Cognition Abilities in Patients with Different Multiple Sclerosis Subtypes. *J. Int. Neuropsychol. Soc.* **2017**, *23*, 653–664. [CrossRef]

29. Patil, I.; Young, L.; Sinay, V.; Gleichgerrcht, E. Elevated moral condemnation of third-PARTY violations in multiple sclerosis patients. *Soc. Neurosci.* **2017**, *12*, 308–329. [CrossRef]

30. Mickens, M.N.; Perrin, P.B.; Aguayo, A.; Rabago, B.; Macias-Islas, M.; Arango-Lasprilla, J. Mediational Model of Multiple Sclerosis Impairments, Family Needs, and Caregiver Mental Health in Guadalajara, Mexico. *Behav. Neurol.* **2018**. [CrossRef]

31. Langdon, D.W. Cognition in multiple sclerosis. *Curr. Opin. Neurol.* **2011**, *24*, 244–249. [CrossRef]

32. Benedict, R.H.; Cookfair, D.; Gavett, R.; Gunther, M.; Munschauer, F.; Garg, N.; Weinstock-Guttman, B. Validity of the Minimal Assessment of Cognitive Function in Multiple Sclerosis (MACFIMS). *J. Int. Neuropsychol. Soc.* **2006**, *12*, 549–558. [CrossRef]

33. Deloire, M.S.; Ruet, A.; Hamel, D.; Bonnet, M.; Dousset, V.; Brochet, B. MRI predictors of cognitive outcome in early multiple sclerosis. *Neurology* **2011**, *76*, 1161–1167. [CrossRef] [PubMed]

34. Cotter, J.; Firth, J.; Enzinger, C.; Kontopantelis, E.; Yung, A.R.; Elliott, R.; Drake, R.J. Social cognition in multiple sclerosis: A systematic review and meta-analysis. *Neurology* **2016**, *87*, 1727–1736. [CrossRef] [PubMed]

35. Ruano, L.; Portaccio, E.; Goretti, B.; Niccolai, C.; Severo, M.; Patti, F.; Cilia, S.; Gallo, P.; Grossi, P.; Ghezzi, A.; et al. Age and disability drive cognitive impairment in multiple sclerosis across disease subtypes. *Mult. Scler.* **2017**, *23*, 1258–1267. [CrossRef]

36. Trenova, A.G.; Slavov, G.S.; Manova, M.G.; Aksentieva, J.B.; Miteva, L.D.; Stanilova, S.A. Cognitive impairment in multiple sclerosis. *Folia Med.* **2016**, *58*, 157–163. [CrossRef] [PubMed]
37. Ciampi, E.; Uribe-San-Martin, R.; Vásquez, M.; Ruiz-Tagle, A.; Labbe, T.; Cruz, J.P.; Lillo, P.; Slachevsky, A.; Reyes, D.; Reyes, A.; et al. Relationship between Social Cognition and traditional cognitive impairment in Progressive Multiple Sclerosis and possible implicated neuroanatomical regions. *Mult. Scler. Relat. Disord.* **2018**, *20*, 122–128. [CrossRef] [PubMed]
38. Ntoskou, K.; Messinis, L.; Nasios, G.; Martzoukou, M.; Makris, G.; Panagiotopoulos, E.; Papathanasopoulos, P. Cognitive and Language Deficits in Multiple Sclerosis: Comparison of Relapsing Remitting and Secondary Progressive Subtypes. *Open Neurol. J.* **2018**, *12*, 19–30. [CrossRef] [PubMed]
39. Lezak, M.D.; Howieson, D.B.; Bigler, E.D.; Tranel, D. *Neuropsychological Assessment*, 5th ed.; Oxford University Press: New York, NY, USA, 2012.
40. Thornton, A.E.; Raz, N.; Tucke, K.A. Memory in multiple sclerosis: Contextual encoding defi cits. *J. Int. Neuropsychol. Soc.* **2002**, *8*, 395–409. [CrossRef] [PubMed]
41. Renell, P.G.; Jensen, F.; Henry, J.D. Prospective memory in multiple sclerosis. *J. Int. Neuropsychol. Soc.* **2007**, *13*, 410–416.
42. Sachdev, P.S.; Blacker, D.; Blazer, D.G.; Ganguli, M.; Jeste, D.V.; Paulsen, J.S.; Petersen, R.C. Classifying neurocognitive disorders: The DSM-5 approach. *Nat. Rev. Neurol.* **2014**, *10*, 634–642. [CrossRef] [PubMed]
43. Silva, P.H.R.; Spedo, C.T.; Baldassarini, C.R.; Benini, C.D.; Ferreira, D.A.; Barreira, A.A.; Leoni, R.F. Brain functional and effective connectivity underlying the information processing speed assessed by the Symbol Digit Modalities Test. *Neuroimage* **2019**, *184*, 761–770. [CrossRef]
44. Costa, S.L.; Genova, H.M.; DeLuca, J.; Chiaravalloti, N.D. Information processing speed in multiple sclerosis: Past, present, and future. *Mult. Scler. J.* **2016**, *23*, 772–789. [CrossRef] [PubMed]
45. Grzegorski, T.; Losy, J. Cognitive impairment in multiple sclerosis. *Rev. Neurosci.* **2017**, *7*, 1139–1151.
46. Van Schependom, J.; D'hooghe, M.B.; Cleynhens, K.; D'hooge, M.; Haelewyck, M.C.; De Keyser, J.; Nagels, G. Reduced information processing speed as primum movens for cognitive decline in MS. *Mult. Scler.* **2015**, *21*, 83. [CrossRef] [PubMed]
47. Leavitt, V.M.; Wylie, G.; Krch, D.; Chiaravalloti, N.; DeLuca, J.; Sumowski, J.F. Does slowed processing speed account for executive deficits in multiple sclerosis Evidence from neuropsychological performance and structural neuroimaging. *Rehabil. Psychol.* **2014**, *59*, 422–428. [CrossRef]
48. Prakash, R.S.; Snook, E.M.; Lewis, J.M.; Motl, R.W.; Kramer, A.F. Cognitive impairments in relapsing-remitting multiple sclerosis: A meta-analysis. *Mult. Scler.* **2008**, *14*, 1250–1261. [CrossRef]
49. Frith, C.D.; Frith, U. Social cognition in humans. *Curr. Biol.* **2007**, *17*, R724–R732. [CrossRef]
50. De Bruin, L.; Strijbos, D. Direct social perception, mindreading and Bayesian predictive coding. *Conscious Cogn.* **2015**, *36*, 565–570. [CrossRef]
51. Singer, T.; Lamm, C. The social neuroscience of empathy. *Ann. N. Y. Acad. Sci.* **2009**, *1156*, 81–96. [CrossRef]
52. Ruggieri, V.L. Empathy, social cognition and autism spectrum disorders. *Rev. Neurol.* **2013**, *56*, S13–S21.
53. Baron-Cohen, S. Without a theory of mind one cannot participate in a conversation. *Cognition* **1988**, *29*, 83–84. [CrossRef]
54. Rovira, À.; Wattjes, M.P.; Tintoré, M.; Tur, C.; Yousry, T.A.; Sormani, M.P.; De Stefano, N.; Filippi, M.; Auger, C.; Rocca, M.A.; et al. Evidence-based guidelines: MAGNIMS consensus guidelines on the use of MRI in multiple sclerosis-clinical implementation in the diagnostic process. *Nat. Rev. Neurol.* **2015**, *11*, 471–482. [CrossRef] [PubMed]
55. Wattjes, M.P.; Rovira, À.; Miller, D.; Yousry, T.A.; Sormani, M.P.; de Stefano, M.P.; Tintoré, M.; Auger, C.; Tur, C.; Filippi, M.; et al. Evidence-based guidelines: MAGNIMS consensus guidelines on the use of MRI in multiple sclerosis—Establishing disease prognosis and monitoring patients. *Nat. Rev. Neurol.* **2015**, *11*, 597–606.
56. Beatty, W.W.; Goodkin, D.E. Screening for cognitive impairment in multiple sclerosis. An evaluation of the Mini-Mental State Examination. *Arch. Neurol.* **1990**, *47*, 297–301. [CrossRef] [PubMed]
57. Rao, S.M. *Neuropsychological Screening Battery for Multiple Sclerosis*; National Multiple Sclerosis Society: New York, NY, USA, 1991.
58. Langdon, D.W.; Amato, M.P.; Boringa, J.; Brochet, B.; Foley, F.; Fredrikson, S.; Hämäläinen, P.; Hartung, H.-P.; Krupp, L.; Penner, I.K.; et al. Recommendations for a Brief International Cognitive Assessment for Multiple Sclerosis (BICAMS). *MSJ* **2012**, *18*, 891–898. [CrossRef]

59. Benedict, R.; DeLuca, J.; Phillips, G.; LaRocca, N.; Hudson, L.D.; Rudick, R.; Multiple Sclerosis Outcome Assessments Consortium. Validity of the Symbol Digit Modalities Test as a cognition performance outcome measure formultiple sclerosis. *Mult. Scler. J.* **2017**, *23*, 721–733. [CrossRef] [PubMed]

60. Delis, D.C.; Kramer, J.H.; Kaplan, E.; Ober, B.A. *California Verbal Learning Test*, 2nd ed.; Psychological Corporation: San Antonio, TX, USA, 2000.

61. Gronwall, D. Paced auditory serial addition task: A measure of recovery from concussion. *Percept. Motor Skills* **1977**, *44*, 363–373. [CrossRef]

62. Cutter, G.R.; Baier, M.S.; Rudick, R.A.; Cookfair, D.L.; Fischer, J.S.; Petkau, J.; Syndulko, K.; Weinshenker, B.G.; Antel, J.P.; Confavreux, C.; et al. Development of a Multiple Sclerosis Functional Composite as a clinical trial outcome measure. *Brain* **1999**, *122*, 101–112. [CrossRef]

63. Fischer, J.S.; Rudick, R.A.; Cutter, G.R.; Reingold, S.C. The Multiple Sclerosis Functional Composite Measure (MSFC): An integrated approach to MS clinical outcome assessment. National MS Society Clinical Outcomes Assessment Task Force. *Mult. Scler.* **1999**, *5*, 244–250. [CrossRef]

64. Friesen, W.V.; Ekman, P. *Friesen Pictures of Facial Affect*; Consulting Psychologists Press: Palo Alto, CA, USA, 1976.

65. Funkiewiez, A.; Bertoux, M.; de Souza, L.C.; Lévy, R.; Dubois, B. The sea (social cognition and emotional assessment): A clinical neuropsychological tool for early diagnosis of frontal variant of frontotemporal lobar degeneration. *Neuropsychology* **2012**, *1*, 81–90. [CrossRef]

66. Bertoux, M.; Volle, E.; de Souza, L.C.; Funkiewiez, A.; Dubois, B.; Habert, M.O. Neural correlates of the mini-SEA (Social cognition and Emotional Assessment) in behavioral variant frontotemporal dementia. *Brain Imaging Behav.* **2014**, *1*, 1–6. [CrossRef]

67. Di Filippo, M.; Portaccio, E.; Mancini, A.; Calabresi, P. Multiple sclerosis and cognition: Synaptic failure and network dysfunction. *Nat. Rev. Neurosci.* **2018**, *19*, 599–609. [CrossRef]

68. Zivadinov, R.; Sepcic, J.; Nasuelli, D.; De Masi, R.; Bragadin, L.M.; Tommasi, M.; Zambito-Marsala, S.; Moretti, R.; Bratina, A.; Ukmar, M.; et al. A longitudinal study of brain atrophy and cognitive disturbances in the early phase of relapsing-remitting multiple sclerosis. *J. Neurol. Neurosurg. Psychiatry* **2001**, *70*, 773–780. [CrossRef] [PubMed]

69. Smith, S.M.; Zhang, Y.; Jenkinson, M.; Chen, J.; Matthews, P.M.; Federico, A.; de Stefano, N. Accurate, robust and automated longitudinal and cross-sectional brain change analysis. *NeuroImage* **2002**, *17*, 479–489. [CrossRef] [PubMed]

70. Smith, S.M.; Jenkinson, M.; Woolrich, M.W.; Beckmann, C.F.; Behrens, T.E.J.; Johansen-Berg, H.; Bannister, P.R.; de Luca, M.; Drobnjak, I.; Flitney, D.E.; et al. Advances in functional and structural MR image analysis and implementation as FSL. *NeuroImage* **2004**, *23*, 208–219. [CrossRef] [PubMed]

71. Geurts, J.G.; Calabrese, M.; Fisher, E.; Rudick, R.A. Measurement and clinical effect of grey matter pathology in multiple sclerosis. *Lancet Neurol.* **2012**, *11*, 1082–1092. [CrossRef]

72. Figueira, F.F.; Santos, V.S.; Figueira, G.M.A.; Da Silva, Â.C.M. Corpus callosum index: A practical method for long-term follow-up in multiple sclerosis. *Arq. Neuropsiquiatr.* **2007**, *65*, 931–935. [CrossRef]

73. Yaldizli, Ö.; Penner, I.K.; Frontzek, K.; Naegelin, Y.; Amann, M.; Papadopoulou, A.; Sprenger, T.; Kuhle, J.; Calabrese, P.; Radü, E.W.; et al. The relationship between total and regional corpus callosum atrophy, cognitive impairment and fatigue in multiple sclerosis patients. *Mult. Scler.* **2014**, *3*, 356–364. [CrossRef] [PubMed]

74. Uribe-San-Martín, R.; Ciampi, E.; Di Giacomo, R.; Vásquez, M.; Cárcamo, C.; Godoy, J.; Lo Russo, G.; Tassi, L. Corpus callosum atrophy and post-surgical seizures in temporal lobe epilepsy associated with hippocampal sclerosis. *Epilepsy Res.* **2018**, *142*, 29–35. [CrossRef] [PubMed]

75. Butzkueven, H.; Kolbe, S.C.; Jolley, D.J.; Brown, J.Y.; Cook, M.J.; van der Mei, I.A.; Groom, P.S.; Carey, J.; Eckholdt, J.; Rubio, J.P.; et al. Validation of linear cerebral atrophy markers in multiple sclerosis. *J. Clin. Neurosci.* **2008**, *15*, 130–137. [CrossRef]

76. Lycke, J.; Wikkelso, C.; Bergh, A.C.; Jacobsson, L.; Andersen, O. Regional cerebral blood flow in multiple sclerosis masured by single photon emission tomography with technetium-99m hexamethylpropyleneamine oxime. *Eur. Neurol.* **1993**, *33*, 163–167. [CrossRef] [PubMed]

77. Roelcke, U.; Kappos, L.; Lechner-Scott, J.; Brunnschweiler, H.; Huber, S.; Ammann, W.; Plohmann, A.; Dellas, S.; Maguire, R.P.; Missimer, J.; et al. Reduced glucose metabolism in the frontal cortex and basal ganglia of multiple sclerosis patients with fatigue a 18F-fl uorodeoxyglucose positron emission tomography study. *Neurology* **1997**, *48*, 1566–1571. [CrossRef]

78. Labbé, T.; Ciampi, E.; Cruz, J.P.; Zurita, M.; Uribe, S.; Cárcamo, C. Functional magnetic resonance imaging in the study of multiple sclerosis. *Rev. Neurol.* **2018**, *67*, 91–98.

79. Meijer, K.A.; Muhlert, N.; Cercignani, M.; Sethi, V.; Ron, M.A.; Thompson, A.J.; Miller, D.H.; Chard, D.; Geurts, J.J.; Ciccarelli, O. White matter tract abnormalities are associated with cognitive dysfunction in secondary progressive multiple sclerosis. *Mult. Scler.* **2016**, *22*, 1429–1437. [CrossRef]

80. Giorgio, A.; De Stefano, N. Advanced Structural and Functional Brain MRI in Multiple Sclerosis. *Semin. Neurol.* **2016**, *36*, 163–176. [CrossRef]

81. Calabrese, M.; Agosta, F.; Rinaldi, F.; Mattisi, I.; Grossi, P.; Favaretto, A.; Atzori, M.; Bernardi, V.; Barachino, L.; Rinaldi, L.; et al. Cortical lesions and atrophy associated with cognitive impairment in relapsing-remitting multiple sclerosis. *Arch. Neurol.* **2009**, *66*, 1144–1150. [CrossRef] [PubMed]

82. Summers, M.M.; Fisniku, L.K.; Anderson, V.M.; Miller, D.H.; Cipolotti, I.; Ron, M. Cognitive impairment in relapsing remitting multiple sclerosis can be predicted by imaging performed several years earlier. *Mult. Scler.* **2008**, *14*, 197–204. [CrossRef] [PubMed]

83. Tekok-Kilic, A.; Benedict, R.H.; Weinstock-Gutman, B.; Dwyer, M.G.; Carone, D.; Srinivasaraghavan, B.; Yella, V.; Abdelrahman, N.; Munschauer, F.; Bakshi, R.; et al. Independent contributions of cortical grey matter atrophy and ventricle enlargement for predicting neuropsychological impairment in multiple sclerosis. *Neurology* **2007**, *36*, 1294–1300.

84. Steenwijk, M.D.; Geurts, J.J.G.; Daams, M.; Tijms, B.M.; Wink, A.M.; Balk, L.J.; Tewarie, P.K.; Uitdehaag, B.M.J.; Barkhof, F.; Vrenken, H.; et al. Cortical atrophy patterns in multiple sclerosis are non-random and clinically relevant. *Brain* **2016**, *139*, 115–126. [CrossRef]

85. Kern, K.C.; Gold, S.M.; Lee, B.; Montag, M.; Horsfall, J.; O'Connor, M.F.; Sicotte, N.L. Thalamic-hippocampal-prefrontal disruption in relapsing-remitting multiple sclerosis. *Neuroimage Clin.* **2014**, *8*, 440–447. [CrossRef]

86. Zivadinov, R.; de, M.R.; Nasuelli, D.; Bragadin, L.M.; Ukmar, M.; Pozzi-Mucelli, R.S.; Grop, A.; Cazzato, G.; Zorzon, M. MRI techniques and cognitive impairment in the early phase of relapsing-remitting multiple sclerosis. *Neuroradiology* **2001**, *43*, 272–278. [CrossRef]

87. Sumowski, J.F.; Leavitt, V.M.; Rocca, M.A.; Inglese, M.; Riccitelli, G.; Buyukturkoglu, K.; Meani, A.; Filippi, M. Mesial temporal lobe and subcortical grey matter volumes differentially predict memory across stages of multiple sclerosis. *Mult. Scler.* **2018**, *24*, 675–678. [CrossRef] [PubMed]

88. Planche, V.; Ruet, A.; Coupé, P.; Lamargue-Hamel, D.; Deloire, M.; Pereira, B.; Manjon, J.V.; Munsch, F.; Moscufo, N.; Meier, D.S.; et al. Hippocampal microstructural damage correlates with memory impairment in clinically isolated syndrome suggestive of multiple sclerosis. *Mult. Scler.* **2017**, *23*, 1214–1224. [CrossRef] [PubMed]

89. Aladro, Y.; López-Alvarez, L.; Sánchez-Reyes, J.M.; Hernández-Tamames, J.A.; Melero, H.; Rubio-Fernández, S.; Thuissard, I.; Cerezo-García, M. Relationship between episodic memory and volume of the brain regions of two functional cortical memory systems in multiple sclerosis. *J. Neurol.* **2018**, *265*, 2182–2189. [CrossRef] [PubMed]

90. Benedict, R.H.; Bakshi, R.; Simon, J.H.; Priore, R.; Miller, C.; Munschauer, F. Frontal cortex atrophy predicts cognitive impairment in multiple sclerosis. *J. Neuropsych. Clin. Neurosci.* **2002**, *14*, 44–51. [CrossRef]

91. Houtchens, M.K.; Benedict, R.H.; Kiliiany, R.; Sharma, J.; Jaisani, Z.; Singh, B.; Weinstock-Guttman, B.; Guttmann, C.R.; Bakshi, R. Thalamic atrophy and cognition in multiple sclerosis. *Neurology* **2007**, *69*, 1213–1223. [CrossRef]

92. Sicotte, N.L.; Kern, K.C.; Giesser, B.S.; Arshanapalli, A.; Schultz, A.; Montag, M.; Wang, H.; Bookheimer, S.Y. Regional hippocampal atrophy in multiple sclerosis. *Brain* **2008**, *131*, 1134–1141. [CrossRef]

93. González Torre, J.A.; Cruz Gómez, Á.J.; Belenguer, A.; Sanchis-Segura, C.; Ávila, C.; Forn, C. Hippocampal dysfunction is associated with memory impairment in multiple sclerosis: A volumetric and functional connectivity study. *Mult. Scler.* **2017**, *23*, 1854–1863. [CrossRef]

94. Minagar, A.; Barnett, M.H.; Benedict, R.H.B.; Pelletier, D.; Pirko, I.; Sahraian, M.A.; Frohman, E.; Zivadinov, R. The thalamus and multiple sclerosis: Modern views on pathologic, imaging, and clinical aspects. *Neurology* **2013**, *80*, 210–219. [CrossRef]

95. Ruet, A.; Hamel, D.; Deloire, M.S.; Charré-Morin, J.; Saubusse, A.; Brochet, B. Information processing speed impairment and cerebellar dysfunction in relapsing-remitting multiple sclerosis. *J. Neurol. Sci.* **2014**, *347*, 246–250. [CrossRef]

96. Moroso, A.; Ruet, A.; Lamargue-Hamel, D.; Munsch, F.; Deloire, M.; Coup, P.; Ouallet, J.C.; Planche, V.; Moscufo, N.; Meier, D.S.; et al. Posterior lobules of the cerebellum and information processing speed at various stages of multiple sclerosis. *J. Neurol. Neurosurg. Psychiatry* **2017**, *88*, 146–151.

97. Foong, J.; Rozewicz, L.; Quaghebeur, G.; Davie, C.A.; Kartsounis, L.D.; Thompson, A.J.; Miller, D.H.; Ron, M.A. Executive function in multiple sclerosis. The role of frontal lobe pathology. *Brain* **1997**, *120*, 15–26. [CrossRef]

98. Muhlert, N.; Sethi, V.; Schneider, T.; Daga, P.; Cipolotti, L.; Haroon, H.A.; Parker, G.J.M.; Ourselin, S.; Wheeler-Kingshott, C.A.M.; Miller, D.H.; et al. Diffusion MRI-based cortical complexity alterations associated with executive function in multiple sclerosis. *J. Magn. Reson. Imaging* **2013**, *38*, 54–63.

99. Weygandt, M.; Wakonig, K.; Behrens, J.; Meyer-Arndt, L.; Söder, E.; Brandt, A.U.; Bellmann-Strobl, J.; Ruprecht, K.; Gold, S.M.; Haynes, J.-D.; et al. Brain activity, regional gray matter loss, and decision-making in multiple sclerosis. *Mult. Scler.* **2017**, *24*, 1163–1173. [CrossRef]

100. Koini, M.; Filippi, M.; Rocca, M.A.; Yousry, T.; Ciccarelli, O.; Tedeschi, G.; Gallo, A.; Ropele, S.; Valsasina, P.; Riccitelli, G.; et al. Correlates of Executive Functions in Multiple Sclerosis Based on Structural and Functional MR Imaging: Insights from a Multicenter Study. *Radiology* **2016**, *280*, 869–879. [CrossRef] [PubMed]

101. Matias-Guiu, J.A.; Cortés-Martínez, A.; Montero, P.; Pytel, V.; Moreno-Ramos, T.; Jorquera, M.; Yus, M.; Arrazola, J.; Matías-Guiu, J. Structural MRI correlates of PASAT performance in multiple sclerosis. *BMC Neurol.* **2018**, *20*, 214. [CrossRef] [PubMed]

102. Bellmann-Strobl, J.; Wuerfel, J.; Aktas, O.; Dorr, J.; Wernecke, K.D.; Zipp, F.; Paul, F. Poor PASAT performance correlates with MRI contrast enhancement in multiple sclerosis. *Neurology* **2009**, *73*, 1624–1627. [CrossRef]

103. Pardini, M.; Uccelli, A.; Grafman, J.H.; Yaldizli, O.; Mancardi, G.L.; Roccatagliata, L. Isolated cognitive relapses in multiple sclerosis. *J. Neurol. Neurosurg. Psychiatry* **2014**, *85*, 1035–1037. [CrossRef] [PubMed]

104. Jehna, M.; Langkammer, C.; Wallner-Blazek, M.; Neuper, C.; Loitfelder, M.; Ropele, S.; Fuchs, S.; Khalil, M.; Pluta-Fuerst, A.; Fazekas, F.; et al. Cognitively preserved MS patients demonstrate functional differences in processing neutral and emotional faces. *Brain Imaging Behav.* **2011**, *5*, 241–251. [CrossRef]

105. Mike, A.; Strammer, E.; Aradi, M.; Orsi, G.; Perlaki, G.; Hajnal, A.; Sandor, J.; Banati, M.; Illes, E.; Zaitsev, A.; et al. Disconnection mechanism and regional cortical atrophy contribute to impaired processing of facial expressions and theory of mind in multiple sclerosis: A structural MRI study. *PLoS ONE* **2013**, *8*, e82422. [CrossRef]

106. Calabrese, P.; Penner, I.K. Cognitive dysfunctions in multiple sclerosis "a multiple disconnection syndrome". *J. Neurol.* **2007**, *254*, 18–21. [CrossRef]

107. Henry, A.; Tourbah, A.; Chaunu, M.; Rumbach, L.; Montreuil, M.; Bakchine, S. Social cognition impairments in relapsing-remitting multiple sclerosis. *J. Int. Neuropsychol. Soc.* **2011**, *17*, 1122–1131. [CrossRef] [PubMed]

108. Batista, S.; d'Almeida, O.C.; Afonso, A.; Freitas, S.; Macário, C.; Sousa, L.; Castelo-Branco, M.; Santana, I.; Cunha, L. Impairment of social cognition in multiple sclerosis: Amygdala atrophy is the main predictor. *Mult. Scler.* **2017**, *23*, 1358–1366. [CrossRef] [PubMed]

109. Chalah, M.A.; Ayache, S.S. Deficits in Social Cognition: An Unveiled Signature of Multiple Sclerosis. *J. Int. Neuropsychol. Soc.* **2017**, *23*, 266–286. [CrossRef] [PubMed]

110. Benedict, R.H.; Hulst, H.E.; Bergsland, N.; Schoonheim, M.M.; Dwyer, M.G.; Weinstock-Guttman, B.; Geurts, J.J.; Zivadinov, R. Clinical significance of atrophy and white matter mean diffusivity within the thalamus of multiple sclerosis patients. *Mult. Scler.* **2013**, *19*, 1478–1484. [CrossRef] [PubMed]

111. Schoonheim, M.M.; Hulst, H.E.; Brandt, R.B.; Strik, M.; Wink, A.M.; Uitdehaag, B.M.J.; Barkhof, F.; Geurts, J.J.G. Thalamus structure and function determine severity of cognitive impairment in multiple sclerosis. *Neurology* **2015**, *84*, 776–783. [CrossRef] [PubMed]

112. Bisecco, A.; Rocca, M.A.; Pagani, E.; Mancini, L.; Enzinger, C.; Gallo, A.; Vrenken, H.; Stromillo, M.L.; Copetti, M.; Thomas, D.L.; et al. Connectivity-based parcellation of the thalamus in multiple sclerosis and its implications for cognitive impairment: A multicenter study. *Hum. Brain Mapp.* **2015**, *36*, 2809–2825. [CrossRef]

113. Nelson, F.; Akhtar, M.A.; Zúñiga, E.; Perez, C.A.; Hasan, K.M.; Wilken, J.; Wolinsky, J.S.; Narayana, P.A.; Steinberg, J.L. Novel fMRI working memory paradigm accurately detects cognitive impairment in multiple sclerosis. *Mult. Scler.* **2016**, *23*, 836–847. [CrossRef]

114. Eijlers, A.J.; Meijer, K.A.; Wassenaar, T.M.; Steenwijk, M.D.; Uitdehaag, B.M.; Barkhof, F.; Wink, A.M.; Geurts, J.J.; Schoonheim, M.M. Increased default-mode network centrality in cognitively impaired multiple sclerosis patients. *Neurology* **2017**, *88*, 952–960. [CrossRef]

115. Campbell, J.; Langdon, D.; Cercignani, M.; Rashid, W. A randomised controlled trial of efficacy of cognitive rehabilitation in multiple sclerosis: A cognitive, behavioural, and MRI study. *Neural Plast.* **2016**, *2016*, 4292585. [CrossRef]

116. Pinter, D.; Beckmann, C.; Koini, M.; Pirker, E.; Filippini, N.; Pichler, A.; Fuchs, S.; Fazekas, F.; Enzinger, C. Reproducibility of resting state connectivity in patients with stable multiple sclerosis. *PLoS ONE* **2016**, *11*, e0152158. [CrossRef]

117. Boutiere, C.; Rey, C.; Zaaraoui, W.; Le Troter, A.; Rico, A.; Crespy, L.; Achard, S.; Reuter, F.; Pariollaud, F.; Wirsich, J.; et al. Improvement of spasticity following intermittent theta burst stimulation in multiple sclerosis is associated with modulation of resting-state functional connectivity of the primary motor cortices. *Mult. Scler.* **2017**, *23*, 855–863. [CrossRef] [PubMed]

118. Pareto, D.; Sastre-Garriga, J.; Alonso, J.; Galán, I.; Arévalo, M.J.; Renom, M.; Montalban, X.; Rovira, À. Classic Block Design "Pseudo"-Resting-State fMRI Changes After a Neurorehabilitation Program in Patients with Multiple Sclerosis. *J. Neuroimaging* **2018**, *28*, 313–319. [CrossRef]

119. Fisher, R.L.; Priore, R.L.; Jacobs, L.D.; Cookfair, D.L.; Rudick, R.A.; Herndon, R.M.; Richert, J.R.; Salazar, A.M. Neuropsychological effects of interferón beta 1 a in relapsing multiple sclerosis. *Ann. Neurol.* **2000**, *48*, 885–892. [CrossRef]

120. Patti, F.; Amato, M.P.; Bastianello, S.; Caniatti, L.; Di Monte, E.; Ferrazza, P.; Goretti, B.; Gallo, P.; Brescia Morra, V.; Lo Fermo, S.; et al. Effects of immunomodulatory treatment with subcutaneous interferon beta-1a on cognitive decline in mildly disabled patients with relapsing-remitting multiple sclerosis. *Mult. Scler.* **2010**, *16*, 68–77. [CrossRef] [PubMed]

121. Patti, F.; Morra, V.B.; Amato, M.P.; Trojano, M.; Bastianello, S.; Tola, M.R.; Cottone, S.; Plant, A.; Picconi, O. Subcutaneous interferon β-1a may protect against cognitive impairment in patients with relapsing-remitting multiple sclerosis: 5-year follow-up of the COGIMUS study. *PLoS ONE* **2013**, *8*, e74111. [CrossRef] [PubMed]

122. Pliskin, N.H.; Hamer, D.P.; Goldstein, D.S.; Towle, V.L.; Reder, A.T.; Noronha, A.; Arnason, B.G. Improved delayed visual reproduction test performance in multiple sclerosis patients receiving interferon beta-1b. *Neurology* **1996**, *47*, 1463–1468. [CrossRef] [PubMed]

123. Edan, G.; Kappos, L.; Montalbán, X.; Polman, C.H.; Freedman, M.S.; Hartung, H.-P.; Miller, D.; Barkhof, F.; Herrmann, J.; Lanius, V.; et al. Longterm impact of interferon beta-1b in patients with CIS: 8-year follow-up of BENEFIT. *J. Neurol. Neurosurg. Psychiatry* **2014**, *85*, 1183–1189. [CrossRef]

124. Weinstein, A.; Schwid, S.I.; Schiffer, R.B.; McDermott, M.P.; Giang, D.W.; Goodman, A.D. Neuropsychologic status in multiple sclerosis after treatment with glatiramer. *Arch. Neurol.* **1999**, *56*, 319–324. [CrossRef]

125. Weinstock-Guttman, B.; Galetta, S.L.; Giovannoni, G.; Havrdova, E.; Hutchinson, M.; Kappos, L.; O'Connor, P.W.; Phillips, J.T.; Polman, C.; Stuart, W.H.; et al. Additional efficacy endpoints from pivotal natalizumab trials in relapsing-remitting MS. *J. Neurol.* **2012**, *259*, 898–905. [CrossRef]

126. Jacques, F.H.; Harel, B.T.; Schembri, A.J.; Paquette, C.; Bilodeau, B.; Kalinowski, P.; Roy, R. Cognitive evolution in natalizumab-treated multiple sclerosis patients. *MSJ* **2016**, *2*. [CrossRef]

127. Riepl, E.; Pfeuffer, S.; Ruck, T.; Lohmannt, H.; Wiendl, H.; Meuth, S.G.; Johnen, A. Alemtuzumab improves cognitive proccesing speed in active multiple sclerosis—A longitudinal observational study. *Front. Neurol.* **2018**, *8*, 730. [CrossRef] [PubMed]

128. Hauser, S.L.; Bar-Or, A.; Comi, G.; Giovannoni, G.; Hartung, H.-P.; Hemmer, B.; Lublin, F.; Montalban, X.; Rammohan, K.W.; Selmaj, K.; et al. Ocrelizumab versus Interferon Beta-1a in Relapsing Multiple Sclerosis. *N. Engl. J. Med.* **2017**, *376*, 221–234. [CrossRef] [PubMed]

129. Krupp, L.B.; Christodoulou, C.; Melville, P.; Scherl, W.F.; MacAllister, W.S.; Elkins, L.E. Donepezil improved memory in multiple sclerosis in a randomized clinical trial. *Neurology* **2004**, *63*, 1579–1585. [CrossRef] [PubMed]
130. Krupp, L.B.; Christodoulou, C.; Melville, P.; Scherl, W.F.; Pai, L.Y.; Muenz, L.R.; He, D.; Benedict, R.H.; Goodman, A.; Rizvi, S.; et al. Multicenter randomized clinical trial of donepezil for memory impairment in multiple sclerosis. *Neurology* **2011**, *76*, 1500–1507. [CrossRef] [PubMed]
131. Lovera, J.F.; Frohman, E.; Brown, T.; Bandari, D.; Nguyen, L.; Yadav, V.; Stuve, O.; Karman, J.; Bogardus, K.; Heimburger, G.; et al. Memantine for cognitive impairment in multiple sclerosis: A randomized placebo-controlled trial. *Mult. Scler.* **2010**, *16*, 715–723. [CrossRef] [PubMed]
132. Sumowski, J.F.; Chiaravalloti, N.; Erlanger, D.; Kaushik, T.; Benedict, R.H.B.; DeLuca, J. L-amphetamine improves memory in MS patients with objective memory impairment. *Mult. Scler.* **2011**, *17*, 1141–1145. [CrossRef] [PubMed]
133. Broicher, S.D.; Filli, L.; Geisseler, O.; Germann, N.; Zörner, B.; Brugger, P.; Linnebank, M. Positive effects of fampridine on cognition, fatigue and depression in patients with multiple sclerosis over 2 years. *J. Neurol.* **2018**, *265*, 1016–1025. [CrossRef] [PubMed]
134. Pavsic, K.; Pelicon, K.; Ledinek, A.H.; Sega, S. Short-term impact of fampridine on motor and cognitive functions, mood and quality of life among multiple sclerosis patients. *Clin. Neurol. Neurosurg.* **2015**, *139*, 35–40. [CrossRef] [PubMed]
135. Ford-Johnson, L.; DeLuca, J.; Zhang, J.; Elovic, E.; Lengenfelder, J.; Chiaravalloti, N.D. Cognitive effects of modafinil in patients with multiple sclerosis: A clinical trial. *Rehabil. Psychol.* **2016**, *61*, 82–91. [CrossRef]
136. Millera, E.; Morelc, A.; Redlickaa, J.; Millera, I.; Salukc, J. Pharmacological and Non-pharmacological Therapies of Cognitive Impairment in Multiple Sclerosis. *Curr. Neuropharmacol.* **2018**, *16*, 475–483. [CrossRef]
137. Chiaravalloti, N.D.; Moore, N.B.; Nikelshpur, O.M.; DeLuca, J. An RCT to treat learning impairment in multiple sclerosis: The MEMREHAB trial. *Neurology* **2013**, *81*, 2066–2072. [CrossRef] [PubMed]
138. Amato, M.P.; Goretti, B.; Viterbo, R.G.; Portaccio, E.; Niccolai, C.; Hakiki, B.; Iaffaldano, P.; Trojano, M. Computer-assisted rehabilitation of attention in patients with multiple sclerosis: Results of a randomized, double-blind trial. *Mult. Scler. J.* **2014**, *20*, 91–98. [CrossRef] [PubMed]
139. De Giglio, L.; De Luca, F.; Prosperini, L.; Borriello, G.; Bianchi, V.; Pantano, P.; Pozzilli, C. A low-cost cognitive rehabilitation with a commercial video game improves sustained attention and executive functions in multiple sclerosis: A pilot study. *Neurorehabil. Neural Repair.* **2015**, *29*, 453–461. [CrossRef] [PubMed]
140. Goverover, Y.; Chiaravalloti, N.D.; O'Brien, A.R.; DeLuca, J. Evidenced-Based Cognitive Rehabilitation for Persons with Multiple Sclerosis: An Updated Review of the Literature From 2007 to 2016. *Arch. Phys. Med. Rehabil.* **2018**, *99*, 390–407. [CrossRef]
141. Carter, A.; Daley, A.; Humphreys, L.; Snowdon, N.; Woodroofe, N.; Petty, J.; Roalfet, Al.; Tosh, J.; Sharrack, B.; Saxton, J. Pragmatic intervention for increasing self-directed exercise behaviour and improving important health outcomes in people with multiple sclerosis: A randomised controlled trial. *Mult. Scler.* **2014**, *20*, 1112–1122. [CrossRef]
142. Briken, S.; Gold, S.M.; Patra, S.; Vettorazzi, E.; Harbs, D.; Tallner, A.; Ketels, G.; Schulz, K.H.; Heesen, C. Effects of exercise on fitness and cognition in progressive MS: A randomized, controlled pilot trial. *Mult. Scler.* **2014**, *20*, 382–390. [CrossRef] [PubMed]
143. Sandroff, B.M.; Motl, R.W.; Scudder, M.R.; DeLuca, J. Systematic, Evidence-Based Review of Exercise, Physical Activity, and Physical Fitness Effects on Cognition in Persons with Multiple Sclerosis. *Neuropsychol. Rev.* **2016**, *26*, 271–294. [CrossRef]
144. Cramer, H.; Lauche, R.; Azizi, H.; Dobos, G. ; Langhorst J Yoga for Multiple Sclerosis: A Systematic Review and Meta-Analysis. *PLoS ONE* **2014**, *9*, e112414. [CrossRef]

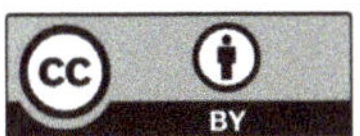

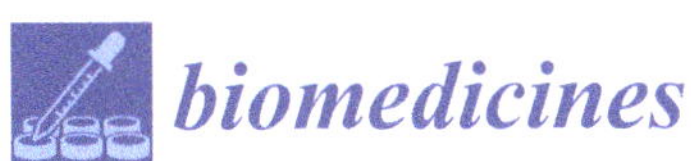 *biomedicines*

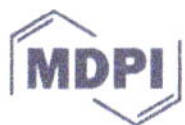

Review

Monoclonal Antibodies in Multiple Sclerosis: Present and Future

Natalia V. Voge and Enrique Alvarez *

Rocky Mountain Multiple Sclerosis Center at the University of Colorado, Department of Neurology, University of Colorado School of Medicine, Academic Office 1, Mail Stop B-185, 12631 East 17th Avenue, Aurora, CO 80045, USA; natalia.voge@ucdenver.edu
* Correspondence: Enrique.Alvarez@ucdenver.edu; Tel.: +1-(303)-724-2187

Received: 9 February 2019; Accepted: 11 March 2019; Published: 14 March 2019

Abstract: The global incidence of multiple sclerosis (MS) appears to be increasing. Although it may not be associated with a high mortality rate, this disease has a high morbidity rate which affects the quality of life of patients and reduces their ability to do their activities of daily living. Thankfully, the development of novel disease modifying therapies continues to increase. Monoclonal antibodies (MABs) have become a mainstay of MS treatment and they are likely to continue to be developed for the treatment of this disease. Specifically, MABs have proven to be some of the most efficacious treatments at reducing relapses and the inflammation in MS patients, including the first treatment for primary progressive MS and are being explored as reparative/remyelinating agents as well. These relatively new treatments will be reviewed here to help evaluate their efficacy, adverse events, immunogenicity, and benefit-risk ratios in the treatment of the diverse spectrum of MS. The focus will be on MABs that are currently approved or may be approved in the near future.

Keywords: monoclonal antibodies; anti-CD20; Ocrevus; Rituxan; Tysabri; multiple sclerosis; clinical trial; disease modifying therapy

---

1. Introduction

Monoclonal antibodies (MABs) are one of the preferred treatments for multiple sclerosis (MS) due to their target specificity and usually high efficacy [1]. These have usually targeted the immune system, which plays a key role in the pathogenesis of MS, especially during the early inflammatory stages. MABs bind very specifically to epitopes or parts of larger proteins (antigens) that allow them to mediate their effects on very specific pathways. In MS, MABs are able to more specifically neutralize key immune players that negatively impact the central nervous system. Because of their specificity, they tend to have few off target effects and less drug–drug interactions minimizing their side effects, which tend to arise from their downstream effects on the immune system and reactions to the drugs themselves, although this problem has been greatly reduced with the advent of humanized MABs [1,2].

Therapeutic MABs were originally developed from non-human species such as mice. The first MAB to be approved was muromonab-CD3 (Orthoclone OKT3) which targeted the CD3 surface protein of T lymphocytes to help prevent organ rejection in 1985 [3]. Reactions to murine MABs were soon associated with the development of antidrug antibodies (ADAs) against the murine-based protein with repeated exposures [4]. In order to reduce the potential immunogenicity of murine MABs, chimeric mouse-human antibodies were developed (Figure 1). This occurs by inserting the antigen-specific variable domain of a mouse antibody on the constant domains of a human antibody, producing antibodies that are up to 65% humanized [5,6]. Humanized antibodies that contain human light and heavy chains but retaining murine hypervariable regions being greater than 90% humanized will be developed. Transgenic mouse strains, which express human variable domains, have allowed the production of MABs with a reduced immunogenic potential, making them "fully humanized" and with properties similar to any human antibody [7]. These antibodies can be further modified to change their properties, for example by altering the glycosylation at amino acid N297 to increase their antigen-dependent cellular cytotoxicity (ADCC).

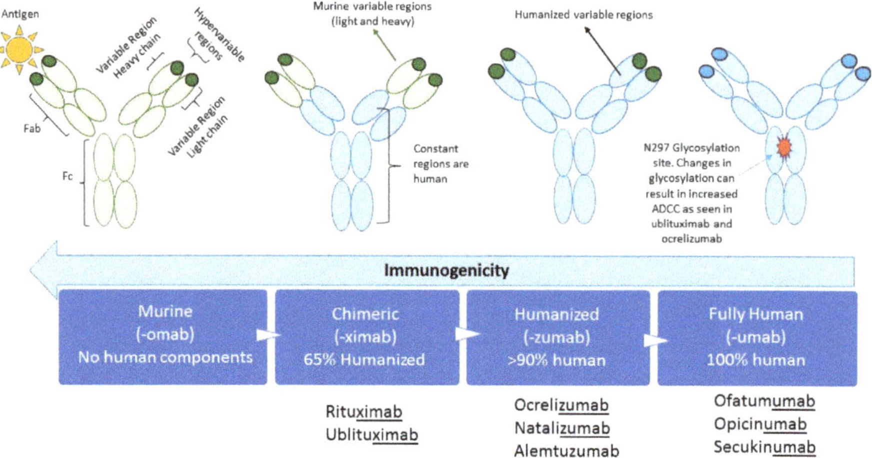

Figure 1. Bioengineering techniques have resulted in progressively more humanized antibodies. The figure shows the different fractions of the monoclonal antibodies and whether they represent mouse (green) or human (blue) sequences. As the sequences become more humanized their immunogenicity decreases. Glycosylation occurs at amino acid N297 and affects ADCC. Fragment antigen binding (Fab), Fragment crystallizable (Fc), Antigen-dependent cellular cytotoxicity (ADCC).

Natalizumab was the first MAB to be approved by the United States Food and Drug Administration (FDA) for the treatment of MS in 2004 [8], heralding the age of MABs for the treatment of MS. Other MABs have followed including alemtuzumab and ocrelizumab. Rituximab and ofatumumab have been used off label in the treatment of MS and ublituximab and ofatumumab are undergoing Phase III studies for approval in MS.

Opicinumab targets leucine-rich repeat and immunoglobulin domain-containing neurite outgrowth inhibitor receptor-interacting protein 1 (LINGO-1) [9], the remyelinating/reparative MAB that has been the most studied in MS. It has undergone phase II trials with mixed results and is currently being evaluated in another phase II study (AFFINITY). The MABs previously listed will be the focus of this review and other treatments completing phase II studies in MS can be found in Table 1; including some preliminary compounds in phase II such as Elezanumab, VAY736, and the HERV-W Env Antagonist GNbAC1.

In the past decade, several MABs were developed in an attempt to find a more efficacious and safe therapeutic option for MS patients; rigorous clinical trials have demonstrated lack of efficacy of as well as serious adverse events from some of them. For example, daclizumab (Zinbryta) [10] binds CD25, a subunit of the IL-2 receptor, was approved in 2016 for the treatment of MS, but was voluntarily withdrawn from the market due to reports of encephalitis in March 2018. Additionally, MABs that have been withdrawn or discontinued from further testing are listed in Table 2.

Table 1. Monoclonal antibodies currently on the market or being evaluated in phase II/III studies.

	Therapeutic Monoclonal Antibodies				
MAB	**Composition**	**Target**	**Mechanism of Action**	**Administration**	**FDA Approval Date for MS**
Alemtuzumab	Humanized MAB IgGk	CD52	ADCC	Intravenous	November 2014
Elezanumab [11]	Fully human MAB	RGMa	Binds and neutralizes RGMa which modulates T cell responses and dendritic cells in CNS lesions	Intravenous	N/A
GNbAC1 [12]	Humanized IgG4 MAB	Envelope protein of HERV-W MSRV	Targets the envelope protein of HERV-W MSRV, which may play a critical role in multiple sclerosis	Intravenous	N/A
Natalizumab	Humanized monoclonal IgG1	Cell adhesion molecule α4-integrin	Preventing lymphocyte transport across the blood brain barrier	Intravenous	November 2004 and reapproved on June 2006
Ocrelizumab	Humanized IgG1	Phosphorylated glycoprotein CD20 on B lymphocytes	ADCC > CDC	Intravenous	March 2017
Ofatumumab	Fully humanized IgG1	CD20	CDC > ADCC	Subcutaneous	N/A
Opicinumab	Humanized MAB	Targets LINGO-1	Allows OPCs to differentiate into mature OLG for remyelination	Intravenous	N/A
Ublituximab	Chimeric IgG1 MAB	CD20	CDC and ADCC	Intravenous	N/A
Rituximab	Chimeric (murine/human) MAB	CD20	CDC and ADCC	Intravenous	N/A
VAY736 [13]	Defucosylated, human IgG1 MAB	Targets the receptor for BAFF-R	ADCC and blockade of BAFF:BAFF-R signaling that drives B cell differentiation, proliferation and survival	Intravenous	N/A

Abbreviations: monoclonal antibody (MAB), multiple sclerosis (MS), not applicable (N/A), envelope protein (Env), human endogenous multiple sclerosis-associated retrovirus (HERV-W MSRV), cluster of differentiation (CD), complement-dependent cytotoxicity (CDC), antibody-dependent cellular cytotoxicity (ADCC), T helper (Th), Leucine-rich repeat and immunoglobulin domain-containing neurite outgrowth inhibitor receptor-interacting protein 1 (LINGO-1), oligodendrocyte precursor cells (OPCs), oligodendrocytes (OLGs), repulsive guidance molecule A (RGMa), B cell activating factor of the TNF family (BAFF-R).

Table 2. Examples of MAB therapies that have been discontinued from further clinical trials due to lack of efficacy or serious adverse events in the treatment of multiple sclerosis.

MAB	Composition	Target/Mechanism	Withdrawn
Atacicept [14]	Fully humanized recombinant fusion protein containing the extracellular ligand-binding portion of the human TACI receptor	Binds to the cytokines BLyS and APRIL, involved in B-cell differentiation, maturation, and survival.	Increases relapse rates in multiple sclerosis reflected on an increase in annualized relapse rates.
Daclizumab [15]	Humanized IgG1 MAB	CD25, which is attached to the Tac epitope on the alpha chain of CD25 (IL-2 receptor) on activated lymphocytes	Post-marketing vigilance helped to detect secondary autoimmune events, including inflammatory encephalitis in 12 patients worldwide leading to at least 3 deaths where an interaction with the drug could not be ruled out.
Muromonab [16]	Chimeric MAB, first MAB to ever be approved	Inhibition of CD3 receptor	High toxicity made it unlikely to be a preferred treatment for MS.
Secukinumab [17]	Humanized IgG1kappa MAB	IL-17 receptor, inhibits proinflammatory IL-17A	Discontinued due to the development of a fully-human anti IL-17 MAB with better potential
Tabalumab [18]	Selective and fully human IgG4 MAB	Neutralization of membrane-bound and soluble B-cell activating factor (BAFF)	Results from phase 2 clinical trials in patients with RMS, showed no evidence of reduction Gd-enhancing lesions versus placebo, further analysis were discontinued.
Ustekinumab [19]	Fully humanized IgG1 MAB	Targets subunit P40 on cytokines IL-12 and IL-23 preventing them from differentiating and activating Th1 cells	Discontinued after phase 2 trials for low/lack of efficacy.
Vatelizumab [20]	Fully humanized MAB that targets VLA-2, a collagen binding integrin expressed on activated lymphocytes	Preventing the crossing of inflammatory cells into the brain, reducing inflammation and tested on RMS	Primary efficacy endpoint was not met after phase 2a and 2b studies halting further development for MS.

Abbreviations: transmembrane activator and calcium modulator and cyclophilin-ligand interactor (TACI), B-lymphocyte stimulator, also known as TNFSF20 (BLyS), a proliferation-inducing ligand, also known as TNFSF13 (APRIL), monoclonal antibody (MAB), T activation (Tac), cluster of differentiation (CD), interleukin (IL-), B-cell activating factor (BAFF), relapsing multiple sclerosis (RMS), gadolinium (Gd), T helper (Th), very late antigen-2 (VLA-2; also known as integrin $\alpha 2\beta 1$).

Although the MABs have some of the best proven efficacy in the treatment of MS, side effects remain a concern for some providers and patients alike. Figure 2 shows how these MABs affect the pathophysiology of MS and their efficacy is described below for each MAB. The incomplete understanding of the immune system and how alterations to it can lead to infections, other autoimmune conditions, and possibly neoplasms is something that we will learn with experience, especially as we look to prescribe these treatments to our patients for many years. Additionally, the relatively unpredictable events secondary to MABs leading to immune reactions, including serum sickness and anaphylaxis, can be reduced by humanizing MABs as described above. Infusion-related reactions (IRRs) can be common and are more likely related to cytokine release syndrome (CRS) than to reactions to the MABs themselves. CRS can be a serious adverse event but is more common in conditions where the target lymphocytes are in high abundance. For example, CRS is much more common and severe in the treatment of B-cell lymphomas than in the treatment of MS with anti-CD20 MABs. CRS manifestations include a wide clinical spectrum, which can vary from mild flu-like symptoms, to life-threatening manifestations including progression to uncontrolled systemic inflammatory response, vascular leakage, disseminated intravascular coagulation and multi-organ system failure [21,22]. Although CRS or milder versions of it have the highest incidence during the first infusion, they can occur with later infusions as well. These IRRs tend to occur during or soon after the infusions. Even some of the fully humanized MABs can be immunogenic, causing anaphylaxis or serum sickness in later infusions [23]. Pretreatment with steroids, acetaminophen, and/or an antihistaminic prior to infusion can reduce IRRs and CRS and are often used prior to medications that cause lymphocyte destruction.

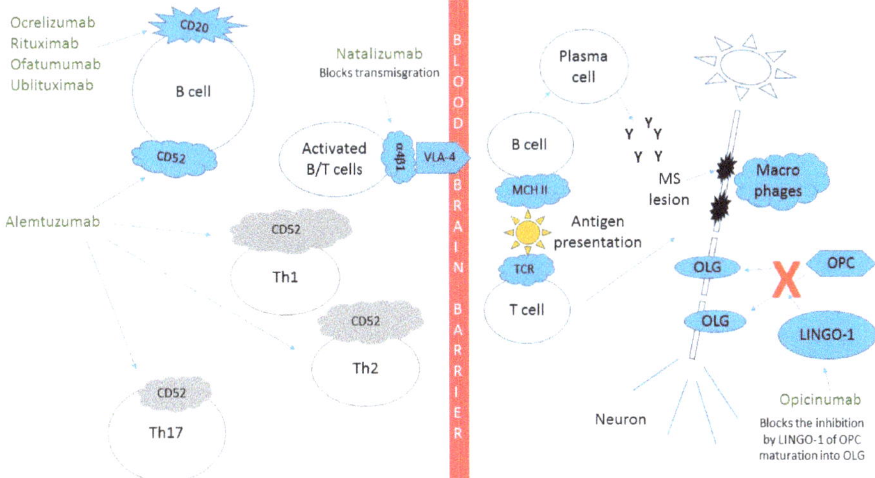

Figure 2. Mechanism of action of monoclonal antibodies in the treatment of multiple sclerosis. Ocrelizumab, rituximab, ofatumumab and ublituximab target CD20 expressing cells. Natalizumab targets transmigration of lymphocytes through the blood brain barrier. Alemtuzumab targets CD52 expressing cells. Opicinumab helps OPC differentiate into myelin producing OLGs. Cluster of differentiation (CD), T helper cells (Th), Leucine rich repeat and Immunoglobin-like domain-containing protein 1 (LINGO-1), oligodendrocyte (OLG), oligodendrocyte precursor cell (OPC).

Clinical evidence of continued disease activity, side effects, ease of administration, and costs are some of the aspects to consider when switching a patient to/from MAB therapies. Understanding the mechanism of action, how to monitor for adverse events and developing strategies for evaluating treatment failure are important tenants of personalized medicine and help to provide the safest treatment for patients with MS.

1.1. Natalizumab (Tysabri™)

Natalizumab was the first MAB approved by the FDA in 2004 for the treatment of MS (Table 1). Although it was temporarily withdrawn from the market due to cases of progressive multifocal leukoencephalopathy (PML), it was returned to the US market in 2006 after development of a risk evaluation and mitigation strategy (REMS) program to monitor the cases of PML [24] It is a recombinant humanized MAB to integrin α-4, which forms a heterodimer with β1. By binding the α4β1 integrin on the surface of activated inflammatory lymphocytes and monocytes, natalizumab blocks the interaction with VCAM-1 on endothelial cells preventing these inflammatory cells' entry into the central nervous system (Figure 2).

Natalizumab has shown great efficacy in the treatment of patients with MS. In the AFFIRM study, natalizumab reduced the annualized relapse rate (ARR) by 68% compared with placebo at one year, and with a significant reduction of 42% in the cumulative probability of sustained 3 months disability progression over two years [25]. Additionally, there was an 83% reduction in new or enlarging T2 lesions with a 92% reduction in contrast-enhancing lesions in the natalizumab group as compared to placebo.

Natalizumab is well tolerated at therapeutic doses with a very low rate of infusion reactions. It has been documented that anti-natalizumab neutralizing antibodies decrease free and cell-bound drug levels [26]. These develop and persist for at least 42 days after treatment in approximately 6% of natalizumab-treated patients [25,27]. Persistence of anti-natalizumab antibodies has been associated with reduced efficacy and increased incidence of IRRs [25,27].

The most serious adverse event consist of the brain infection PML caused by the John Cunningham virus (JCV). The risk of PML has been associated with prior chemotherapy and immunosuppressant use as well as amount of time on the drug. Additionally, a positive stratify JCV titer has been associated with higher risk of PML and this increases with higher titers. The index to assess PML risk consist in measurement of antibodies to JCV. Patients with a positive index have a higher risk of PML, which increases particularly in patients with an index >1.5 [24].

A routine monitoring strategy of the JCV titer should be part of the drug monitoring strategy for natalizumab (usually every 6 months) along with routine basic laboratories including a comprehensive metabolic panel and complete cell count with differential. In JCV seronegative patients, the benefits of natalizumab treatment still greatly outweigh the potential risks of PML [28,29] Clinical and neuroimaging follow-ups are recommended for disease activity monitoring and detection of side effects.

Other documented adverse events (AEs) with natalizumab include infections with herpes virus [27,30] and is contraindicated in patients that are severely immunocompromised. Melanoma risk may be higher in at risk-patients [31]. Liver injury can occur in patients with no previous history of liver disease, although rarely [32]. Hypereosinophilia may occur during treatment with this MAB [33].

1.2. Ocrelizumab (Ocrevus™)

Ocrelizumab is a cytotoxic recombinant humanized MAB that targets CD20 on circulating B-lymphocytes (Table 1, Figure 2). Ocrelizumab was the first anti-CD20 treatment approved for use in MS patients, although rituximab had been used off-label previously. In comparison to rituximab, ocrelizumab has a modified Fc region with enhanced ADCC [34]. As a humanized molecule, ocrelizumab is expected to be less immunogenic and might thus have fewer IRRs than rituximab [35]. Ocrelizumab reduces CD20 counts after infusion with a median time for B-cell counts to return to baseline of 72 weeks [36]. CD19 counts are often used instead of CD20 cell counts for monitoring these medications since both proteins are expressed in nearly the same cell populations and due to concerns that CD20 could be masked by a bound drug not allowing detection of cells but that did not lyse [36].

In relapsing MS, ocrelizumab showed efficacy superiority over interferon Beta-1a (IFN-β1a). The ARR was significantly reduced by 46% and 47% in the two OPERA studies [37]. Additionally, contrast enhancing lesions decreased by 94% and 95% and new or newly enlarging T2 lesions decreased by 77% and 83%. Confirmed disability progression at 12 weeks decreased by 40% in a pooled analysis of both studies.

In primary progressive MS, ocrelizumab reduced the confirmed disability progression at 12 weeks by 24% over placebo. T2-weighted lesion volume decreased by 3.4% in ocrelizumab-treated patients but increased 7.4% with a placebo. The brain volume loss in ocrelizumab-treated patients was 0.90% versus 1.09% with placebo ($p = 0.02$) [34].

Common adverse events include IRRs, which is the reason that premedication is recommended with methylprednisolone, acetaminophen and diphenhydramine. Although common, these are rarely serious. Additionally, nasopharyngitis (14.8%), upper respiratory tract infections (15.2%) [37], headache, and urinary tract infections have been seen in patients treated with ocrelizumab. An increased risk of neoplasms, particularly breast cancer were noted and will need to be studied more to understand if this was indeed related to ocrelizumab. It is recommended that vaccinations be administered at least six weeks prior to starting ocrelizumab, with avoidance of live or live attenuated vaccines during treatment [38,39]. Ocrelizumab is contraindicated in patients with active hepatitis B infections, thus patients should be screened prior to starting treatment. PML has been reported when transitioning from natalizumab or fingolimod, but should be regularly monitored for in patients on ocrelizumab long term [40]. Additionally, patients should have standardized monitoring during treatment with ocrelizumab, including immunoglobulin G levels, as these levels can decrease placing patients at increased risk of infection if their levels drop to very low levels [38].

1.3. Rituximab (Rituxan™)

Rituximab is a chimeric MAB that binds to CD20 and lyses B cells via complement-dependent cytotoxicity (CDC) and ADCC (Table 1) [1,41,42]. It achieves a >95% depletion of B cells, which is sustained at week 24. By 48 weeks, B cells remain at 30.7% of baseline [43]. After the initial infusion, a depletion of T cells is observed in CSF in addition to the expected decrease in B cells [41,44,45].

Rituximab, commonly prescribed off-label, is very effective in relapsing MS [43]. In the HERMES phase II study, patients in the rituximab group had a significant reduction in total number of contrast enhancing lesions over 24 weeks versus placebo (mean number 0.5 versus 5.5; relative reduction 91%). The proportion of patients in the rituximab group with relapses was decreased at week 24 (14.5% vs. 34.3%, $p = 0.02$) and week 48 (20.3% vs. 40.0%, $p = 0.04$) [43]. The OLYMPUS study in primary progressive MS failed to show a reduction in the confirmed progression of disability at 12 weeks, but did find a significant reduction of 48% in those aged <51 and of 59% in those with enhancing lesions at baseline [46].

Rituximab caused more IRRs within 24 h after the first infusion versus placebo [43]. Adverse reactions include serum sickness, PML, neutropenic fever, sinusitis, nasopharyngitis, upper respiratory infection, urinary tract infection, reactivation of hepatitis B virus, cardiac arrhythmias, cytopenias and malignancies, which have been associated with chronic B-cell depletion, among other less frequently reported [41,47]. Serious AEs were predominantly reported in patients >55 years of age [47]. The development of anti-chimeric neutralizing antibodies secondary to treatment with rituximab is reported in 26% of patients treated in progressive MS and in 37% in RRMS patients, which is partially the reason for the development of less immunogenic humanized MABs [48]. Recommended patient monitoring is similar to that with ocrelizumab.

1.4. Ofatumumab

Ofatumumab is currently being evaluated in phase 3 clinical trials for the treatment of relapsing MS (Table 1). Ofatumumab is a fully humanized MAB, which binds to the human CD20 antigen inducing B-cell lysis through ADCC and CDC. Its target epitope is located in a different cellular site than rituximab and ocrelizumab [49,50].

A small phase II study was completed which showed a reduction in new MRI lesions of 99% for all dose groups versus placebo by 24 weeks [50]. The MIRROR study, which compared ofatumumab to placebo in a phase IIB trial using subcutaneous dosing, showed a reduction in cumulative new gadolinium lesions of 65% for all dose groups when compared to placebo ($p < 0.001$). For all doses of >30 mg a reduction of >90% new brain lesions was seen over a 12 week period. The most common adverse event was injection related reactions at the first dose, which decreased in subsequent doses [49].

Observed adverse events included rash and urticaria, infusion reactions, pruritus, headaches, nasopharyngitis, hypersensitivity and dyspnea [50,51]. None of the patients developed human anti-human antibodies. Marginal changes in IgG, IgA, and IgM were observed [50]. Monitoring is similar to that with ocrelizumab.

1.5. Ublituximab

Ublituximab is a novel glycoengineered chimeric MAB antiCD20 therapy that is currently in phase III studies (ULTIMATE) (Table 1). Glycoenginering allows it to have enhanced affinity for Fc γ RIIIa receptors, eliciting increased ADCC. At week 4, a 99% B cell depletion was observed and maintained up to week 24 after treatment [52]. One particular benefit is that the infusion time duration is typically between 1 and 2 h.

Results from a phase II study with a median duration of 11 months, showed that ublituximab at week 24 has an ARR of 0.05 and a reduction in new T2 lesion volume of 7.67% compared to baseline. Additionally at week 24, 98% of participants were relapse free, no subjects had a contrast enhancing lesion, 84% did not have any new/enlarging T2 lesion, and 93% did not have confirmed disability progression at 24 weeks resulting in 76% of subjects meeting criteria for no evidence of disease activity [52].

No grade 3–4 AEs were observed, all IRRs reported were levels 1 and 2. Some adverse reactions reported include mild/moderate IRRs, fatigue, headache, numbness, common colds, dizziness, nausea/vomiting, and upper respiratory infection [52]. Monitoring is similar to that with ocrelizumab.

1.6. Alemtuzumab (Lemtrada™)

Alemtuzumab is a humanized anti-CD52 cytolytic MAB which targets the surface of lymphocytes and monocytes predominantly by ADCC. The repopulation of B cells occurs within 6 weeks of treatment, but T cells take longer to normalize at 9–12 months after a course of treatment [53,54]. This provides a long pharmacodynamic effect allowing the medication to be administered intravenously over two treatment courses. The first treatment consist of 12 mg/day on 5 consecutive days with the second on 3 consecutive days administered 12 months after the first treatment [53,54].

As a first line treatment, alemtuzumab in CARE-MS 1 showed an ARR of 54%, a non-significant reduction in sustained accumulation of disability, a 17% reduction in new or enlarging T2 lesion, a 63% reduction in contrast enhancing lesions, and a 42% reduction in brain parenchymal atrophy compared with IFN-β1a [53]. In CARE-MS 2, alemtuzumab showed an ARR of 50%, a non-significant reduction in sustained accumulation of disability, a 32% reduction in new or enlarging T2 lesion, a 61% reduction in contrast enhancing lesions, and a non-significant reduction in brain parenchymal atrophy compared with IFN-β1a [54]. Over 5 years, it lowered the risk of sustained accumulation of disability by 72% compared with IFN-β1a ($p < 0.0001$) and reduced the number of relapses by 69% over IFN-β1a ($p < 0.0001$) [54]. Both studies were performed in a non-blinded fashion, meaning patients knew if they were under the experimental arm of the trial and being prescribed this MAB. This approach was adopted due to the severity of the IRRs, nonetheless, blinded neurologists performed the efficacy assessments [55].

Adverse events have created the need for a REMS program. For example, recently the FDA issued a warning about elevated risk of stroke and artery damage, for this reason a black box label was added to the U.S. product label [56]. Patients can develop other autoimmune conditions such as thyroid disease (40.7%) [57], as well as immune thrombocytopenia, autoimmune hemolytic anemia, and anti-glomerular basement membrane disease [53,54]. Additionally, there has been an increased risk of malignancies such as thyroid cancer, melanoma, and lymphoproliferative disorders. IRRs are also common (>90%) [53,58], including rare cases of serum sickness and anaphylaxis. Over time, infections (>71%) can also occur including nasopharyngitis, urinary tract infections, upper respiratory tract infections, herpes viral infection, and fungal infections [59]. The monitoring labs that constitute the REMS program include complete blood count with differential, serum creatinine, urinalysis with microscopy, which should be performed monthly, and thyroid function tests, which should be done every 3 months, until 48 months after the last infusion [60].

1.7. Opicinumab

It is encouraging to see new MABs being developed for repair/remyelination of lesions in MS patients. Opicinumab is a fully humanized MAB that targets LINGO-1. By inhibiting LINGO-1, oligodendrocyte precursor cells (OPCs) can differentiate into mature oligodendrocytes (OLCs) and allow for remyelination of damaged plaques (Table 1, Figure 2) [9,38,61].

Opicinumab was evaluated in a phase II study (RENEW) as an add-on in patients with optic neuritis where it did not differ significantly in remyelination rates when compared to placebo at week 24. However, there was a small improvement of 9.1 milliseconds on full field visual evoked responses in the per protocol analysis that was not significant in the intention to treat analysis [9]. Subgroup analysis showed an improvement for baseline age ≥33 years of −14.17 milliseconds suggesting a greater benefit in older patients [62].

Another phase II study (SYNERGY) evaluated the efficacy of coadministration of opicinumab with IFN-β1a. The primary end point was the percentage of patients with an improvement over at least 3 months on a multicomponent endpoint comprising the expanded disability status scale, timed 25 foot walk, 9-hole peg test, and a 3-s paced auditory serial addition test. The percentage of improvement was 51.6% for placebo, 51.1% for 3 mg/kg opicinumab, 65.6% for 10 mg/kg, 68.8% for 30 mg/kg, and 41.2% for 100 mg/kg. In summary, there was an increased percentage of remyelination with opicinumab at 10 and 30 mg/kg when compared to placebo [63]. An additional study is underway (AFFINITY), which looks at patients that did better in SYNERGY, and includes those with disease activity of less than 21 years and that meet certain criteria on magnetization transfer ratio and diffusion tensor imaging on magnetic resonance scans.

Opicinumab has been well tolerated, adverse events have been similarly reported among groups treated with opicinumab and placebo [62,63]. However, some mild hypersensitivity reactions have been reported [61].

2. New Horizons and Future Trends for Therapeutic Monoclonal Antibodies

MABs have become a mainstay of MS treatment and they are likely to continue to be developed and optimized for the treatment of this disease, such as analyzing the safety of faster infusion times and administration by subcutaneous routes. MABs are some of the most effective therapies for relapsing MS without the side effects associated with chemotherapeutic agents. Additionally, new MABS are being developed to help repair the damage/disability that has already occurred, which is promising. New advancements in bioengineering are being incorporated to antibodies that are more humanized to help optimize their effectiveness and improve their tolerability and safety. The newer MABs that are being developed (Table 1) are based on lessons learned from past studies and drug development programs of drugs that have already been approved (Table 1) or stopped (Table 2). Overall, it is expected that MABs will continue to be a preferred therapy for MS in the foreseeable future.

Author Contributions: N.V.V. and E.A. designed and wrote this paper.

Funding: This research received no external funding.

Conflicts of Interest: E.A. consulted for Biogen, Celgene, EMD Serono, Genzyme, Genentech, Novartis, and TG pharmaceuticals, received research funding from Acorda, Biogen, Genentech, Novartis, and Rocky Mountain MS Center. N.V.V., nothing to disclose.

References

1. Wootla, B.; Watzlawik, J.O.; Stavropoulos, N.; Wittenberg, N.J.; Dasari, H.; Abdelrahim, M.A.; Henley, J.R.; Oh, S.H.; Warrington, A.E.; Rodriguez, M. Recent Advances in Monoclonal Antibody Therapies for Multiple Sclerosis. *Expert Opin. Biol. Ther.* **2016**, *16*, 827–839. [CrossRef] [PubMed]
2. Steinman, L.; Carlson, C.M. Monoclonal Antibody Therapy in Multiple Sclerosis. *Pract. Neurol.* **2018**, 28–31.
3. Smith, S.L. Ten years of Orthoclone OKT3 (muromonab-CD3): A review. *J. Transpl. Coord.* **1996**, *6*, 109–121. [CrossRef] [PubMed]
4. Ober, R.J.; Radu, C.G.; Ghetie, V.; Ward, E.S. Differences in promiscuity for antibody-FcRn interactions across species: Implications for therapeutic antibodies. *Int. Immunol.* **2001**, *13*, 1551–1559. [CrossRef] [PubMed]
5. Buss, N.A.; Henderson, S.J.; McFarlane, M.; Shenton, J.M.; de Haan, L. Monoclonal antibody therapeutics: History and future. *Curr. Opin. Pharmacol.* **2012**, *12*, 615–622. [CrossRef] [PubMed]
6. Morrison, S.L.; Johnson, M.J.; Herzenberg, L.A.; Oi, V.T. Chimeric human antibody molecules: Mouse antigen-binding domains with human constant region domains. *Proc. Natl. Acad. Sci. USA* **1984**, *81*, 6851–6855. [CrossRef]
7. Lonberg, N. Fully human antibodies from transgenic mouse and phage display platforms. *Curr. Opin. Immunol.* **2008**, *20*, 450–459. [CrossRef]
8. Yaldizli, Ö.; Putzki, N. Natalizumab in the treatment of multiple sclerosis. *Ther. Adv. Neurol. Disord.* **2009**, *2*, 115–128. [CrossRef]
9. Cadavid, D.; Balcer, L.; Galetta, S.; Aktas, O.; Ziemssen, T.; Vanopdenbosch, L.; Frederiksen, J.; Skeen, M.; Jaffe, G.J.; Butzkueven, H.; et al. Safety and efficacy of opicinumab in acute optic neuritis (RENEW): A randomised, placebo-controlled, phase 2 trial. *Lancet Neurol.* **2017**, *16*, 189–199. [CrossRef]
10. Giovannoni, G.; Gold, R.; Selmaj, K.; Havrdova, E.; Montalban, X.; Radue, E.W.; Stefoski, D.; McNeill, M.; Amaravadi, L.; Sweetser, M.; et al. Daclizumab high-yield process in relapsing-remitting multiple sclerosis (selection): A multicentre, randomised, double-blind extension trial. *Lancet Neurol.* **2014**, *13*, 472–481. [CrossRef]
11. Cree, B.; Rosebraugh, M.; Barger, B.; Ziemann, A. A Phase 1, Multiple-Dose Study of Elezanumab (ABT-555) in Patients with Relapsing Forms of Multiple Sclerosis. In Proceedings of the European Committee for Treatment and Research in Multiple Sclerosis Conference, Berlin, Germay, 11 October 2018.
12. Curtin, F.; Perron, H.; Kromminga, A.; Porchet, H.; Lang, A.B. Preclinical and early clinical development of gnbac1, a humanized igg4 monoclonal antibody targeting endogenous retroviral msrv-env protein. *MAbs* **2015**, *7*, 265–275. [CrossRef] [PubMed]
13. Dörner, T.; Posch, M.; Wagner, F.; Hüser, A.; Fischer, T.; Mooney, L.; Petricoul, O.; Maguire, P.; Pal, P.; Doucet, J.; et al. THU0313 Double-Blind, Randomized Study of VAY736 Single Dose Treatment in Patients with Primary Sjögren's Syndrome (PSS). *Ann. Rheum. Dis.* **2016**, *75*, 300–301. [CrossRef]
14. Bible, E. Multiple sclerosis: Atacicept increases relapse rates in multiple sclerosis. *Nat. Rev. Neurol.* **2014**, *10*, 182. [CrossRef]
15. EMA Recommends Immediate Suspension and Recall of Multiple Sclerosis Medicine Zinbryta. Available online: https://www.ema.europa.eu/en/news/ema-recommends-immediate-suspension-recall-multiple-sclerosis-medicine-zinbryta (accessed on 12 March 2019).
16. Weinshenker, B.G.; Bass, B.; Karlik, S.; Ebers, G.C.; Rice, G.P. An open trial of OKT3 in patients with multiple sclerosis. *Neurology* **1991**, *41*, 1047–1052. [CrossRef]
17. Havrdová, E.; Belova, A.; Goloborodko, A.; Tisserant, A.; Wright, A.; Wallstroem, E.; Garren, H.; Maguire, R.P.; Johns, D.R. Activity of secukinumab, an anti-IL-17A antibody, on brain lesions in RRMS: Results from a randomized, proof-of-concept study. *J. Neurol.* **2016**, *263*, 1287–1295. [CrossRef]
18. Silk, M.; Nantz, E. Efficacy and Safety of Tabalumab in Patients with Relapsing-Remitting Multiple Sclerosis: A Randomized, Double-Blind, Placebo-Controlled Study (P3.397). *Neurology* **2018**, *90*.
19. Segal, B.M.; Constantinescu, C.S.; Raychaudhuri, A.; Kim, L.; Fidelus-Gort, R.; Kasper, L.H.; Ustekinumab, M.S.I. Repeated subcutaneous injections of IL12/23 p40 neutralising antibody, ustekinumab, in patients with relapsing-remitting multiple sclerosis: A phase II, double-blind, placebo-controlled, randomised, dose-ranging study. *Lancet Neurol.* **2008**, *7*, 796–804. [CrossRef]
20. Vatelizumab. Available online: https://multiplesclerosisnewstoday.com/vatelizumab-gbr-500 (accessed on 1 February 2019).

21. Wing, M.G.; Moreau, T.; Greenwood, J.; Smith, R.M.; Hale, G.; Isaacs, J.; Waldmann, H.; Lachmann, P.J.; Compston, A. Mechanism of first-dose cytokine-release syndrome by CAMPATH 1-H: Involvement of CD16 (FcgammaRIII) and CD11a/CD18 (LFA-1) on NK cells. *J. Clin. Investig.* **1996**, *98*, 2819–2826. [CrossRef]

22. Klinger, M.; Brandl, C.; Zugmaier, G.; Hijazi, Y.; Bargou, R.C.; Topp, M.S.; Gokbuget, N.; Neumann, S.; Goebeler, M.; Viardot, A.; et al. Immunopharmacologic response of patients with B-lineage acute lymphoblastic leukemia to continuous infusion of T cell-engaging CD19/CD3-bispecific BiTE antibody blinatumomab. *Blood* **2012**, *119*, 6226–6233. [CrossRef]

23. Del Boccio, P.; Rossi, C.; di Ioia, M.; Cicalini, I.; Sacchetta, P.; Pieragostino, D. Integration of metabolomics and proteomics in multiple sclerosis: From biomarkers discovery to personalized medicine. *Proteom. Clin. Appl.* **2016**, *10*, 470–484. [CrossRef]

24. McGuigan, C.; Craner, M.; Guadagno, J.; Kapoor, R.; Mazibrada, G.; Molyneux, P.; Nicholas, R.; Palace, J.; Pearson, O.R.; Rog, D.; et al. Stratification and monitoring of natalizumab-associated progressive multifocal leukoencephalopathy risk: Recommendations from an expert group. *J. Neurol. Neurosurg. Psychiatry* **2016**, *87*, 117–125. [CrossRef] [PubMed]

25. Polman, C.H.; O'Connor, P.W.; Havrdova, E.; Hutchinson, M.; Kappos, L.; Miller, D.H.; Phillips, J.T.; Lublin, F.D.; Giovannoni, G.; Wajgt, A.; et al. A randomized, placebo-controlled trial of natalizumab for relapsing multiple sclerosis. *N. Engl. J. Med.* **2006**, *354*, 899–910. [CrossRef] [PubMed]

26. Sehr, T.; Proschmann, U.; Thomas, K.; Marggraf, M.; Straube, E.; Reichmann, H.; Chan, A.; Ziemssen, T. New insights into the pharmacokinetics and pharmacodynamics of natalizumab treatment for patients with multiple sclerosis, obtained from clinical and in vitro studies. *J. Neuroinflamm.* **2016**, *13*, 164. [CrossRef]

27. Rudick, R.A.; Stuart, W.H.; Calabresi, P.A.; Confavreux, C.; Galetta, S.L.; Radue, E.W.; Lublin, F.D.; Weinstock-Guttman, B.; Wynn, D.R.; Lynn, F.; et al. Natalizumab plus interferon beta-1a for relapsing multiple sclerosis. *N. Engl. J. Med.* **2006**, *354*, 911–923. [CrossRef]

28. Walker, A.; Watson, C.; Alexopoulos, S.T.; Deniz, B.; Arnold, R.; Bates, D. A benefit–risk analysis of natalizumab in the treatment of patients with multiple sclerosis when considering the risk of progressive multifocal leukoencephalopathy. *Curr. Med. Res. Opin.* **2014**, *30*, 629–635. [CrossRef]

29. Thompson, J.P.; Noyes, K.; Dorsey, E.R.; Schwid, S.R.; Holloway, R.G. Quantitative risk-benefit analysis of natalizumab. *Neurology* **2008**, *71*, 357–364. [CrossRef]

30. Bloomgren, G.; Richman, S.; Hotermans, C.; Subramanyam, M.; Goelz, S.; Natarajan, A.; Lee, S.; Plavina, T.; Scanlon, J.V.; Sandrock, A.; et al. Risk of natalizumab-associated progressive multifocal leukoencephalopathy. *N. Engl. J. Med.* **2012**, *366*, 1870–1880. [CrossRef] [PubMed]

31. Mullen, J.T.; Vartanian, T.K.; Atkins, M.B. Melanoma Complicating Treatment with Natalizumab for Multiple Sclerosis. *N. Engl. J. Med.* **2008**, *358*, 647–648. [CrossRef] [PubMed]

32. Bezabeh, S.; Flowers, C.M.; Kortepeter, C.; Avigan, M. Clinically significant liver injury in patients treated with natalizumab. *Aliment. Pharmacol. Ther.* **2010**, *31*, 1028–1035. [CrossRef] [PubMed]

33. Abbas, M.; Lalive, P.H.; Chofflon, M.; Simon, H.-U.; Chizzolini, C.; Ribi, C. Hypereosinophilia in patients with multiple sclerosis treated with natalizumab. *Neurology* **2011**, *77*, 1561–1564. [CrossRef]

34. Montalban, X.; Hauser, S.L.; Kappos, L.; Arnold, D.L.; Bar-Or, A.; Comi, G.; de Seze, J.; Giovannoni, G.; Hartung, H.P.; Hemmer, B.; et al. Ocrelizumab versus Placebo in Primary Progressive Multiple Sclerosis. *N. Engl. J. Med.* **2017**, *376*, 209–220. [CrossRef] [PubMed]

35. Sorensen, P.S.; Blinkenberg, M. The potential role for ocrelizumab in the treatment of multiple sclerosis: Current evidence and future prospects. *Ther. Adv. Neurol. Disord.* **2016**, *9*, 44–52. [CrossRef] [PubMed]

36. Pasic, I.; Lipton, J.H. Current approach to the treatment of chronic myeloid leukaemia. *Leuk. Res.* **2017**, *55*, 65–78. [CrossRef] [PubMed]

37. Hauser, S.L.; Bar-Or, A.; Comi, G.; Giovannoni, G.; Hartung, H.-P.; Hemmer, B.; Lublin, F.; Montalban, X.; Rammohan, K.W.; Selmaj, K.; et al. Ocrelizumab versus Interferon Beta-1a in Relapsing Multiple Sclerosis. *N. Engl. J. Med.* **2017**, *376*, 221–234. [CrossRef] [PubMed]

38. Calabresi, P.A. B-Cell Depletion—A Frontier in Monoclonal Antibodies for Multiple Sclerosis. *N. Engl. J. Med.* **2017**, *376*, 280–282. [CrossRef] [PubMed]

39. Kappos, L.; Li, D.; Calabresi, P.A.; O'Connor, P.; Bar-Or, A.; Barkhof, F.; Yin, M.; Leppert, D.; Glanzman, R.; Tinbergen, J.; et al. Ocrelizumab in relapsing-remitting multiple sclerosis: A phase 2, randomised, placebo-controlled, multicentre trial. *Lancet* **2011**, *378*, 1779–1787. [CrossRef]

40. Diem, L.; Nedeltchev, K.; Kahles, T.; Achtnichts, L.; Findling, O. Long-term evaluation of NEDA-3 status in relapsing-remitting multiple sclerosis patients after switching from natalizumab to fingolimod. *Ther. Adv. Neurol. Disord.* **2018**, *11*. [CrossRef] [PubMed]

41. He, D.; Guo, R.; Zhang, F.; Zhang, C.; Dong, S.; Zhou, H. Rituximab for relapsing-remitting multiple sclerosis. *Cochrane Database Syst. Rev.* **2013**. [CrossRef] [PubMed]

42. Di Gaetano, N.; Cittera, E.; Nota, R.; Vecchi, A.; Grieco, V.; Scanziani, E.; Botto, M.; Introna, M.; Golay, J. Complement Activation Determines the Therapeutic Activity of Rituximab In Vivo. *J. Immunol.* **2003**, *171*, 1581–1587. [CrossRef]

43. Hauser, S.L.; Waubant, E.; Arnold, D.L.; Vollmer, T.; Antel, J.; Fox, R.J.; Bar-Or, A.; Panzara, M.; Sarkar, N.; Agarwal, S.; et al. B-cell depletion with rituximab in relapsing-remitting multiple sclerosis. *N. Engl. J. Med.* **2008**, *358*, 676–688. [CrossRef]

44. Bar-Or, A.; Calabresi, P.A.; Arnold, D.; Markowitz, C.; Shafer, S.; Kasper, L.H.; Waubant, E.; Gazda, S.; Fox, R.J.; Panzara, M.; et al. Rituximab in relapsing-remitting multiple sclerosis: A 72-week, open-label, phase I trial. *Ann. Neurol.* **2008**, *63*, 395–400. [CrossRef] [PubMed]

45. Cross, A.H.; Stark, J.L.; Lauber, J.; Ramsbottom, M.J.; Lyons, J.A. Rituximab reduces B cells and T cells in cerebrospinal fluid of multiple sclerosis patients. *J. Neuroimmunol.* **2006**, *180*, 63–70. [CrossRef] [PubMed]

46. Hawker, K.; O'Connor, P.; Freedman, M.S.; Calabresi, P.A.; Antel, J.; Simon, J.; Hauser, S.; Waubant, E.; Vollmer, T.; Panitch, H.; et al. Rituximab in patients with primary progressive multiple sclerosis: Results of a randomized double-blind placebo-controlled multicenter trial. *Ann. Neurol.* **2009**, *66*, 460–471. [CrossRef]

47. Memon, A.B.; Javed, A.; Caon, C.; Srivastawa, S.; Bao, F.; Bernitsas, E.; Chorostecki, J.; Tselis, A.; Seraji-Bozorgzad, N.; Khan, O. Long-term safety of rituximab induced peripheral B-cell depletion in autoimmune neurological diseases. *PLoS ONE* **2018**, *13*, e0190425. [CrossRef] [PubMed]

48. Dunn, N.; Juto, A.; Ryner, M.; Manouchehrinia, A.; Piccoli, L.; Fink, K.; Piehl, F.; Fogdell-Hahn, A. Rituximab in multiple sclerosis: Frequency and clinical relevance of anti-drug antibodies. *Mult. Scler. J.* **2018**, *24*, 1224–1233. [CrossRef]

49. Bar-Or, A.; Grove, R.A.; Austin, D.J.; Tolson, J.M.; VanMeter, S.A.; Lewis, E.W.; Derosier, F.J.; Lopez, M.C.; Kavanagh, S.T.; Miller, A.E.; et al. Subcutaneous ofatumumab in patients with relapsing-remitting multiple sclerosis: The MIRROR study. *Neurology* **2018**, *90*, e1805–e1814. [CrossRef] [PubMed]

50. Sorensen, P.S.; Lisby, S.; Grove, R.; Derosier, F.; Shackelford, S.; Havrdova, E.; Drulovic, J.; Filippi, M. Safety and efficacy of ofatumumab in relapsing-remitting multiple sclerosis: A phase 2 study. *Neurology* **2014**, *82*, 573–581. [CrossRef]

51. Kurrasch, R.; Brown, J.C.; Chu, M.; Craigen, J.; Overend, P.; Patel, B.; Wolfe, S.; Chang, D.J. Subcutaneously administered ofatumumab in rheumatoid arthritis: A phase I/II study of safety, tolerability, pharmacokinetics, and pharmacodynamics. *J. Rheumatol.* **2013**, *40*, 1089–1096. [CrossRef] [PubMed]

52. Inglese, M.; Petracca, M.; Cocozza, S.; Wray, S.; Racke, M.; Shubin, R.; Twyman, C.; Eubanks, J.L.; Mok, K.; Weiss, M.; Fox, E. Final MRI results at 6 months from a Phase 2 Multicenter Study of Ublituximab, A Novel Glycoengineered Anti-CD20 Monoclonal Antibody, In Patients With Relapsing Forms of Multiple Sclerosis (RMS), Demonstrates Complete Elimination of Gd-Enhancing Lesions. In Proceedings of the AAN Enterprises, Los Angeles, CA, USA, 21–27 April 2018.

53. Cohen, J.A.; Coles, A.J.; Arnold, D.L.; Confavreux, C.; Fox, E.J.; Hartung, H.P.; Havrdova, E.; Selmaj, K.W.; Weiner, H.L.; Fisher, E.; et al. Alemtuzumab versus interferon beta 1a as first-line treatment for patients with relapsing-remitting multiple sclerosis: A randomised controlled phase 3 trial. *Lancet* **2012**, *380*, 1819–1828. [CrossRef]

54. Coles, A.J.; Twyman, C.L.; Arnold, D.L.; Cohen, J.A.; Confavreux, C.; Fox, E.J.; Hartung, H.P.; Havrdova, E.; Selmaj, K.W.; Weiner, H.L.; et al. Alemtuzumab for patients with relapsing multiple sclerosis after disease-modifying therapy: A randomised controlled phase 3 trial. *Lancet* **2012**, *380*, 1829–1839. [CrossRef]

55. Coles, A.J.; Compston, A. Product licences for alemtuzumab and multiple sclerosis. *Lancet* **2014**, *383*, 867–868. [CrossRef]

56. FDA. FDA Warns about Rare but Serious Risks of Stroke and Blood Vessel Wall Tears with Multiple Sclerosis Drug Lemtrada (Alemtuzumab). Available online: https://www.fda.gov/Drugs/DrugSafety/ucm624247.htm (accessed on 3 July 2019).

57. Decallonne, B.; Bartholome, E.; Delvaux, V.; D'Haeseleer, M.; El Sankari, S.; Seeldrayers, P.; Van Wijmeersch, B.; Daumerie, C. Thyroid disorders in alemtuzumab-treated multiple sclerosis patients: A Belgian consensus on diagnosis and management. *Acta Neurol. Belg.* **2018**, *118*, 153–159. [CrossRef] [PubMed]

58. LaCasce, A.S.; Castells, M.C.; Burstein, H.J.; Meyerhardt, J.A. Infusion-Related Reactions to Therapeutic Monoclonal Antibodies Used for Cancer Therapy. Available online: https://www.uptodate.com/contents/infusion-related-reactions-to-therapeutic-monoclonal-antibodies-used-for-cancer-therapy (accessed on 6 February 2019).

59. Daniels, G.H.; Vladic, A.; Brinar, V.; Zavalishin, I.; Valente, W.; Oyuela, P.; Palmer, J.; Margolin, D.H.; Hollenstein, J. Alemtuzumab-related thyroid dysfunction in a phase 2 trial of patients with relapsing-remitting multiple sclerosis. *J. Clin. Endocrinol. Metab.* **2014**, *99*, 80–89. [CrossRef] [PubMed]

60. Van Den Neste, E.; Cazin, B.; Janssens, A.; Gonzalez-Barca, E.; Terol, M.J.; Levy, V.; Perez de Oteyza, J.; Zachee, P.; Saunders, A.; de Frias, M.; et al. Acadesine for patients with relapsed/refractory chronic lymphocytic leukemia (cll): A multicenter phase i/ii study. *Cancer Chemother. Pharmacol.* **2013**, *71*, 581–591. [CrossRef]

61. McCroskery, P.; Selmaj, K.; Fernandez, O.; Grimaldi, L.M.E.; Silber, E.; Pardo, G.; Freedman, S.M.; Zhang, Y.; Xu, L.; Cadavid, D.; et al. Safety and Tolerability of Opicinumab in Relapsing Multiple Sclerosis: The Phase 2b SYNERGY Trial (P5.369). *Neurology* **2017**, *88*.

62. Cadavid, D.; Balcer, L.; Galetta, S.; Aktas, O.; Ziemssen, T.; Vanopdenbosch, L.J.; Leocani, L.; Freedman, M.S.; Plant, G.T.; Preiningerova, J.L.; et al. Predictors of response to opicinumab in acute optic neuritis. *Ann. Clin. Transl. Neurol.* **2018**, *5*, 1154–1162. [CrossRef] [PubMed]

63. Mellion, M.; Edwards, K.R.; Hupperts, R.; Drulović, J.; Montalban, X.; Hartung, H.-P.; Brochet, B.; Calabresi, P.A.; Rudick, R.; Ibrahim, A.; et al. Efficacy Results from the Phase 2b SYNERGY Study: Treatment of Disabling Multiple Sclerosis with the Anti-LINGO-1 Monoclonal Antibody Opicinumab (S33.004). *Neurology* **2017**, *88*, S33.004.

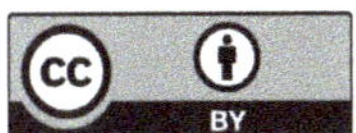

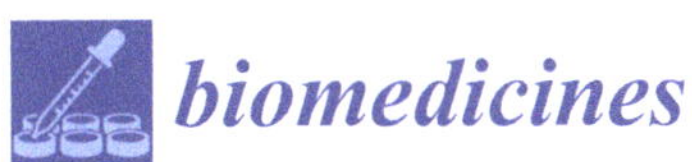 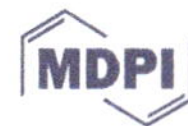

Review

Daclizumab: Mechanisms of Action, Therapeutic Efficacy, Adverse Events and Its Uncovering the Potential Role of Innate Immune System Recruitment as a Treatment Strategy for Relapsing Multiple Sclerosis

Stanley L. Cohan [1,*], **Elisabeth B. Lucassen** [1], **Meghan C. Romba** [1] **and Stefanie N. Linch** [2]

[1]   Providence Multiple Sclerosis Center, Providence Brain and Spine Institute, Portland, OR 97225, USA; elisabeth.lucassen@providence.org (E.B.L.); meghan.romba@providence.org (M.C.R.)

[2]   Providence Health and Services, Regional Research Department, Portland, OR 97213, USA; stefanie.linch@providence.org

*   Correspondence: Stanley.Cohan@Providence.org; Tel.: +1-503-216-1150

Received: 22 January 2019; Accepted: 6 March 2019; Published: 11 March 2019

Abstract: Daclizumab (DAC) is a humanized, monoclonal antibody that blocks CD25, a critical element of the high-affinity interleukin-2 receptor (IL-2R). DAC HYP blockade of CD25 inhibits effector T cell activation, regulatory T cell expansion and survival, and activation-induced T-cell apoptosis. Because CD25 blockade reduces IL-2 consumption by effector T cells, it increases IL-2 bioavailability allowing for greater interaction with the intermediate-affinity IL-2R, and therefore drives the expansion of CD56^{bright} natural killer (NK) cells. Furthermore, there appears to be a direct correlation between CD56^{bright} NK cell expansion and DAC HYP efficacy in reducing relapses and MRI evidence of disease activity in patients with RMS in phase II and phase III double-blind, placebo- and active comparator-controlled trials. Therapeutic efficacy was maintained during open-label extension studies. However, treatment was associated with an increased risk of rare adverse events, including cutaneous inflammation, autoimmune hepatitis, central nervous system Drug Reaction with Eosinophilia Systemic Symptoms (DRESS) syndrome, and autoimmune Glial Fibrillary Acidic Protein (GFAP) alpha immunoglobulin-associated encephalitis. As a result, DAC HYP was removed from clinical use in 2018. The lingering importance of DAC is that its use led to a deeper understanding of the underappreciated role of innate immunity in the potential treatment of autoimmune disease.

Keywords: daclizumab; relapsing multiple sclerosis; CD25; innate immune system; interleukin-2; drug reaction with eosinophilia systemic symptoms; DRESS; autoimmunity

---

1. Introduction

Daclizumab (DAC) is a humanized monoclonal antibody that blocks CD25, the α-subunit of the high-affinity interleukin-2 receptor (IL-2R-HA). DAC was initially developed as an intravenous therapy (Zenapax, Hoffman-LaRoche, Nutley, New Jersey) to prevent transplant organ rejection and to treat T cell leukemia and severe uveitis [1–4]. Subcutaneous DAC, often referred to as DAC High Yield Process (DAC HYP; Zinbryta, Biogen, Cambridge MA and AbbVie, Chicago II), demonstrated efficacy in reducing both clinical and MRI measures of disease activity in patients with relapsing forms of multiple sclerosis (RMS) and was approved to treat RMS in 2016 [5–8]. Unfortunately, secondary autoimmune disease directed primarily against the central nervous system (CNS), liver, and skin resulted in serious adverse events (SAE) leading to its withdrawal in 2018. However, investigations of its mechanisms of therapeutic action and immunomodulatory activity have revealed insights into heretofore underappreciated relationships between innate and adaptive immunity in autoimmune diseases, particularly RMS. Future exploitation of these relationships may provide further therapeutic opportunities. This review will discuss known and proposed, direct and indirect effects of DAC HYP upon the immune system and how these effects are potentially related to its therapeutic impact in RMS. To better appreciate the multiple mechanisms by which DAC may impact autoimmunity, a brief description of the major immune system components that it is believed to affect, and the downstream impact of those actions, will be reviewed.

2. Immunologic Background for DAC Efficacy

2.1. IL-2 and IL-2R Signaling

IL-2 is a trophic cytokine expressed predominantly by activated T cells, which occurs upon cognate antigen recognition by the T cell receptor. While IL-2 promotes proliferation and survival of both activated effector and naïve T cells, it also promotes the expansion of regulatory T cells (T_{reg} cells), and some authors have reported that IL-2 activation may also promote apoptosis of antigen-activated T cells, thereby contributing to the maintenance of immune homeostasis [9–15]. Although most IL-2 is produced by activated T cells, it is also produced by myeloid dendritic cells (mDC) and macrophages [16,17].

IL-2 activity is primarily mediated through binding to the IL-2 high-affinity receptor (IL-2R-HA), which, in addition to IL-2, is comprised of three subunits: the α-subunit (CD25), the β-subunit (CD122), and the common γ-chain subunit (CD132), as shown in Figure 1. CD122 and CD132 can also combine to form an intermediate-affinity IL-2R (IL-2R-IA). CD132 is expressed on all lymphoid cells, whereas CD122 is constitutively expressed on natural killer (NK) and CD8 memory T cells, and can be induced on naïve T cells following antigen recognition. CD25 expression is much more tightly restricted; it is absent on naïve and memory cells, but is induced following antigen activation [17,18]. Furthermore, CD25 is constitutively expressed at very high levels on T_{reg} cells and is vital for the development and peripheral maintenance of the T_{reg} cell population [19]. It is also expressed on mDC, which may assist in T cell activation by using CD25 to "trans-present" IL-2 to a CD25-deficient IL-2R expressed on recently activated T cells, thus converting it to the IL-2R-HA [20].

Although both CD122 and CD132 are constitutively expressed on lymphocytes, IL-2 must be bound to CD25 to recruit these subunits to form the IL-2R-HA complex [21,22]. While IL-2 can also bind and signal through the IL-2R-IA, receptor affinity increases 1000-fold following its association with CD25 [18]. Furthermore, in the absence of CD25, the IL-2R-IA requires up to 50 times the IL-2 available at basal physiological states [23]. IL-2 bound to the IL-2R-HA results in rapid internalization and degradation of the high-affinity receptor complex. This latter step, terminating IL-2-induced T cell activation via the intracellular domain of CD122, may be initiated by activation of the intracellular domain of the CD132 portion of the IL-2R, thereby regulating IL-2 effects [24–26]. Subsequently, CD25 can be recycled back to the surface of the cell for future engagement with CD122, CD132, and IL-2 [27,28].

2.2. Innate Lymphoid Cells (ILC)

Innate lymphoid cells (ILC) arise from a hematopoietic CD34$^+$ cell line, which is considered the common progenitor for all ILC [29]. Multiple subsets of ILC have been identified, of which several are relevant to the potential immunoregulatory actions of DAC: group 1, which includes ILC1 and CD56^{bright} NK cells; group 2, comprised of ILC2, to which we will return later; and group 3, which includes ILC3 and pro-inflammatory lymphoid tissue inducer (LTi) cells [30–33]. NK cells constitutively express CD122 and CD132. Notably, CD56^{bright} NK cells have 10-fold greater expression of CD122 relative to the pro-inflammatory CD56^{dim} NK cells [34]. IL-2 stimulation of the IL-2R-IA has been reported to drive ILC toward anti-inflammatory CD56^{bright} NK cell production, possibly at the expense of the pro-inflammatory LTi cell pathway [11,35,36].

There is considerable evidence to support a role for CD56[bright] NK cells in auto-regulation and tolerance. CD56[bright] NK cells can destroy activated immune cells through direct contact, including autologous antigen-activated CD4[+] and CD8[+] T cells, which play a critical role in autoimmune responses [34,37,38]. In support of this concept, reduced CD56[bright] NK cell cytotoxicity was observed in patients with MS as early as the 1980s [39–42]. Subsequently, investigators demonstrated that CD56[bright] NK cells are directly cytotoxic to auto-antigen-specific T cells [34,38]. Of note and expanded upon below, there is a strong correlation between DAC-induced up-regulation of CD56[bright] NK cells and the therapeutic efficacy of DAC HYP in RMS [34,43,44].

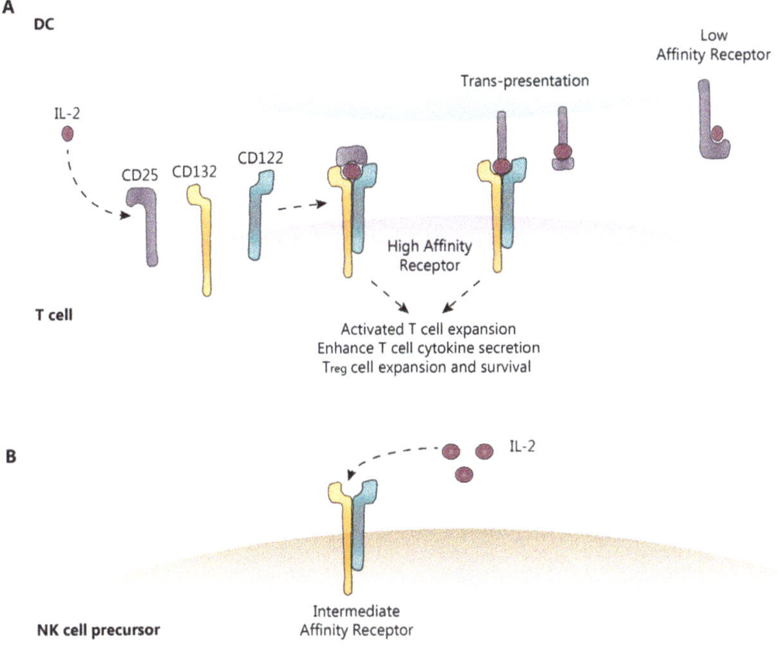

Figure 1. IL-2 receptor (IL-2R) subunits. (**A**) CD25 (α-subunit) is the low-affinity IL-2R and is expressed on activated T cells, T_reg cells, and mDC. Once IL-2 is bound to CD25 on the cell surface, CD132 (γ) and CD122 (β) are recruited to form the high-affinity IL-2R. CD132 and CD122 are the only subunits capable of intracellular signaling. (**B**) Other cell types such as NK cells express the intermediate-affinity IL-2R, comprised of CD132 and CD122 only. This receptor requires elevated levels of IL-2 for signaling, such as those found in a local draining lymph node, due to reduced binding affinity for IL-2. DC-dendritic cell; IL-2-interleukin-2; NK-natural killer. Dotted lines show the sequence of events following IL-2 binding to its receptor.

3. DAC Mechanisms of Action: Known and Proposed

DAC reversibly binds to CD25, preventing the interaction of IL-2 with the IL-2R-HA, leaving more IL-2 available to induce IL-2R-IA signaling. As noted above, the IL-2R requires CD25 to render it high-affinity. By blocking the formation of IL-2R-HA, DAC blocks IL-2 consumption by activated effector T cells, causing a moderate decrease in the frequency of CD4[+] and CD8[+] T cells in the periphery and increasing the availability of IL-2 to interact with the IL-2R-IA [34,37,43,45]. As might be expected with a reduction in IL-2 consumption, IL-2 concentrations in the serum were elevated following DAC treatment by approximately 50% [46]. Because expansion of T_reg cells is dependent upon IL-2 interaction with the IL-2R-HA, as predicted, DAC treatment also resulted in a 50–60% decrease in peripheral T_{reg} cells [37,46–48], as shown in Figure 2. By blocking the IL-2R-HA, DAC may also potentially prevent activation-induced T cell apoptosis, paradoxically inhibiting auto-regulation by allowing the survival of activated effector T cells recognizing "self" antigens [10,11]. DAC HYP administration has also been reported to normalize previously elevated intrathecal CD4+, CD8+ and HLA-DR-expressing CD4+ T cells and B cells in patients with RMS [35]. In some patients, the effect of DAC on effector T and T_{reg} cells may not be adequately compensated for by CD56[bright] NK cell expansion, as is observed in patients with spontaneously occurring autoimmunity due to genetic variants that delete CD25 [49,50]. These resultant autoimmunity-promoting circumstances may also explain, in part, the paradoxical increase risk of autoimmune adverse events (AE) observed in some DAC HYP-treated RMS patients (see below).

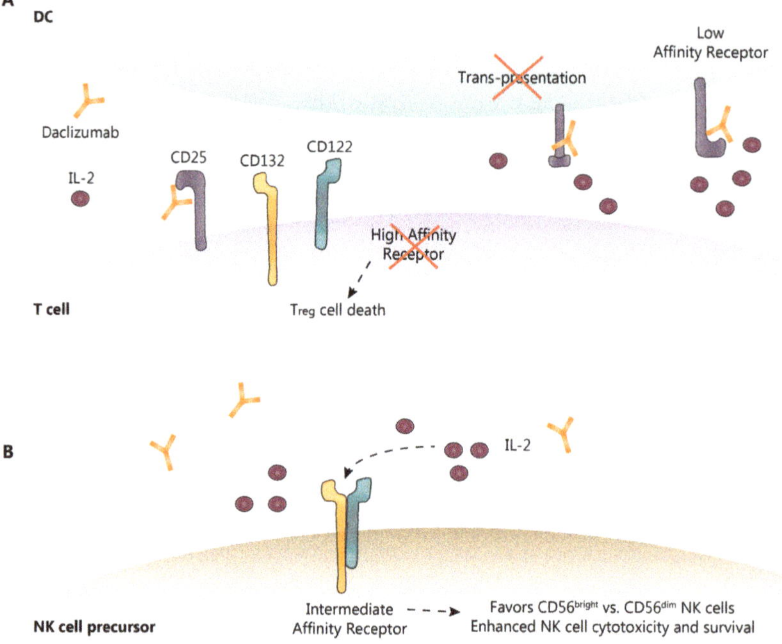

Figure 2. Known and proposed DAC mechanisms of action. (**A**) DAC binds to CD25 blocking its association with CD132 and CD122. This prevents trans-presentation of CD25 from mDC to T cells and ultimately results in effector T cell and T_{reg} cell death; (**B**) As a result of CD25 blockade, serum IL-2 levels are elevated allowing for NK cell activation through the intermediate-affinity receptor, CD132 and CD122, and promoting CD56[bright] NK cell cytotoxicity and survival. DC-dendritic cell; IL-2-interleukin-2; NK-natural killer. Dotted lines show the sequence of events following IL-2 binding to its receptor.

Although part of the anti-inflammatory activity of DAC is through selective inhibition of IL-2-driven effector T cell activation and expansion, it is evident that this does not entirely account for its therapeutic efficacy [37]. Innate immune components also play an essential role in auto-tolerance and autoimmunity. As mentioned above, CD56[bright] NK cells from multiple sclerosis patients exhibit reduced cytotoxicity. This is important because CD56[bright] NK cells are believed to be directly cytotoxic to auto-antigen activated T cells [34,38]. CD56[bright] NK cells also express high levels of cell surface IL-2R-IA, and IL-2 activation of the IL-2R-IA through DAC resulted in CD56[bright] NK cell expansion, which was abolished by IL-2 inhibition [37]. IL-2 may also enhance CD56^{bright} NK cell maturation and reduce NK cell death, and further increase NK cell cytotoxicity, through enhanced killing efficiency [37,51] as shown in Figure 2. In prospective clinical studies, DAC HYP treatment resulted in an expansion of CD56^{bright} NK cells in up to 90% of DAC HYP-treated patients, with a 5-fold elevation of CD56^{bright} NK cell counts seen by 52 weeks of treatment that was sustained thereafter [44]. By blocking consumption of IL-2 by the IL-2R-HA, IL-2 levels increase systemically, thereby increasing the bioavailability of IL-2 to interact with the IL-2R-IA and preferentially promoting the expansion of anti-inflammatory CD56^{bright} NK cells via CD122 intracellular signaling [52].

It has also been reported that DAC reduces the expansion of pro-inflammatory LTi, as shown in Figure 3 [34]. By orienting the innate CD34^{+} progenitor cell line away from the pro-inflammatory LTi cell line, DAC may indirectly reduce the formation or activity of meningeal lymphoid follicle-like structures, which have been observed overlying cortical areas of demyelination [53–55]. Consistent with this concept, DAC HYP administration reportedly normalized previously elevated LTi cell numbers in the spinal fluid of patients with RMS [35]. One study found that the total number of ILC was reduced in DAC HYP-treated patients; however, this remains controversial and has not been replicated by subsequent research [31,35,36,56,57].

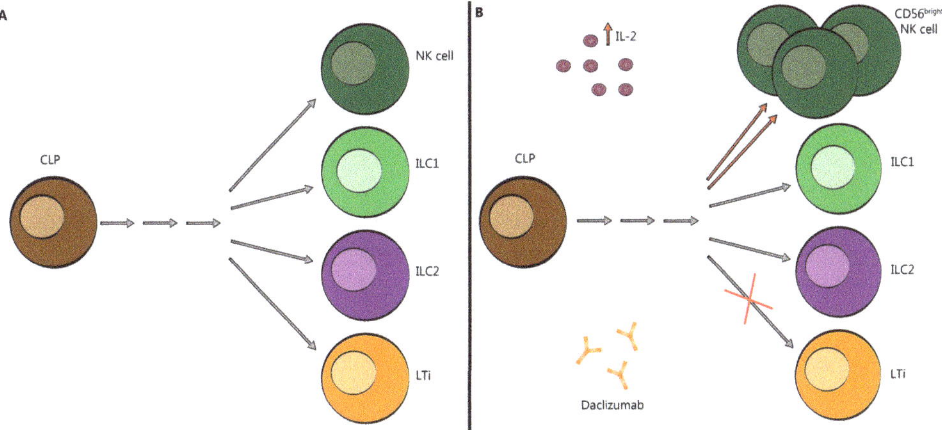

Figure 3. Innate Lymphoid Cells skewed toward CD56^{bright} NK cells following DAC treatment. (**A**) DAC binds to CD25 blocking association with CD132 and CD122. This prevents trans-presentation of CD25 from mDC to T cells and results in effector T cell and T$_{reg}$ cell death. (**B**) As a result of CD25 blockade, serum IL-2 levels are elevated allowing for NK cell activation through the intermediate-affinity receptor, CD132 and CD122, and promoting CD56^{bright} NK cell cytotoxicity and survival (red arrows). It may also redirect the commitment of LTi cells (red ×). CLP-common lymphoid progenitor; NK-natural killer; ILC-innate lymphoid cell; LTi-lymphoid tissue-inducer cell; IL-2-interleukin-2. Grey arrows indicate a series of differentiation steps not depicted in this figure.

Because CD25 is also expressed on mDC, which may use CD25 to "trans-present" IL-2 to CD25-deficient T cells, it is possible that may block mDC potentiation of IL-2R-HA signaling on effector T cells, as shown in Figure 2a [20]. There is also some preclinical evidence to suggest that the modulation of cytokine production by mDC may also be a target of DAC therapy [58]. Further research is needed to confirm these reported effects of DAC on mDC.

In summary, activated effector T cell expansion is dependent upon IL-2 interaction with IL-2R-HA expressed on the cell surface. To perform as a high-affinity receptor, the IL-2R requires CD25, which is blocked by DAC, reducing IL-2 utilization by T cells. This drives IL-2 towards IL-2R-IA and CD56^{bright} NK cell expansion, which destroy activated effector T cells by direct contact. As will become evident from the paragraphs that follow, there is a direct correlation between the DAC-induced decrease in activated effector T cells and CD56^{bright} NK cell expansion with both clinical and MRI efficacy of DAC. However, there is also a reduction in T$_{reg}$ cells, and possibly a decrease in activated T cell apoptosis, both of which may paradoxically promote the up-regulation of heightened autoimmunity, leading to SAE which will be discussed further below.

4. Pharmacokinetics and Pharmacodynamics of DAC HYP

Initial studies of DAC HYP in healthy adult subjects (ages 18–65) showed that the maximum serum concentration (C$_{max}$) was 7 days while the t$^{1/2}$ of elimination was 24 days [59]. In a subsequent study in adults with RMS, C$_{max}$ was achieved in 5–7 days, and the t$^{1/2}$ of elimination was approximately 21 days after the last injection [60]. Maximum CD25 saturation by DAC HYP was reached by 7 h and was sustained as long as DAC HYP serum concentration was 5.0 mcg/mL or higher. Baseline CD25 saturation was achieved in approximately 24 weeks following DAC HYP discontinuation, in parallel with a serum DAC HYP concentration of 1.0 mcg/mL or less. During treatment with DAC HYP (150 mg every 4 weeks), maximum CD56^{bright} NK cell level is reached by approximately 36 weeks, achieving a maximum 5-fold increase over baseline [47]. For patients treated with 300 mg DAC HYP, the changes in NK cell and T$_{reg}$ frequency were nearly identical; no other results were reported separately for this group [47].

Several other studies examined various immune parameters in pooled DAC HYP-treated patients (150 mg and 300 mg) from the SELECT, SELECTION, and DECIDE trials. Following DAC HYP cessation, in both 150 mg DAC HYP alone and pooled (150 mg and 300 mg) DAC HYP groups CD56^{bright} NK cells return to pre-treatment levels by 24 weeks after the last injection. In parallel with increased CD56^{bright} NK cells, serum IL-2 levels increased by roughly 50% within 4 weeks of DAC HYP treatment and T$_{reg}$ cell counts fell by 50–60% within 4 days of a 150 mg DAC HYP injection and returned to pre-treatment levels approximately 20 weeks after the last DAC HYP injection [34,44,46,47]. CD4$^+$ and CD8$^+$ T lymphocyte counts were decreased by 7–10% after 52 weeks and by 15–18% after 96 weeks of DAC HYP treatment [7]. Importantly, there was also a roughly 25% decrease in HLA-DR2-expressing activated effector CD4$^+$ T cells, in DAC HYP treatment in patients with RMS in both the 150 mg and 300 mg groups similarly [61]. This coincides with the timing of maximum inflammatory lesion reductions observed in the CHOICE study and provides further evidence of the down-regulation of the pro-inflammatory activity of DAC HYP [5].

5. DAC Efficacy: Controlled Clinical Trial Data

As noted in the section on mechanisms of action, DAC administration expands immunoregulatory CD56^{bright} natural killer cells, reduces whole blood and intrathecal pro-inflammatory T cells and T$_{reg}$ cells. Based on its immunologic effects, subcutaneous use of DAC HYP was approved by the United States Food and Drug Administration for RMS in May 2016 and the European Medicines Agency (EMA) in July 2016 [62].

Several small open-label studies evaluating intravenous DAC in RMS demonstrated improvement in several outcome measures [43,63,64]. Due to cell-mediated toxicities reported with intravenous DAC preparations, it was subsequently reformulated to DAC HYP, facilitating subcutaneous administration [59]. CHOICE was a randomized phase II double-blind, placebo-controlled trial in which DAC HYP was an add-on therapy to interferon beta (IFNβ) versus placebo plus IFNβ. CHOICE demonstrated that DAC HYP administered at 2 mg/kg with IFNβ resulted in a 72% decrease in the number of contrast-enhancing lesions relative to IFNβ with placebo ($p = 0.004$) [5], as shown in Table 1.

Table 1. Selected Clinical and MRI Outcomes of DAC HYP Treatment in RMS Controlled Trials.

	CHOICE		SELECT			Clinical Trials SELECTION			DECIDE	
	DAC [1]	pl	150 mg	300 mg	pl	Continuous [2]	Switch [3]	Washout [4]	DAC	IFNβ
Parameters										
ARR	0.27	0.41	0.21	0.23	0.46	0.165	0.179 ****	0.302	0.22	0.39
Risk Reduction, %	34		54 ****	50 ***					45 ***	
PPRF, %	52	55	81 ****	80 ***	64	86.4	82.4 ****	75.9	67	51
CDP, %										
12 weeks	NR	NR	6*	8	13	7	8 ****	10	16	20
24 weeks	NR	NR	NR	NR	NR	NR	NR	NR	13 *	18
New Gd+	1.32 **	4.75	0.3 ****	0.2 ****	1.4	0.2	0.2 ****	0.2	0.4 ***	1.0
Reduction, %	72		79	86			NR	NR	NR	60	
T2 Lesions										
New/enlarging	1.1 **	3.4	2.4 ****	1.7 ****	8.1	1.2	2.1 ****	3.3	4.3	9.4
Reduction, %	68		70	79					54 ***	
Volume change, %	ND		−11.1 ****	−12.5 ****	−27.3	−6.9	−8.1 ****	−3.1	0.2 ***	8.6
Brain Volume, % change	NR	NR	−0.79	−0.70	−0.74	−0.536	−0.830	−0.551	−0.559 ***	−0.585 ***
NEDA%	NR	NR	NR	NR	NR	NR	NR	NR	13 ***	22

DAC—daclizumab; HYP—high-yield process; pl—placebo; RMS—relapsing forms of multiple sclerosis; ARR—annualized relapse rate; CDP—confirmed disability progression; PPRF—proportion of patients relapse-free; Gd+—gadolinium-enhancing lesions; IFNβ—interferon beta-1a; NR—not reported; ND—no difference. [1] Data reported are for patients receiving high-dose DAC (2 mg/kg); both DAC and placebo received IFNβ; [2] Continuous-patients receiving DAC HYP 150 or 300 mg every 4 weeks during SELECT continued their same dose of DAC HYP through additional 52 weeks of SELECTION; [3] Switch-patients receiving placebo during SELECT were placed on either 150 or 300 mg DAC HYP for the 52 weeks of SELECTION; [4] Washout-patients receiving either 150 or 300 mg of DAC HYP during SELECT were placed on placebo for 20 weeks followed by resumption of their previous dose of DAC HYP administered during SELECT; **** $p < 0.0001$; *** $p < 0.001$; ** $p < 0.01$; * $p < 0.05$.

DAC HYP was subsequently studied in two large, pivotal phase III clinical trials in patients with RMS; a 52-week placebo-controlled trial (SELECT) and an active comparator trial (DECIDE) of DAC HYP versus IFNβ. The primary endpoint of the SELECT and DECIDE trials was the annualized relapse rate (ARR). Secondary and tertiary outcomes measured include: impact on 3 month confirmed disability progression, T2 lesion burden and gadolinium-enhancing (Gd$^+$) lesions, safety, measurement of markers of immune activity; and in DECIDE, changes in cognitive status and patient-reported outcomes [6,7,65].

5.1. SELECT

In SELECT, patients with RMS were randomized 1:1:1 to subcutaneous DAC HYP 150 mg, DAC HYP 300 mg, or placebo every four weeks for 52 weeks. The primary endpoint was met with a 54% relative reduction in ARR (95% CI 33–68%; $p < 0.0001$) in the group treated with DAC HYP 150 mg (ARR 0.21) and 50% reduction (95% CI 28–65%; $p < 0.0001$) in those treated with DAC HYP 300 mg (ARR 0.23) in comparison to placebo (ARR 0.46). At 52 weeks, the three-month sustained disability progression decreased by 57% in the DAC HYP 150 mg group and 43% in the DAC HYP 300 mg group compared to placebo [7], as shown in Table 1.

Subcutaneous DAC HYP also demonstrated effects on brain MRI measures in SELECT. There was a statistically significant relative decrease in the number of Gd$^+$ lesions ($p < 0.0001$) at week 52, with a 69% reduction in the DAC HYP 150 mg group versus 78% reduction in the DAC HYP 300 mg group compared to placebo. The number of new/newly enlarging T2 hyperintense lesions were also significantly reduced at week 52 ($p < 0.0001$) in the 150 mg group by 70% versus 79% in the 300 mg group compared to placebo [7], as shown in Table 1. The mean percentage of brain volume loss was not significantly different between the treatment arms in SELECT. Exploratory studies performed in SELECT demonstrated a strong correlation between early increases in CD56^{bright}NK cells and decrease in new and enlarging T2 lesions at 24 and 52 weeks of DAC HYP treatment, and DAC HYP patients in the highest CD56bright NK cell quartile had 62% fewer new and enlarging T2 lesions than those in the lowest quartile [44].

5.2. SELECTION

SELECTION was a double-blind extension of SELECT, designed to further assess the risks of AE associated with prolonged DAC HYP therapy (52 weeks), the impact of discontinuing DAC HYP, and to determine if early efficacy was sustained. Placebo-treated patients in SELECT were randomized 1:1 to initiate either 150 mg or 300 mg DAC HYP subcutaneously every four weeks ("Switch" in Table 1). The patients who received DAC HYP during SELECT either continued the same medication dose through SELECTION for a total of 104 weeks of continuous therapy, or underwent a blinded, placebo-treated washout that lasted for a total of 20 weeks, followed by resumption of their prior DAC HYP dose for the remaining 32 weeks of their participation in SELECTION [8]. Therapeutic efficacy achieved by DAC HYP therapy in SELECT was measured by: ARR, proportion of patients experiencing a relapse (PPRF), 12-week confirmed disability worsening, number of new Gd$^+$ lesions, number of new and enlarging T2 lesions, volume of T2 lesions, mean and total T1 lesion volume was sustained by week 52 of SELECTION (104 weeks of total DAC HYP therapy).

For patients treated with placebo in SELECT, treatment with DAC HYP during SELECTION resulted in a statistically significant decrease in ARR, the proportion of patients having relapses, the number of Gd$^+$ enhancing lesions, new and enlarging T2, and the volume of T2 lesions. No significant differences were observed in T1 lesion measurements or whole brain volume, as shown in Table 1. For DAC HYP-treated patients in SELECT who underwent the 20-week washout period in SELECTION, clinical and MRI end-points were similar after 52 weeks in SELECTION to those patients who received DAC HYP for the entire 52 weeks in SELECTION, as shown in Table 1. By the end of the washout period, CD56^{bright} NK counts had returned to baseline values, but at the conclusion of SELECTION (32 weeks of DAC HYP treatment), CD56^{bright} NK numbers were similar to those found in patients who had been continuously treated with DAC HYP through the 104 weeks of SELECT and SELECTION.

5.3. DECIDE

DECIDE was a double-blind and double-dummy, active-comparator, phase III study, and compared efficacy in patients with RMS, randomized 1:1 to either subcutaneous DAC HYP 150 mg every four weeks plus weekly intramuscular placebo, or to IFNβ (30 µg, intramuscularly) once weekly, and placebo subcutaneously every four weeks, for up to 144 weeks [6]. The primary end point was met with a 45% reduction in annualized relapse rate (ARR 0.22) in the DAC HYP treated group compared to the IFNβ group (ARR 0.32) $p < 0.001$. The DAC HYP group also demonstrated a significant reduction in the annualized rate of severe relapses (38% reduction, $p = 0.002$). The number of patients who remained relapse-free at week 144 was 67% in the DAC HYP group and 51% in the IFNβ group. Three-month confirmed disability progression measured at week 144 revealed a 16% relative risk reduction in the DAC HYP cohort compared to IFNβ, which did not reach statistical significance. However, the risk of 24-week confirmed disability worsening demonstrated DAC HYP significantly reduced disability worsening by 27% compared to IFNβ ($p = 0.03$)

There was a 75% relative decrease ($p < 0.001$) in new Gd$^+$ lesions and a 54% relative reduction ($p < 0.001$) in the number of new or newly enlarged T2 hyperintense brain MRI lesions over a 96-week period in patients treated with DAC HYP compared to IFNβ ($p < 0.001$). There was also a statistically significant decrease in brain volume loss in DAC HYP versus IFNβ treated patients after two years of treatment ($p < 0.01$). No evidence of disease activity (NEDA) over 96 weeks, as measured by no relapses, no disability progression, no new/enlarged T2 or Gd$^+$ lesions, was seen in 22% of DAC HYP and 13% of IFNβ-treated patients ($p < 0.001$).

Investigators also observed a 7–10% drop in total CD4$^+$ and CD8$^+$ T lymphocyte counts over 52 weeks in the DAC HYP treated group in SELECT versus 15–18% over 96 weeks among the DAC HYP treated group in the DECIDE trial. The ratio of CD4$^+$ to CD8$^+$ T cells remained stable in the DAC HYP group in both SELECT and DECIDE. No correlation was found between the reduced CD4$^+$ and CD8$^+$ T cells and the infection rate in the DECIDE trial [6].

A tertiary outcome in DECIDE was the assessment of cognitive outcomes, as measured by changes in the orally administered Symbol Digit Modalities Test (SDMT). At 96 weeks, there was a significantly greater ($p = 0.0274$) improvement from baseline SDMT in DAC HYP-treated patients compared to IFNβ treated patients [65]. Furthermore, a significantly greater number of DAC HYP-treated patients experienced clinically meaningful improvement ($p = 0.0366$) and a significantly smaller number of patients experienced a clinically-meaningful decline ($p = 0.0103$) in their SDMT scores.

5.4. SELECTED

SELECTED was a single-armed open-label extension trial of DAC HYP 150 mg, for which any patient completing SELECT and SELECTION qualified [66]. Although the primary outcomes dealt with AE (see below), adjusted ARR was calculated every six months from the time the patient received their first dose of DAC HYP dose in either SELECT or SELECTION up to 144 weeks; changes in the number of new/enlarging T2 lesions and brain volume (percentage) compared to baseline, were obtained on yearly MRI scans. ARR varied from 0.21 in patients having received DAC HYP for 0–24 weeks and gradually declined to 0.15 in patients receiving DAC HYP for 121–144 weeks. The adjusted mean number of new/enlarging T2 lesions was 1.96 after year 1, 1.62 at year 2 and 1.26 at year 3. The annualized median decrease in brain volume from the first dose of DAC HYP was 0.77 at year 1, 0.57 at year 2, and 0.32 at year 3. As in all single arm open-label studies, efficacy outcomes may have been affected by selection bias arising from dropout of poor responders, and subjects with AE.

5.5. Patient-Reported Outcomes

The DAC HYP treatment groups in both SELECT and DECIDE demonstrated significant benefits in patient-reported outcomes, when utilizing the 29-item Multiple Sclerosis Impact Scale (MSIS-29), which evaluates the impact of MS on physical (PHYS) and psychological health (psychological impact scale), as well as EuroQol 5-Dimensions (EQ-5D), which is used to examine overall health status using five domains. In SELECT, there was a significant improvement in MSIS-29 PHYS score at week 52 in the subcutaneous DAC HYP 150 mg compared with placebo ($p = 0.00082$), but not with the DAC HYP 300 mg group. There was also a statistically significant benefit for subcutaneous DAC HYP 150 mg for EQ-5D index ($p = 0.0091$) compared to placebo in SELECT.

In DECIDE, DAC HYP 150mg treated patients showed a greater improvement compared to IFNβ at 96 weeks in regards to MSIS-29 PHYS ($p < 0.001$), MSIS-29 psychological impact scale ($p = 0.04$), and EQ-5D index ($p = 0.005$). Clinically meaningful worsening was defined as an increase in $\geq$7.5 points in the patient-reported outcomes at 96 weeks. As measured by MSIS-29 physical subscale, worsening was 19% in the DAC HYP group versus 23% in the interferon IFNβ group (NS). DECIDE also demonstrated a greater improvement in Multiple Sclerosis Functional Composite (MSFC) at 96 weeks in patients treated with DAC HYP compared to IFNβ in DECIDE ($p < 0.001$) [6].

6. Adverse Events with DAC: Prospective Clinical Trial Data

6.1. SELECT

In the randomized, double-blind, placebo-controlled SELECT trial, SAE excluding relapse was similar between groups, as shown in Table 2. Nine (2%) patients treated with DAC HYP developed serious infections, one of whom discontinued treatment, while six resumed treatment after the resolution of infection. No placebo-treated patients had serious infections. The frequency of oral herpes and herpes zoster infections was similar in all groups.

Table 2. Adverse Event Incidence for DAC treated patients in Controlled Trials of DAC HYP.

			Clinical Trials				
	SELECT			SELECTION		DECIDE	SELECTED
			Continuous [1]	Switch [2]	Washout [3]		
DAC Dose	150 mg	300 mg	150 mg, 300 mg	150 mg, 300 mg	150 mg, 300 mg	150 mg	150 mg
AE							
Infection (%)	104 (50)	112 (54)	36 (42),36 (41)	34 (40), 31 (37)	34 (40), 38 (43)	595 (65)	205 (50)
Serious Infection (%)	6 (3)	3 (1)	2 (2), 2 (2)	3 (3), 1 (1)	3 (3), 2 (2)	40 (4)	13 (3)
Hepatic TA (%)	NR	NR	NR	NR	NR	144 (16)	61 (15)
AST/ALT:							
1–3× ULN (%)	54 (26)	62 (30)	30 (35), 30 (34)	23 (27), 22 (26)	21 (24), 26 (30)	NR	NR
3–5× ULN (%)	7 (3)	6 (3)	1 (1), 5 (6)	0, 2 (2)	2 (2), 0	96 (10)	37 (9)
>5× ULN (%)	9 (4)	8 (4)	0, 3 (3)	1 (1), 1 (1)	2 (2), 4 (5)	59 (6)	18 (4)
Hepatic SAE (%)	NR	NR	0, 0	0, 0	0, 1 (<1)	6 (1)	5 (1)
Malignancy (%)	1 (<1)	2 (<1)	0, 0	0, 1 (1)	0, 0	7 (1)	4 (1)
Death (%)	1 (<1)	0	0, 0	0, 0	0, 1 (<1)	1 (<1)	0

DAC—daclizumab; HYP—high-yield process; TA—transaminases; AST—aspartate aminotransferase; ALT—alanine aminotransferase; AE—adverse events; ULN—upper limit of normal; NR—not reported. [1] Continuous-patients receiving DAC HYP 150 or 300 mg every 4 weeks during SELECT continued their same dose of DAC HYP through additional 52 weeks of SELECTION; [2] Switch-patients receiving placebo during SELECT were placed on either 150 or 300 mg DAC HYP for the 52 weeks of SELECTION; [3] Washout-patients receiving either 150 or 300 mg of DAC HYP during SELECT were placed on placebo for 20 weeks followed by resumption of their previous dose of DAC HYP administered during SELECT.

Four malignancies were reported during the trial, including two cervical carcinomas (one in the placebo, one in DAC HYP 150 mg) and two melanomas in the DAC HYP 300 mg group. Two patients in the DAC HYP 150 mg group and three in the DAC HYP 300 mg group, had serious cutaneous events, including rash, atopic and allergic dermatitis, ex-foliative dermatitis, and erythema nodosum, as shown in Table 3. While recovering from a serious rash, one DAC HYP (150 mg) patient died due to a psoas abscess. No serious cutaneous events were seen in the placebo group. More patients in the DAC HYP groups had liver transaminase increases of greater than five times the upper limit of normal (>5× ULN). These increases had a median onset at 308 (±SD) treatment days. Continued DAC HYP dosing did not increase recovery time of transaminase abnormalities, and 7/17 patients with elevated alanine aminotransferase levels >5× ULN continued or resumed DAC HYP after enzyme recovery, and did not experience a recurrence of liver function test abnormalities in the five months that followed [7].

Table 3. Cutaneous AE Incidence for DAC treated patients in Controlled Trials of DAC HYP.

	SELECT		Continuous [1]	Clinical Trials SELECTION Switch [2]	Washout [3]	DECIDE	SELECTED	Post Approval [4]
DAC Dose	150 mg	300 mg	150 mg, 300 mg	150 mg, 300 mg	150 mg, 300 mg	150 mg	150 mg	
Cutaneous Events								
AE (%)	38 (18)	45 (22)	15 (17), 21 (24)	17 (20), 11 (13)	19 (22), 16 (18)	344 (37)	114 (28)	23 (77)
SAE (%)	2 (<1)	3 (<1)	0, 3 (3)	2 (2), 0	1 (1), 0	14 (2)	8 (2)	6 (19)

DAC-daclizumab; HYP-high-yield process; AE-adverse event; SAE-serious adverse event. [1] Continuous-patients receiving DAC HYP 150 or 300 mg every 4 weeks during SELECT continued their same dose of DAC HYP through additional 52 weeks of SELECTION; [2] Switch-patients receiving placebo during SELECT were placed on either 150 or 300 mg DAC HYP for the 52 weeks of SELECTION; [3] Washout-patients receiving either 150 or 300 mg of DAC HYP during SELECT were placed on placebo for 20 weeks followed by resumption of their previous dose of DAC HYP administered during SELECT; [4] Cortese et al., open-label study.

6.2. SELECTION

In the multicenter, randomized, double-blind SELECT extension trial (SELECTION), frequencies of AEs and SAEs were similar between the patients switched from placebo to DAC HYP treatment and the continuous DAC HYP treatment groups, as shown in Table 2. Infections were reported in 42% of patients; 3% were considered serious infections. The only serious infection occurring in more than one patient was bronchitis. All infections were resolved with standard-of-care.

Breast cancer was reported in one (<1%) patient, which investigators did not believe was treatment-related. Cutaneous events occurred in up to 24% of patients as shown in Table 3. Serious cutaneous events were reported in six (1%) patients. These events included drug eruption, eczema, pityriasis rubra pilaris, exfoliative dermatitis, and urticaria. Alanine or aspartate aminotransferase levels of >5× ULN were observed in 11 patients (2%) and resolved in a median of 84.5 days. Of these patients, 10 resumed DAC HYP without recurrence; one did not resume treatment. One patient died due to autoimmune hepatitis following re-initiation of 300 mg DAC HYP; this was confirmed by liver histology upon autopsy. The contribution of DAC HYP could not be ruled out [8].

6.3. DECIDE

In the double-blind, active-controlled, randomized phase III DECIDE trial comparing DAC HYP 150 mg with IFNβ weekly injections, the overall incidence of AEs was similar among all groups, leading to discontinuation in 14% of DAC HYP-treated patients and 9% in the IFNβ treated group, as shown in Table 2. SAEs (excluding relapse) occurred in 15% of the patients treated with DAC HYP and in 10% of those treated with IFNβ. One patient in the DAC HYP group and four in the IFNβ died, but none of these deaths was considered to be related to study treatment according to investigators.

Infections occurred in 65% of DAC HYP patients and 57% of IFNβ patients. Five DAC HYP patients (1%) and three (<1%) IFNβ patients discontinued treatment due to infection. Common infections included nasopharyngitis (25% in DAC HYP group; 21% in IFNβ group), upper respiratory infection (16% and 13%, respectively), and urinary tract infection (UTI; 10% and 11%, respectively). The incidence of herpes virus infections, including herpes zoster, was similar in both treatment groups. Serious infections were reported in 4% of patients in the DAC HYP group and in 2% of the IFNβ group, including UTI, cellulitis, appendicitis, pneumonia, and viral infection. There were no reported cases of progressive multifocal leukoencephalopathy or infectious encephalitis.

Malignancies were found in seven DAC HYP patients and eight IFNβ patients, and no deaths related to treatment [6]. Cutaneous events occurred in 37% of DAC HYP patients and 19% of IFNβ patients, leading to treatment discontinuation in 5% and 1% of patients, respectively, as shown in Table 3. The most frequent cutaneous events were rash (7% in DAC HYP and 3% in IFNβ) and eczema (4% and 1%, respectively). Serious cutaneous events were observed in 2% of DAC HYP patients and <1% of IFNβ patients, and included dermatitis and angioedema. Hepatic events occurred in 16% of DAC HYP- and 14% of IFNβ-treated patients (serious events in 1% and <1%, respectively). Transaminase elevations >5× ULN occurred in 6% of DAC HYP and 3% of IFNβ patients. Elevations of transaminase levels were more common during the first year of IFNβ treatment, but were distributed evenly throughout DAC HYP treatment.

6.4. SELECTED

In SELECTED, the open-label DAC HYP extension study, SAEs (not including MS relapse) occurred in 16%. Discontinuation of treatment due to AEs including MS relapse occurred in 12% of patients, as shown in Table 2. The most common AEs (not including MS relapse) included nasopharyngitis and upper respiratory infection (both 12%). The most common SAEs (not including MS relapse) included elevated hepatic enzymes, ulcerative colitis, pneumonia, and UTI (<1% for each). Infections were observed in 50% of patients; 3% were considered serious. The infection incidence did not increase over time, and less than 1% of discontinuations were as a result of infection. Serious infections included UTI, pneumonia, and bronchitis. There were two reports of opportunistic infection—vulvovaginal candidiasis and pulmonary tuberculosis.

Malignancies were reported in four (1%) patients and included breast cancer, basal cell carcinoma, anal cancer, and a pulmonary carcinoid tumor. Investigators believed the anal cancer and pulmonary carcinoma cases were related to DAC HYP treatment, though there was no observed pattern in malignancies [66]. Cutaneous events occurred in 28% of patients, with the most frequent cutaneous AEs being rash (7%), allergic dermatitis (5%), and eczema (3%). Cutaneous events in 3% of patients led to treatment discontinuation as shown in Table 3. Serious cutaneous events occurred in 2% of patients: urticaria was reported in two patients; and Stevens–Johnson Syndrome (SJS) in one case, which was not validated by a dermatologist and did not meet standard SJS diagnostic criteria. Drug-related hepatic disorders were found in 15% of patients, only 1% of which were serious.

Gastrointestinal AEs were observed in 16% of patients, six (1%) of which were serious inflammatory gastrointestinal events, including ulcerative colitis (three patients), and colitis, Crohn's disease, and hemorrhagic enterocolitis (one patient each). Overall the safety profile in the SELECTED open-label extension was felt to be comparable to that observed in the SELECT trial, and the risks associated with DAC HYP did not appear to increase with longer durations of therapy [66].

7. Adverse Events: DAC HYP Post-Marketing

7.1. Cutaneous Events

A prospective open-label study evaluated the risk of development of cutaneous AEs over a 42-month period, as shown in Table 3 [67]. Twenty-three participants (77%) developed new or recurring cutaneous AEs. The majority of cutaneous eruptions presented with localized eczematous and in some cases progressive patches. All moderate to severe rashes (6/23) had psoriaform features, which persisted in later stages. Six patients developed mucosal lesions, the most common of which were recurring aphthous ulcers. Non-eczematous facial rashes included eyelid edema with erythema or diffuse facial erythema. Scalp involvement resembling seborrheic dermatitis was observed in six patients. Eight patients presented cyclic exacerbations of skin symptoms. Skin manifestations developed in most patients within the first 12 months of treatment, and commonly recurred two weeks after DAC HYP injection. There was no correlation between duration of DAC HYP treatment and rash development, and was not associated with MS disease course or with efficacy of DAC HYP therapy in suppressing CNS inflammation. However, a predisposing factor was a prior history of eczema or seborrheic dermatitis.

Biopsies from eight patients showed features of eczematous dermatitis, including scattered CD25$^+$ and T$_{reg}$ FOXP3$^+$ cells. A consistent finding, most notable in moderate and severe rashes, was a robust population of CD56$^+$ cells, but the degree of CD56$^+$ infiltration did not correlate with the degree of expansion of this cell population in peripheral blood.

The cyclic pattern of eruptions and/or their temporal relationship to DAC HYP dosing in 8/31 patients (25.8%), including three patients with severe cutaneous AEs, led the authors to conclude that these events may be drug-related, and that by altering normal immune networks, DAC HYP could induce adverse cutaneous reactions resulting in the expansion of CD56$^+$ cells, the hallmark of DAC HYP-related skin inflammation. As previously noted, CD56^{bright} NK cells are part of the ILC lineage, and ILC are strategically placed at pathogen entry locations such as skin and mucous membranes. Since DAC typically skews differentiation of common ILC precursors toward CD56^{bright} NK cells, DAC-driven changes in ILC differentiation, while beneficial for CNS inflammatory disease, might in some patients lead paradoxically to enhanced skin reactivity. Because DAC prevents the expansion of T$_{reg}$ cells, this may further contribute to heightened skin reactivity in affected patients [67]. Contrary to most of the literature on drug-induced cutaneous and systemic reactions, which has been attributed to the adaptive immune system, SAE to DAC HYP might suggest a larger role for CD56^{bright} NK cells and the innate immune system in this process [68–70]. Further study in this area is warranted.

7.2. Drug Reaction with Eosinophilia and Systemic Symptoms (DRESS Syndrome)

The EMA reported on March 6, 2018 that four DAC HYP-treated patients developed exanthema/skin reactions with the involvement of other organs and eosinophilia, and five additional patients developed multi-organ failure that were possibly immune-mediated and later recognized as DRESS syndrome. DRESS is a life-threatening syndrome manifesting with cutaneous lesions and internal organ involvement; it has a 10% mortality rate. The time of onset of DRESS varies, typically from 2 and 12 weeks following drug exposure, though diagnosis may be missed or unnoticed due to its rare and varied presentation [71]. Typical features include eosinophilia, fever, extensive cutaneous lesions, atypical lymphocytosis, lymphadenopathy, hepatic injury, and renal failure. Lung, cardiac, and CNS involvement with meningitis and/or encephalitis may also occur, including brain edema, rhombencephalitis, and high cerebrospinal fluid (CSF) cell count [71,72]. Brain biopsy in one case contained demyelinating lesions showing conspicuous inflammation, and an abundance of T cells, plasma cells, eosinophils and eosinophilic/lymphocytic/plasma cellular meningitis, leading to a diagnosis of DAC-induced DRESS syndrome of the CNS. In marked contrast to typical DRESS syndrome, DAC-induced DRESS appears to occur principally within the CNS. Though CNS DRESS is exceptionally rare and usually presents with a pattern resembling vasculitis, it is likely that five of the patients with CNS complications in the EMA report had CNS DRESS syndrome [72]. Reduced IL-2 consumption due to DAC HYP blockade of IL-2R-HA may increase the opportunity for IL-2 to interact with ILC2 lineage cells, promoting IL-5 secretion and expansion of eosinophils, offering a potential pathway to CNS DRESS in rare cases [73].

7.3. Glial Fibrillary Acidic Protein (GFAP)-α Immunoglobulin (IgG)-Associated Encephalitis and Other Severe Encephalopathy Syndromes

Of the 12 patients with severe encephalopathy syndromes cited in the EMA report, one patient had CNS vasculitis, and several cases were reported as anti-N-methyl-D-aspartate (NMDA) receptor encephalitis. One patient was described who developed GFAP-α IgG-associated encephalitis [74]. This patient presented with behavioral and cognitive changes eight months after starting DAC HYP treatment. CSF contained oligoclonal bands and intrathecal immunoglobulin A (IgA) synthesis. Immunostaining showed GFAP-IgG antibodies in CSF. Although anti-GFAP-IgG may occur in isolation, it has also been in the setting of anti-NMDA receptor encephalitis or CNS vasculitis. Although one-third of cases with GFAP-IgG are paraneoplastic, malignancy was not found with this DAC HYP-treated patient.

As a consequence of these 12 cases of severe encephalopathy, four of which had a fatal outcome, DAC HYP was withdrawn from the market in February 2018. Although the precise mechanisms of these disorders are yet to be illuminated, it is reasonable to postulate that inhibition of T_{reg} cell expansion without an adequate concomitant expansion of immunoregulatory $CD56^{bright}$ NK cells or general immune suppression by depletion of activated effector $CD25^{+}$ T cells may have played a role. These latter cases suggest that redirecting IL-2 away from its high-affinity receptor may reduce activation and expansion of pro-inflammatory effector T cells, but in some cases does so at the expense of T_{reg} cells to such an extent that it may result in severe, paradoxical secondary autoimmune attack on multiple organs, including the CNS [74].

7.4. DAC: Is There a Future?

Although efficacious in controlled trials, the SAE leading to DAC withdrawal may preclude it from ever returning to clinical use. Even in a head-to-head trial against IFN-β, its therapeutic benefit was modest compared to more recently approved medications for the treatment of RMS [75–78]. At perhaps the simplest level, given the immunogenicity of the subcutaneous space, would intravenous administration of DAC have been preferable? Would this have reduced the likelihood of SAE?

The frequency of autoimmune cutaneous AE, and rarer but very serious autoimmune hepatitis and CNS events, including CNS DRESS and anti-NMDA encephalitis, reduce the likelihood of DAC returning as a therapeutic agent. Although SAE are also observed with other RMS medications, these can be prevented through the adoption of risk stratification strategies, such as detection and monitoring for John Cunningham virus infection in patients treated with natalizumab, exclusionary co-morbidities in patients receiving fingolimod or ocrelizumab, or frequent monitoring and early detection of side effects with use of alemtuzumab [79–82]. However, no risk stratification emerged for patients treated with DAC, with the possible exception of a prior history of hepatic disease, psoriasis, or eczema.

The time and expense of additional research to determine biomarkers for risk and efficacy are considerable barriers to pursuing the continued use of DAC. Despite these obstacles, the ability to modify disease activity in RMS, and possibly other autoimmune diseases, via innate immune system expansion should be recognized as a topic of potential scientific and therapeutic importance and thus justify further investigation into the development of biomarkers of risk or modified treatment protocols. If changes in immune cell parameters—the reduction in T_{reg} cell numbers, combined with the modest percentage decrease in $CD4^{+}$ and $CD8^{+}$ T cells and the expansion in $CD56^{bright}$ NK cells—resulting from DAC treatment contribute to autoimmune AE, this data could theoretically be used to develop an index table which might predict risk for developing secondary autoimmune AE. Data obtained from patients in already executed clinical trials and knowledge of their clinical outcomes could be used to develop such an index. However, the calculation of the risk index value in an individual patient would probably require treating them with DAC long enough to obtain steady state T_{reg}, $CD4^{+}/CD8^{+}$ T cell and $CD56^{bright}$ NK cell levels, which in of itself might place the patient at significant risk of an autoimmune AE. At a more complex and expensive level, transcriptomic and microRNA analyses of still stored serum samples from patients treated with DAC in past clinical trials could reveal valid predictive biomarkers for both efficacy and risk susceptibility.

The current standard of care for multiple sclerosis, at least as it pertains to disease process modifying drugs, relies upon adaptive immune system manipulation. This ranges from immune pathway alterations, immune cell expansion and maturation, reducing oxidative stress, immune cell sequestration and/or migration into the CNS, to outright antibody-directed lymphocyte and monocyte destruction. Unfortunately, the opportunity to expand therapeutic immune modulation into the potentially promising innate system arena has, at least for the present, been stymied by the SAE profile that accompanied DAC use in RMS. Targeting innate immune system expansion, without suppressing IL-2-dependent T_{reg} expansion through activation of IL-2R-IA directly via a CD122 agonist, might be employed as a strategy to expand the $CD56^{bright}$NK cell population. Nevertheless, at least for the present, we do not anticipate that the lessons learned from DAC will positively impact the process of future agent development, and instead may discourage attempts at further development of agents targeting innate immune modulation for RMS. Despite these challenges, developing additional strategies to promote innate immune system expansion should be employed in preclinical models of RMS, with the hope of developing novel therapeutic agents targeting innate immune pathways.

8. Conclusions

DAC HYP was efficacious for the treatment of RMS, demonstrating a reduction in relapse rate and disability progression, a reduction in MRI markers of disease activity, and an improvement in patient-reported outcome measures. DAC HYP may reduce autoimmune reactivity by obstructing IL-2 interaction with its high-affinity receptor on lymphoid cells, thus reducing activation and expansion of effector T cell-driven inflammation. However, most of the evidence to date would suggest that the impact of DAC on the innate immune system is largely responsible for its therapeutic efficacy. Unique to RMS therapeutic agents, DAC drives the innate immune system through the expansion of $CD56^{bright}$ NK cells, further reducing T cell-driven auto-reactivity in RMS. Both these actions appear to underlie DAC HYP efficacy in RMS. However, DAC significantly impairs T_{reg} cell expansion, and, possibly, activation-induced T cell apoptosis, both of which depend on IL-2 interacting with its high-affinity receptor on lymphoid lineage cells, and may largely explain the susceptibility of DAC HYP-treated patients to develop the severe secondary autoimmune disorders that resulted in its removal from clinical use in patients with RMS. Hopefully, this will not dissuade future research into the potential utility of innate immune system modulation in the treatment of autoimmune disorders.

Author Contributions: Writing—original draft preparation, S.L.C., E.B.L., M.C.R.; writing—review and editing, S.L.C., E.B.L., M.C.R., and S.N.L.; visualization, S.L.C., E.B.L., S.N.L.

Funding: This research received no external funding.

Conflicts of Interest: S.L.C. has received speaking honoraria from and/or is on advisory boards for: Biogen, Sanofi Genzyme, Roche Genentech, and Novartis, and has received research support from AbbVie, Biogen, MedDay, Novartis, and Sanofi Genzyme; E.B.L. has received speaking honoraria from and/or is on advisory boards for: Biogen, EMD Serono, Sanofi Genzyme, Roche Genentech, and Novartis; S.N.L. has received patent licensing royalties from Galectin Therapeutics; M.C.R. has no disclosures to report.

References

1. Nussenblatt, R.B.; Fortin, E.; Schiffman, R.; Rizzo, L.; Smith, J.; Van Veldhuisen, P.; Sran, P.; Yaffe, A.; Goldman, C.K.; Waldmann, T.A.; et al. Treatment of noninfectious intermediate and posterior uveitis with the humanized anti-Tac mAb: A phase I/II clinical trial. *Proc. Natl. Acad. Sci. USA* **1999**, *96*, 7462–7466. [CrossRef] [PubMed]

2. Waldmann, T.A.; Goldman, C.K.; Bongiovanni, K.F.; Sharrow, S.O.; Davey, M.P.; Cease, K.B.; Greenberg, S.J.; Longo, D.L. Therapy of patients with human T-cell lymphotrophic virus I-induced adult T-cell leukemia with anti-Tac, a monoclonal antibody to the receptor for interleukin-2. *Blood* **1988**, *72*, 1805–1816. [PubMed]

3. Vincenti, F.; Kirkman, R.; Light, S.; Bumgardner, G.; Pescovitz, M.; Halloran, P.; Neylan, J.; Wilkinson, A.; Ekberg, H.; Gaston, R.; et al. Interleukin-2-receptor blockade with daclizumab to prevent acute rejection in renal transplantation. Daclizumab Triple Therapy Study Group. *N. Engl. J. Med.* **1998**, *338*, 161–165. [CrossRef] [PubMed]

4. Bumgardner, G.L.; Hardie, I.; Johnson, R.W.; Lin, A.; Nashan, B.; Pescovitz, M.D.; Ramos, E.; Vincenti, F. Phase III Daclizumab Study Group. Results of 3-year phase III clinical trials with daclizumab prophylaxis for prevention of acute rejection after renal transplantation. *Transplantation* **2001**, *72*, 839–845. [CrossRef] [PubMed]

5. Wynn, D.; Kaufman, M.; Montalban, X.; Vollmer, T.; Simon, J.; Elkins, J.; O'Neill, G.; Neyer, L.; Sheridan, J.; Wang, C.; et al. Daclizumab in active relapsing multiple sclerosis (CHOICE study): A phase 2, randomised, double-blind, placebo-controlled, add-on trial with interferon beta. *Lancet Neurol.* **2010**, *9*, 381–390. [CrossRef]

6. Kappos, L.; Wiendl, H.; Selmaj, K.; Arnold, D.L.; Havrdova, E.; Boyko, A.; Kaufman, M.; Rose, J.; Greenberg, S.; Sweetser, M.; et al. Daclizumab HYP versus Interferon Beta-1a in Relapsing Multiple Sclerosis. *N. Engl. J. Med.* **2015**, *373*, 1418–1428. [CrossRef] [PubMed]

7. Gold, R.; Giovannoni, G.; Selmaj, K.; Havrdova, E.; Montalban, X.; Radue, E.W.; Stefoski, D.; Robinson, R.; Riester, K.; Rana, J.; et al. Daclizumab high-yield process in relapsing-remitting multiple sclerosis (SELECT): A randomised, double-blind, placebo-controlled trial. *Lancet* **2013**, *381*, 2167–2175. [CrossRef]

8. Giovannoni, G.; Gold, R.; Selmaj, K.; Havrdova, E.; Montalban, X.; Radue, E.W.; Stefoski, D.; McNeill, M.; Amaravadi, L.; Sweetser, M.; et al. Daclizumab high-yield process in relapsing-remitting multiple sclerosis (SELECTION): A multicentre, randomised, double-blind extension trial. *Lancet Neurol.* **2014**, *13*, 472–481. [CrossRef]

9. Lenardo, M.J. Interleukin-2 programs mouse alpha beta T lymphocytes for apoptosis. *Nature* **1991**, *353*, 858–861. [CrossRef] [PubMed]

10. Baan, C.C.; Balk, A.H.; van Riemsdijk, I.C.; Vantrimpont, P.J.; Maat, A.P.; Niesters, H.G.; Zondervan, P.E.; van Gelder, T.; Weimar, W. Anti-CD25 monoclonal antibody therapy affects the death signals of graft-infiltrating cells after clinical heart transplantation. *Transplantation* **2003**, *75*, 1704–1710. [CrossRef] [PubMed]

11. Bielekova, B. Daclizumab therapy for multiple sclerosis. *Neurotherapeutics* **2013**, *10*, 55–67. [CrossRef] [PubMed]

12. Richter, G.H.; Mollweide, A.; Hanewinkel, K.; Zobywalski, C.; Burdach, S. CD25 blockade protects T cells from activation-induced cell death (AICD) via maintenance of TOSO expression. *Scand. J. Immunol.* **2009**, *70*, 206–215. [CrossRef] [PubMed]

13. Ku, C.C.; Murakami, M.; Sakamoto, A.; Kappler, J.; Marrack, P. Control of homeostasis of CD8+ memory T cells by opposing cytokines. *Science* **2000**, *288*, 675–678. [CrossRef] [PubMed]

14. Lenardo, M.; Chan, K.M.; Hornung, F.; McFarland, H.; Siegel, R.; Wang, J.; Zheng, L. Mature T lymphocyte apoptosis–immune regulation in a dynamic and unpredictable antigenic environment. *Annu. Rev. Immunol.* **1999**, *17*, 221–253. [CrossRef] [PubMed]

15. Li, X.C.; Demirci, G.; Ferrari-Lacraz, S.; Groves, C.; Coyle, A.; Malek, T.R.; Strom, T.B. IL-15 and IL-2: A matter of life and death for T cells in vivo. *Nat. Med.* **2001**, *7*, 114–118. [CrossRef] [PubMed]

16. Granucci, F.; Feau, S.; Angeli, V.; Trottein, F.; Ricciardi-Castagnoli, P. Early IL-2 production by mouse dendritic cells is the result of microbial-induced priming. *J. Immunol.* **2003**, *170*, 5075–5081. [CrossRef] [PubMed]

17. Malek, T.R. The biology of interleukin-2. *Annu. Rev. Immunol.* **2008**, *26*, 453–479. [CrossRef] [PubMed]

18. Waldmann, T.A. The multi-subunit interleukin-2 receptor. *Annu. Rev. Biochem.* **1989**, *58*, 875–911. [CrossRef] [PubMed]

19. Setoguchi, R.; Hori, S.; Takahashi, T.; Sakaguchi, S. Homeostatic maintenance of natural Foxp3(+) CD25(+) CD4(+) regulatory T cells by interleukin (IL)-2 and induction of autoimmune disease by IL-2 neutralization. *J. Exp. Med.* **2005**, *201*, 723–735. [CrossRef] [PubMed]

20. Wuest, S.C.; Edwan, J.H.; Martin, J.F.; Han, S.; Perry, J.S.; Cartagena, C.M.; Matsuura, E.; Maric, D.; Waldmann, T.A.; Bielekova, B. A role for interleukin-2 trans-presentation in dendritic cell-mediated T cell activation in humans, as revealed by daclizumab therapy. *Nat. Med.* **2011**, *17*, 604–609. [CrossRef] [PubMed]

21. Roessler, E.; Grant, A.; Ju, G.; Tsudo, M.; Sugamura, K.; Waldmann, T.A. Cooperative interactions between the interleukin 2 receptor alpha and beta chains alter the interleukin 2-binding affinity of the receptor subunits. *Proc. Natl. Acad. Sci. USA* **1994**, *91*, 3344–3347. [CrossRef] [PubMed]

22. Takeshita, T.; Asao, H.; Ohtani, K.; Ishii, N.; Kumaki, S.; Tanaka, N.; Munakata, H.; Nakamura, M.; Sugamura, K. Cloning of the gamma chain of the human IL-2 receptor. *Science* **1992**, *257*, 379–382. [CrossRef] [PubMed]

23. Gaffen, S.L. Signaling domains of the interleukin 2 receptor. *Cytokine* **2001**, *14*, 63–77. [CrossRef] [PubMed]

24. Duprez, V.; Cornet, V.; Dautry-Varsat, A. Down-regulation of high affinity interleukin 2 receptors in a human tumor T cell line. Interleukin 2 increases the rate of surface receptor decay. *J. Biol. Chem.* **1988**, *263*, 12860–12865. [PubMed]

25. Fujii, M.; Sugamura, K.; Nakai, S.; Tanaka, Y.; Tozawa, H.; Hinuma, Y. High- and low-affinity interleukin 2 receptors: Distinctive effects of monoclonal antibodies. *J. Immunol.* **1986**, *137*, 1552–1556. [PubMed]

26. Morelon, E.; Dautry-Varsat, A. Endocytosis of the common cytokine receptor gammac chain. Identification of sequences involved in internalization and degradation. *J. Biol. Chem.* **1998**, *273*, 22044–22051. [CrossRef] [PubMed]

27. Hemar, A.; Subtil, A.; Lieb, M.; Morelon, E.; Hellio, R.; Dautry-Varsat, A. Endocytosis of interleukin 2 receptors in human T lymphocytes: Distinct intracellular localization and fate of the receptor alpha, beta, and gamma chains. *J. Cell Biol.* **1995**, *129*, 55–64. [CrossRef] [PubMed]

28. Malek, T.R.; Yu, A.; Scibelli, P.; Lichtenheld, M.G.; Codias, E.K. Broad programming by IL-2 receptor signaling for extended growth to multiple cytokines and functional maturation of antigen-activated T cells. *J. Immunol.* **2001**, *166*, 1675–1683. [CrossRef] [PubMed]

29. Freud, A.G.; Becknell, B.; Roychowdhury, S.; Mao, H.C.; Ferketich, A.K.; Nuovo, G.J.; Hughes, T.L.; Marburger, T.B.; Sung, J.; Baiocchi, R.A.; et al. A human CD34(+) subset resides in lymph nodes and differentiates into CD56bright natural killer cells. *Immunity* **2005**, *22*, 295–304. [CrossRef] [PubMed]

30. Spits, H.; Cupedo, T. Innate lymphoid cells: Emerging insights in development, lineage relationships, and function. *Annu. Rev. Immunol.* **2012**, *30*, 647–675. [CrossRef] [PubMed]

31. Spits, H.; Di Santo, J.P. The expanding family of innate lymphoid cells: Regulators and effectors of immunity and tissue remodeling. *Nat. Immunol.* **2011**, *12*, 21–27. [CrossRef] [PubMed]

32. Artis, D.; Spits, H. The biology of innate lymphoid cells. *Nature* **2015**, *517*, 293–301. [CrossRef] [PubMed]

33. Huang, Q.; Seillet, C.; Belz, G.T. Shaping Innate Lymphoid Cell Diversity. *Front. Immunol.* **2017**, *8*, 1569. [CrossRef] [PubMed]

34. Bielekova, B.; Catalfamo, M.; Reichert-Scrivner, S.; Packer, A.; Cerna, M.; Waldmann, T.A.; McFarland, H.; Henkart, P.A.; Martin, R. Regulatory CD56(bright) natural killer cells mediate immunomodulatory effects of IL-2Ralpha-targeted therapy (daclizumab) in multiple sclerosis. *Proc. Natl. Acad. Sci. USA* **2006**, *103*, 5941–5946. [CrossRef] [PubMed]

35. Lin, Y.C.; Winokur, P.; Blake, A.; Wu, T.; Romm, E.; Bielekova, B. Daclizumab reverses intrathecal immune cell abnormalities in multiple sclerosis. *Ann. Clin. Transl. Neurol.* **2015**, *2*, 445–455. [CrossRef] [PubMed]

36. Perry, J.S.; Han, S.; Xu, Q.; Herman, M.L.; Kennedy, L.B.; Csako, G.; Bielekova, B. Inhibition of LTi cell development by CD25 blockade is associated with decreased intrathecal inflammation in multiple sclerosis. *Sci. Transl. Med.* **2012**, *4*, 145ra106. [CrossRef] [PubMed]

37. Martin, J.F.; Perry, J.S.; Jakhete, N.R.; Wang, X.; Bielekova, B. An IL-2 paradox: Blocking CD25 on T cells induces IL-2-driven activation of CD56(bright) NK cells. *J. Immunol.* **2010**, *185*, 1311–1320. [CrossRef] [PubMed]

38. Xu, W.; Fazekas, G.; Hara, H.; Tabira, T. Mechanism of natural killer (NK) cell regulatory role in experimental autoimmune encephalomyelitis. *J. Neuroimmunol.* **2005**, *163*, 24–30. [CrossRef] [PubMed]

39. Benczur, M.; Petranyi, G.G.; Palffy, G.; Varga, M.; Talas, M.; Kotsy, B.; Foldes, I.; Hollan, S.R. Dysfunction of natural killer cells in multiple sclerosis: A possible pathogenetic factor. *Clin. Exp. Immunol.* **1980**, *39*, 657–662. [PubMed]

40. Merrill, J.; Jondal, M.; Seeley, J.; Ullberg, M.; Siden, A. Decreased NK killing in patients with multiple sclerosis: An analysis on the level of the single effector cell in peripheral blood and cerebrospinal fluid in relation to the activity in the disease. *Clin. Exp. Immunol.* **1982**, *47*, 419–430. [PubMed]

41. Neighbour, P.A.; Grayzel, A.I.; Miller, A.E. Endogenous and interferon-augmented natural killer cell activity of human peripheral blood mononuclear cells in vitro. Studies of patients with multiple sclerosis, systemic lupus erythematosus or rheumatoid arthritis. *Clin. Exp. Immunol.* **1982**, *49*, 11–21. [PubMed]

42. Oger, J.; Kastrukoff, L.F.; Li, D.K.; Paty, D.W. Multiple sclerosis: In relapsing patients, immune functions vary with disease activity as assessed by MRI. *Neurology* **1988**, *38*, 1739–1744. [CrossRef] [PubMed]

43. Bielekova, B.; Howard, T.; Packer, A.N.; Richert, N.; Blevins, G.; Ohayon, J.; Waldmann, T.A.; McFarland, H.F.; Martin, R. Effect of anti-CD25 antibody daclizumab in the inhibition of inflammation and stabilization of disease progression in multiple sclerosis. *Arch. Neurol.* **2009**, *66*, 483–489. [CrossRef] [PubMed]

44. Elkins, J.; Sheridan, J.; Amaravadi, L.; Riester, K.; Selmaj, K.; Bielekova, B.; Parr, E.; Giovannoni, G. CD56(bright) natural killer cells and response to daclizumab HYP in relapsing-remitting MS. *Neurol. NeuroImmunol. Neuroinflamm.* **2015**, *2*, e65. [CrossRef] [PubMed]

45. Oh, U.; Blevins, G.; Griffith, C.; Richert, N.; Maric, D.; Lee, C.R.; McFarland, H.; Jacobson, S. Regulatory T cells are reduced during anti-CD25 antibody treatment of multiple sclerosis. *Arch. Neurol.* **2009**, *66*, 471–479. [CrossRef] [PubMed]

46. Huss, D.J.; Mehta, D.S.; Sharma, A.; You, X.; Riester, K.A.; Sheridan, J.P.; Amaravadi, L.S.; Elkins, J.S.; Fontenot, J.D. In vivo maintenance of human regulatory T cells during CD25 blockade. *J. Immunol.* **2015**, *194*, 84–92. [CrossRef] [PubMed]

47. Diao, L.; Hang, Y.; Othman, A.A.; Mehta, D.; Amaravadi, L.; Nestorov, I.; Tran, J.Q. Population PK-PD analyses of CD25 occupancy, CD56(bright) NK cell expansion, and regulatory T cell reduction by daclizumab HYP in subjects with multiple sclerosis. *Br. J. Clin. Pharmacol.* **2016**, *82*, 1333–1342. [CrossRef] [PubMed]

48. Rech, A.J.; Mick, R.; Martin, S.; Recio, A.; Aqui, N.A.; Powell, D.J., Jr.; Colligon, T.A.; Trosko, J.A.; Leinbach, L.I.; Pletcher, C.H.; et al. CD25 blockade depletes and selectively reprograms regulatory T cells in concert with immunotherapy in cancer patients. *Sci. Transl. Med.* **2012**, *4*, 134ra162. [CrossRef] [PubMed]

49. Roifman, C.M. Human IL-2 receptor alpha chain deficiency. *Pediatr. Res.* **2000**, *48*, 6–11. [CrossRef] [PubMed]

50. Sharfe, N.; Dadi, H.K.; Shahar, M.; Roifman, C.M. Human immune disorder arising from mutation of the alpha chain of the interleukin-2 receptor. *Proc. Natl. Acad. Sci. USA* **1997**, *94*, 3168–3171. [CrossRef] [PubMed]

51. Fehniger, T.A.; Bluman, E.M.; Porter, M.M.; Mrozek, E.; Cooper, M.A.; VanDeusen, J.B.; Frankel, S.R.; Stock, W.; Caligiuri, M.A. Potential mechanisms of human natural killer cell expansion in vivo during low-dose IL-2 therapy. *J. Clin. Investig.* **2000**, *106*, 117–124. [CrossRef] [PubMed]

52. Sheridan, J.P.; Zhang, Y.; Riester, K.; Tang, M.T.; Efros, L.; Shi, J.; Harris, J.; Vexler, V.; Elkins, J.S. Intermediate-affinity interleukin-2 receptor expression predicts CD56(bright) natural killer cell expansion after daclizumab treatment in the CHOICE study of patients with multiple sclerosis. *Mult. Scler.* **2011**, *17*, 1441–1448. [CrossRef] [PubMed]

53. Howell, O.W.; Reeves, C.A.; Nicholas, R.; Carassiti, D.; Radotra, B.; Gentleman, S.M.; Serafini, B.; Aloisi, F.; Roncaroli, F.; Magliozzi, R.; et al. Meningeal inflammation is widespread and linked to cortical pathology in multiple sclerosis. *Brain* **2011**, *134*, 2755–2771. [CrossRef] [PubMed]

54. Magliozzi, R.; Howell, O.; Vora, A.; Serafini, B.; Nicholas, R.; Puopolo, M.; Reynolds, R.; Aloisi, F. Meningeal B-cell follicles in secondary progressive multiple sclerosis associate with early onset of disease and severe cortical pathology. *Brain* **2007**, *130*, 1089–1104. [CrossRef] [PubMed]

55. Serafini, B.; Rosicarelli, B.; Magliozzi, R.; Stigliano, E.; Aloisi, F. Detection of ectopic B-cell follicles with germinal centers in the meninges of patients with secondary progressive multiple sclerosis. *Brain Pathol.* **2004**, *14*, 164–174. [CrossRef] [PubMed]

56. Gillard, G.O.; Saenz, S.A.; Huss, D.J.; Fontenot, J.D. Circulating innate lymphoid cells are unchanged in response to DAC HYP therapy. *J. NeuroImmunol.* **2016**, *294*, 41–45. [CrossRef] [PubMed]

57. Sawa, S.; Cherrier, M.; Lochner, M.; Satoh-Takayama, N.; Fehling, H.J.; Langa, F.; Di Santo, J.P.; Eberl, G. Lineage relationship analysis of RORgammat+ innate lymphoid cells. *Science* **2010**, *330*, 665–669. [CrossRef] [PubMed]

58. Mnasria, K.; Lagaraine, C.; Velge-Roussel, F.; Oueslati, R.; Lebranchu, Y.; Baron, C. Anti-CD25 antibodies affect cytokine synthesis pattern of human dendritic cells and decrease their ability to prime allogeneic CD4+ T cells. *J. Leukoc. Biol.* **2008**, *84*, 460–467. [CrossRef] [PubMed]

59. Othman, A.A.; Tran, J.Q.; Tang, M.T.; Dutta, S. Population pharmacokinetics of daclizumab high-yield process in healthy volunteers: Integrated analysis of intravenous and subcutaneous, single- and multiple-dose administration. *Clin. Pharm.* **2014**, *53*, 907–918. [CrossRef] [PubMed]

60. Tran, J.Q.; Othman, A.A.; Mikulskis, A.; Wolstencroft, P.; Elkins, J. Pharmacokinetics of daclizumab high-yield process with repeated administration of the clinical subcutaneous regimen in patients with relapsing-remitting multiple sclerosis. *Clin. Pharmacol.* **2016**, *8*, 9–13. [CrossRef] [PubMed]

61. Zhang, Y.; McClellan, M.; Efros, L.; Shi, D.; Bielekova, B.; Tang, M.T.; Vexler, V.; Sheridan, J.P. Daclizumab reduces CD25 levels on T cells through monocyte-mediated trogocytosis. *Mult. Scler.* **2014**, *20*, 156–164. [CrossRef] [PubMed]

62. Soelberg Sorensen, P. Safety concerns and risk management of multiple sclerosis therapies. *Acta Neurol. Scand.* **2017**, *136*, 168–186. [CrossRef] [PubMed]

63. Bielekova, B.; Richert, N.; Howard, T.; Blevins, G.; Markovic-Plese, S.; McCartin, J.; Frank, J.A.; Wurfel, J.; Ohayon, J.; Waldmann, T.A.; et al. Humanized anti-CD25 (daclizumab) inhibits disease activity in multiple sclerosis patients failing to respond to interferon beta. *Proc. Natl. Acad. Sci. USA* **2004**, *101*, 8705–8708. [CrossRef] [PubMed]

64. Rose, J.W.; Burns, J.B.; Bjorklund, J.; Klein, J.; Watt, H.E.; Carlson, N.G. Daclizumab phase II trial in relapsing and remitting multiple sclerosis: MRI and clinical results. *Neurology* **2007**, *69*, 785–789. [CrossRef] [PubMed]

65. Benedict, R.H.; Cohan, S.; Lynch, S.G.; Riester, K.; Wang, P.; Castro-Borrero, W.; Elkins, J.; Sabatella, G. Improved cognitive outcomes in patients with relapsing-remitting multiple sclerosis treated with daclizumab beta: Results from the DECIDE study. *Mult. Scler.* **2018**, *24*, 795–804. [CrossRef] [PubMed]

66. Gold, R.; Radue, E.W.; Giovannoni, G.; Selmaj, K.; Havrdova, E.; Stefoski, D.; Sprenger, T.; Montalban, X.; Cohan, S.; Umans, K.; et al. Safety and efficacy of daclizumab in relapsing-remitting multiple sclerosis: 3-year results from the SELECTED open-label extension study. *BMC Neurol.* **2016**, *16*, 117. [CrossRef] [PubMed]

67. Cortese, I.; Ohayon, J.; Fenton, K.; Lee, C.C.; Raffeld, M.; Cowen, E.W.; DiGiovanna, J.J.; Bielekova, B. Cutaneous adverse events in multiple sclerosis patients treated with daclizumab. *Neurology* **2016**, *86*, 847–855. [CrossRef] [PubMed]

68. Zawodniak, A.; Lochmatter, P.; Yerly, D.; Kawabata, T.; Lerch, M.; Yawalkar, N.; Pichler, W.J. In vitro detection of cytotoxic T and NK cells in peripheral blood of patients with various drug-induced skin diseases. *Allergy* **2010**, *65*, 376–384. [CrossRef] [PubMed]

69. Porebski, G. In Vitro Assays in Severe Cutaneous Adverse Drug Reactions: Are They Still Research Tools or Diagnostic Tests Already? *Int. J. Mol. Sci.* **2017**, *18*, 1737. [CrossRef] [PubMed]

70. Peter, J.G.; Lehloenya, R.; Dlamini, S.; Risma, K.; White, K.D.; Konvinse, K.C.; Phillips, E.J. Severe Delayed Cutaneous and Systemic Reactions to Drugs: A Global Perspective on the Science and Art of Current Practice. *J. Allergy Clin. Immunol. Pract.* **2017**, *5*, 547–563. [CrossRef]

71. Scheibe, F.; Metz, I.; Radbruch, H.; Siebert, E.; Wolf, S.; Kohnlein, M.; Harms, L.; Meisel, A. Drug reaction with eosinophilia and systemic symptoms after daclizumab therapy in MS. *Neurol. NeuroImmunol. Neuroinflamm.* **2018**, *5*, e479. [CrossRef] [PubMed]

72. Avasarala, J. DRESS Syndrome and Daclizumab Failure-Were Potentially Dangerous Signs Missed in Clinical Trials? *Drug Target. Insights* **2018**, *12*, 1177392818785136. [CrossRef] [PubMed]

73. Van Gool, F.; Molofsky, A.B.; Morar, M.M.; Rosenzwajg, M.; Liang, H.E.; Klatzmann, D.; Locksley, R.M.; Bluestone, J.A. Interleukin-5-producing group 2 innate lymphoid cells control eosinophilia induced by interleukin-2 therapy. *Blood* **2014**, *124*, 3572–3576. [CrossRef] [PubMed]

74. Luessi, F.; Engel, S.; Spreer, A.; Bittner, S.; Zipp, F. GFAPalpha IgG-associated encephalitis upon daclizumab treatment of MS. *Neurol. NeuroImmunol. Neuroinflamm.* **2018**, *5*, e481. [CrossRef] [PubMed]

75. Polman, C.H.; O'Connor, P.W.; Havrdova, E.; Hutchinson, M.; Kappos, L.; Miller, D.H.; Phillips, J.T.; Lublin, F.D.; Giovannoni, G.; Wajgt, A.; et al. A Randomized, Placebo-Controlled Trial of Natalizumab for Relapsing Multiple Sclerosis. *N. Engl. J. Med.* **2006**, *354*, 899–910. [CrossRef] [PubMed]

76. Kappos, L.; Li, D.; Calabresi, P.A.; O'Connor, P.; Bar-Or, A.; Barkhof, F.; Yin, M.; Leppert, D.; Glanzman, R.; Tinbergen, J.; et al. Ocrelizumab in relapsing-remitting multiple sclerosis: A phase 2, randomised, placebo-controlled, multicentre trial. *Lancet* **2011**, *378*, 1779–1787. [CrossRef]

77. Alemtuzumab vs. Interferon Beta-1a in Early Multiple Sclerosis. *N. Engl. J. Med.* **2008**, *359*, 1786–1801. [CrossRef]

78. Kappos, L.; Radue, E.-W.; O'Connor, P.; Polman, C.; Hohlfeld, R.; Calabresi, P.; Selmaj, K.; Agoropoulou, C.; Leyk, M.; Zhang-Auberson, L.; et al. A Placebo-Controlled Trial of Oral Fingolimod in Relapsing Multiple Sclerosis. *N. Engl. J. Med.* **2010**, *362*, 387–401. [CrossRef] [PubMed]

79. Kappos, L.; Bates, D.; Hartung, H.P.; Havrdova, E.; Miller, D.; Polman, C.H.; Ravnborg, M.; Hauser, S.L.; Rudick, R.A.; Weiner, H.L.; et al. Natalizumab treatment for multiple sclerosis: Recommendations for patient selection and monitoring. *Lancet Neurol.* **2007**, *6*, 431–441. [CrossRef]

80. Ayzenberg, I.; Hoepner, R.; Kleiter, I. Fingolimod for multiple sclerosis and emerging indications: Appropriate patient selection, safety precautions, and special considerations. *Ther. Clin. Risk Manag.* **2016**, *12*, 261–272. [CrossRef] [PubMed]

81. Cossburn, M.; Pace, A.A.; Jones, J.; Ali, R.; Ingram, G.; Baker, K.; Hirst, C.; Zajicek, J.; Scolding, N.; Boggild, M.; et al. Autoimmune disease after alemtuzumab treatment for multiple sclerosis in a multicenter cohort. *Neurology* **2011**, *77*, 573–579. [CrossRef]

82. Montalban, X.; Hauser, S.L.; Kappos, L.; Arnold, D.L.; Bar-Or, A.; Comi, G.; de Seze, J.; Giovannoni, G.; Hartung, H.P.; Hemmer, B.; et al. Ocrelizumab versus Placebo in Primary Progressive Multiple Sclerosis. *N. Engl. J. Med.* **2017**, *376*, 209–220. [CrossRef] [PubMed]

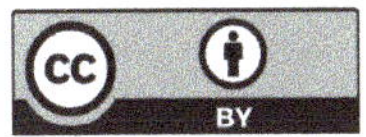

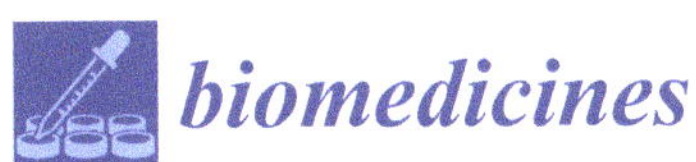 *biomedicines*

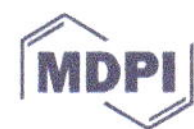

Review

Stem Cell-Based Therapies for Multiple Sclerosis: Current Perspectives

Fernando X. Cuascut * and George J. Hutton *

Baylor College of Medicine, Maxine Mesigner Multiple Sclerosis Center, Houston, TX 77030, USA
* Correspondence: fernando.cuascut@bcm.edu (F.X.C.); ghutton@bcm.edu (G.J.H.);
  Tel.: +1-713-798-2273 (F.X.C. & G.J.H.)

Received: 25 January 2019; Accepted: 25 March 2019; Published: 30 March 2019

Abstract: Multiple sclerosis (MS) is an inflammatory and neurodegenerative autoimmune disease of the central nervous system (CNS). Disease-modifying therapies (DMT) targeting inflammation have been shown to reduce disease activity in patients with relapsing–remitting MS (RRMS). The current therapeutic challenge is to find an effective treatment to halt disease progression and reverse established neural damage. Stem cell-based therapies have emerged to address this dilemma. Several types of stem cells have been considered for clinical use, such as autologous hematopoietic (aHSC), mesenchymal (MSC), neuronal (NSC), human embryonic (hESC), and induced pluripotent (iPSC) stem cells. There is convincing evidence that immunoablation followed by hematopoietic therapy (aHSCT) has a high efficacy for suppressing inflammatory MS activity and improving neurological disability in patients with RRMS. In addition, MSC therapy may be a safe and tolerable treatment, but its clinical value is still under evaluation. Various studies have shown early promising results with other cellular therapies for CNS repair and decreasing inflammation. In this review, we discuss the current knowledge and limitations of different stem cell-based therapies for the treatment of patients with MS.

Keywords: multiple sclerosis; stem cells; autologous hematopoietic; mesenchymal; neuronal; induced pluripotent; human embryonic

---

1. Introduction

Multiple sclerosis is an autoimmune condition characterized by demyelination and the loss of CNS neurons. Active inflammation is most evident in early RRMS. A neurodegenerative process may contribute to disability accumulation during later secondary progressive MS (SPMS) [1]. Available disease-modifying therapies (DMT) for MS have been shown to reduce the number and severity of relapses. Despite the broad range of options, there is still a therapeutic challenge in finding an effective treatment to halt disease progression and to reverse established neural injuries [2,3]. A subgroup of MS patients and those with an aggressive subtype may continue to deteriorate despite the use of DMT [4,5].

In the last 20 years, stem cell transplantation has been considered as a potentially effective therapeutic approach for aggressive MS. At least five types of stem cells have been considered as potential therapeutic approaches: autologous hematopoietic (aHSC), mesenchymal (MSC), neuronal (NSC), induced pluripotent (iPSC), and human embryonic (hESC) [6]. Each of these cell-based therapies works through various mechanisms, including replacing the malfunctioning immune system using immunoablation with high-dose immunosuppressive therapy (HDIT), followed by aHSC administration [7]; modifying the immune response and intrinsic repair mechanisms by alteration of cytokines and trophic factors (MSC) [8,9]; replacing damaged or lost neuronal tissue with NSC or iPSC [10,11]; and providing immunosuppressive and neuroprotective mechanisms (hESC) [12].

In this review, we aim to describe the current knowledge and limitations regarding cell-based approaches for treating MS, and discuss the future considerations that are required to optimize the therapeutic parameters regarding treatment efficacy and safety.

2. Immunoablation Followed by Hematopoietic Stem Cell Transplantation

2.1. The Procedure

Immunoablative therapy followed by aHSC therapy (aHSCT) to manage highly active and treatment-refractory MS has been investigated for the last two decades, following reports of the coincidental improvement of autoimmune disease symptoms in patients undergoing transplantation for hematological malignancies [13,14]. The therapeutic effects of immunoablation followed by aHSC transplantation were initially studied in rats with experimental autoimmune encephalomyelitis (EAE)—a rodent model of central nervous system (CNS) inflammation—showing that the procedure can induce remission, prevent relapses, and enhance the recovery of symptoms [15–17]. As discussed below, one rationale behind this method is to eliminate the abnormal immune system cells using HDIT, gradually developing a "new" and more tolerant immune system after aHSC infusion [18,19]. An alternative explanation is that HDIT produces a radical and long-lasting suppression of the inflammatory MS activity [20–22]. The procedure encompasses a series of steps which includes the mobilization, harvesting, ablative conditioning, and transplantation of aHSC [23,24] (Figure 1). First, hematopoietic stem cell (HSC) are mobilized, typically from peripheral blood, by using either granulocyte colony-stimulating factor (G-CSF) or granulocyte-macrophage colony-stimulating factor (GM-CSF), with or without cyclophosphamide (CY). It is preferred to pretreat with CY due to the potential for either a clinical relapse or worsening of pre-existing symptoms with the administration of G-CSF or GM-CSF alone [25]. The HSC are then harvested and cryopreserved until the patient is ready for transplantation. The HSC can be positively selected for CD34$^+$ cells ex vivo, which theoretically reduces the risk of reinfusing potentially autoreactive lymphocytes. However, there is limited evidence indicating any obvious advantage of CD34$^+$ selection, which increases the technical complexity of the transplant procedure [26]. The next step is to eliminate autoreactive cells (ablative conditioning) with HDIT. Different conditioning regimens have been proposed and classified according to the intensity of the ablation. High-intensity regimens typically consist of a high IV dose of busulfan, combined with a high dose of CY, and anti-thymocyte globulin (ATG) for in vivo T cell depletion. Total body irradiation is no longer used due to its severe toxicity [26]. Intermediate-intensity regimens involve a combination of different chemotherapies, which often include BCNU, cytosine arabinoside, etoposide, and melphalan, with or without ATG, referred to as BEAM. Other modified BEAM regimens have also been utilized with similar results [27] (Table 1). The low-intensity regimens, also referred to as nonmyeloablative, use CY and ATG [28].

Currently, there is a debate regarding which conditioning regimen should be used. For instance, high-intensity regimens are associated with more adverse effects and mortality [29–33]. Conversely, low-intensity regimens are associated with reduced toxicity and require less supportive care, but may be associated with the early reappearance of MRI lesion activity post-transplant [34–37]. It is becoming more acceptable to use BEAM or modified BEAM as an intermediate regimen for ablative conditioning [38]. After the conditioning regimen, the cryopreserved cells are thawed and then infused back into the patient. ATG is administered before or after the HSC infusion, to primarily remove any autoreactive T cells that might have escaped prior conditioning procedures. Subsequently, the patient enters an aplastic phase, characterized by an extremely low level of hematopoietic blood cells, requiring prophylactic treatment with antivirals and antibiotics.

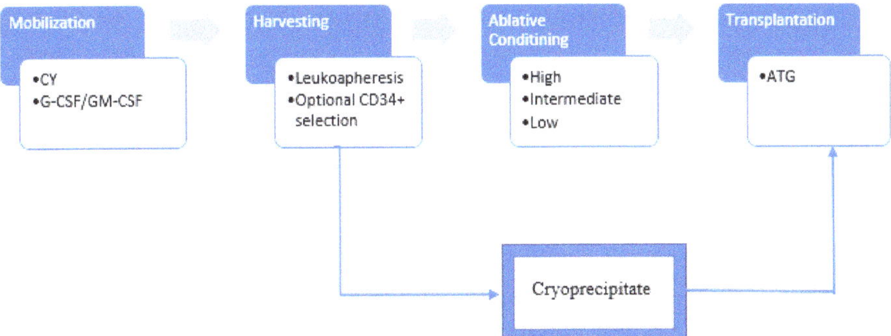

Figure 1. Immunoablation followed by autologous hematopoietic stem cell transplantation. First, HSC are mobilized, typically from peripheral blood, by using granulocyte colony-stimulating factor (G-CSF) or granulocyte-macrophage colony-stimulating factor (GM-CSF), with or without cyclophosphamide (CY). The HSC are then harvested and cryopreserved until the patient is ready for transplantation. The HSC can be positively selected for CD34$^+$ cells ex vivo. The next step is to eliminate autoreactive cells (ablative conditioning) using either a high-, intermediate (BEAM), or low-intensity regimen. After the conditioning regimen, the cryopreserved cells are thawed and then infused back into the patient. Anti-thymocyte globulin (ATG) is administered before or after the aHSC infusion to primarily remove any autoreactive T cells that might have escaped prior conditioning procedures. Subsequently, the patient enters an aplastic phase, characterized by an extremely low level of hematopoietic blood cells requiring prophylactic treatment with antivirals and antibiotics.

Table 1. Immunoablation regimens.

Intensity	Regimen
High	High dose of busulfan combined with cyclophosphamide and ATG
Intermediate	BEAM (BCNU, etoposide, cytosine arabinoside, melphalan) +/− ATG
Low (nonmyeloablative)	Cyclophosphamide and ATG

2.2. Immune Mechanisms

Although the efficacy of aHSCT in MS is increasingly being validated, the immune mechanisms that account for its therapeutic effects are still unclear. There are at least two basic hypotheses to explain its beneficial effects. First, aHSCT is considered to "reset" the immune system by depleting adaptive immune cells and gradually developing a "new" immune system [7,18,19,39,40]. The naïve T cells reemerge over time and undergo a complex T cell receptor (TCR) rearrangement, leading to an augmentation of the T cell repertoire and clonal diversity [18,19,41]. After immune reconstitution, pathogenic CD4+ Th17 lymphocytes are reduced [42]. On the other hand, T cell clones that recognize and react to myelin basic protein (MBP) are initially depleted by the conditioning regimen but reappear over time, although it has not established whether these cells are pathological [41]. The extent to which aHSCT leads to an immune reconfiguration is not completely clear, and demonstrating how the immune system resets to a pre-pathological state is scientifically challenging. However, the characteristics that the immune system acquires following aHCST certainly suggest that it has become alternatively programmed. Conversely, an alternate explanation of the therapeutic benefits of aHSCT might be that the conditioning regimen severely depletes T cell populations for an extended time, thus inducing a state of long-lasting immunosuppression incapable of mounting an autoimmune response of clinical significance [20–22]. Both of the aforementioned hypotheses may have diverse effects that could be beneficial to MS treatment and, when applied alone, either hypothesis is ineffective or less effective at explaining the benefits of the treatment than when applied in combination. Therefore, the reconciliation of these hypotheses should be achieved in order to obtain optimal therapeutic results [43].

2.3. Current Clinical Knowledge

The initial studies using aHSCT to treat MS were performed over two decades ago [13]. Since then, there has been an increasing number of studies looking into this treatment approach. Typically, the primary endpoint is event-free survival (EFS), which is defined as survival without death, or the patient having no evidence of disease activity (NEDA) (i.e., no disability progression, relapse, and/or new lesions on MRI). Earlier studies were conducted mostly in patients with a high level of disability and progressive disease [13,31,44].

For example, a recent retrospective study evaluated the long-term outcomes of patients with MS treated with aHSCT between January 1995 and December 2006 [45]. In this study, the authors established that most patients had progressive MS (78%), mostly with secondary progressive MS (66%). The median Expanded Disability Status Scale (EDSS) score was 6.5, demonstrating moderately advanced disability, on average. The progression-free survival at 5 years was established for the combined group (46%), RRMS subgroup (73%), and the SPMS subgroup (33%). Also, no statistical difference in the risk of progression between primary progressive MS (PPMS) and SPMS was identified. Furthermore, transplant-related mortality (TRM) occurring in the first 100 days after transplantation was 2.8%. The authors concluded that a younger age, RRMS, and fewer prior disease-modifying treatments were associated with better neurological outcomes.

Recent studies have focused on patients with RRMS with an aggressive disease course, given the evidence that aHSCT is most successful in this population [34,36,46–48]. The HALT-MS study, in which only patients with RRMS were enrolled, demonstrated a 5-year event-free survival of 69.2% [49,50]. Similarly, a phase II multicenter single-arm trial of patients with aggressive MS who underwent aHSCT transplantation reported an event-free survival at 3 years of 69.6% [51]. Both groups also demonstrated an improvement of their EDSS by 0.5 points or more at their latest follow-up. An additional large single-center trial using nonmyeloablative aHSCT in patients with RRMS and SPMS showed a 4-year relapse-free survival of 80% and progression-free survival of 87% [52]. The study also showed improved disability scores 2 years after aHSCT, mainly in those with RRMS and mild to moderate disability. This benefit was not seen in patients with severe disability due to progressive MS. These three major studies concluded that either HDIT or a nonmyeloablative regimen followed by aHSCT was effective in inducing long-term sustained remissions and disability improvement.

The safety of aHSCT has dramatically improved through the years. The European Bone Marrow Transplantation (EBMT) Registry analysis of patients treated from 1995 to 2000 showed a TRM of 7.3%, while the TRM from 2001 to2007 was 1.3%, further decreasing to 0.7% during 2008–2016, and most recently down to 0.2% [24,38,45]. This improvement is likely related to the better selection of patients (younger patients with RRMS and exclusion of older patients with advanced disability), increased experience with aHSCT treatment, and decreased use of high-intensity regimens [31]. For example, high-intensity conditioning regimens were associated with life-threatening infections [32,33]. Furthermore, some clinical trials using nonmyeloablative conditioning report no mortality associated with the procedure [52]. A recent meta-analysis found that TRM was close to zero in studies that included patients who were younger, had RRMS rather than SPMS along with a lower baseline EDSS, and whose procedure was performed in more recent years, although there was no significant association of TRM with regimen intensity [53]. The authors pointed out a few limitations that may contribute to their results. Regardless, growing evidence suggests intense conditioning and/or extensive T cell depletion protocols increase morbidity and mortality rate [24].

3. Mesenchymal Stem Cells

3.1. Preclinical Animal Studies with Mesenchymal Stem Cells

Besides aHSC, the use of MSC has emerged as a potential powerful cellular therapy for inflammatory and neurodegenerative diseases of the CNS, including MS [54,55]. The MSC are multipotent, nonhematopoietic cells that have both immunomodulatory and regenerative properties [56]. Typically, MSC are obtained from the bone marrow, but other tissues have been used, including adipose tissue, umbilical cord blood, and placenta [57,58]. For example, bone marrow MSC (BM-MSC) have been shown to reduce inflammatory responses, stimulate neuronal stem cell differentiation, and promote the regeneration of damaged areas in the CNS [59–63]. These effects are thought to be possible due to peripheral paracrine signals and/or the homing of MSC to injured tissue [64,65].

Studies on EAE have revealed the potential beneficial effects of MSC. EAE mice exhibit multifocal inflammation, variable demyelination, and axonal damage in the CNS via immunization with myelin proteins or immunogenic myelin peptides [65]. The EAE animal model has been helpful in explaining the immunobiological basis of tissue damage in MS and identifying potential therapeutic approaches. When BM-MSC are infused into EAE mice, there is a reduction in the severity of the clinical symptoms and diminished immune cell infiltration, demyelination, and axonal damage [59–63]. These therapeutic effects are seen when MSC are injected intravenously (IV), intraventricular (IVT), and even intraperitoneally (IP) [61,66,67]. However, the optimal route for MSC injection is yet to be determined. Moreover, the therapeutic effects are observed when BM-MSC are injected at disease onset or peak, but are not seen if they are administered during the chronic stage of disease [60].

The exact mechanisms by which BM-MSC mediate their beneficial outcomes are still not completely understood. One potential explanation includes the release of anti-inflammatory and neurotrophic molecules that modulate the immune inflammatory responses targeting the CNS. For instance, EAE mice that received an IVT infusion of exogenous BM-MSC exhibited a significant reduction in disease activity that was associated with the suppression of reactive T cells [67]. In a different study, human BM-MSC infusion in EAE mice was associated with decreased inflammatory myelin-specific Th1 cells and increased anti-inflammatory Th2 cells [59]. These results suggest an immunosuppressive reaction to BM-MSC infusion. Interestingly, IV injection of conditioned media used in MSC (MSC-CM) culture was associated with the symptomatic improvement of EAE mice, suggesting that the beneficial effects were produced by extracellular immunomodulatory molecules secreted by MSC [68].

An additional possibility that may explain the therapeutic effects of MSC is their migration to inflamed tissues. Several studies have tried to describe the ability of MSC to migrate to and repair injured tissue [61,69]. For example, intravenously administered MSC were detected in CNS in proportion to the degree of inflammation [69]. However, the data are limited, and the factors that attract MSC to areas of inflammation have not yet been elucidated.

In addition to their immunomodulatory capabilities, MS might have the potential of influencing neuronal stem cell differentiation and promoting remyelination and axonal survival. For example, MSC promote the differentiation of oligodendrocytes and/or neurons from neuronal stem cells in vitro, in preference to astroglial fate [70]. Similarly, brain dissection and histopathological studies of EAE mice treated with MSC infusion showed an increased number of oligodendrocytes, remyelination of white matter, and improved axonal integrity in injured tissue [59].

By contrast, some studies have reported deteriorative responses and the exacerbation of EAE symptoms with MSC treatment [71]. These findings implicate a different immunobiological mechanism from the previously described possibilities. Moreover, ectopic tissue formation when MS were administered via IVT in an EAE model [72] and malignant transformation are a theoretical concern, although not yet reported in humans [73].

Finally, it is unclear which tissues are the optimal source of MSC. Adipose tissue (AT) has been cited as a superior source because AT-MSC are relatively easier to harvest, have a higher availability, and better expansion capabilities ex vivo than BM-MSC [74]. Further studies are warranted to determine the best source.

3.2. Clinical Trials Using Mesenchymal Stem Cells for the Treatment of Multiple Sclerosis

Based on the results of treating EAE, MSC therapy has advanced to clinical trials. The first publication of a clinical trial using MSC in MS patients was in 2007 by Mohyeddin Bonab and colleagues [75]. Their study assessed the safety and efficacy of autologous BM-MSC transplantation in 10 patients with progressive MS. There were no major adverse events reported with a mean follow-up of 19 months. The preliminary report described varying results of EDSS and MRI progression. The authors pointed out the feasibility of MSC therapy to treat MS patients.

Subsequent studies have investigated the potential of MSC therapy in MS patients. These studies have preliminarily shown beneficial results and the safety of the procedure with no major adverse effects reported [76–78]. However, all studies had an open-label design, and varied in the source dose and administration route.

In 2010, a group of experts formed the International Mesenchymal Stem Cells Transplantation Study Group (IMSCTSG) in order to have a consensus protocol on the use of MSC for the treatment of MS [8]. The protocol established a phase I/II clinical trial to evaluate MS patients treated with autologous MSC who have not responded to at least one year of treatment with conventional immunomodulatory therapy. Patients are randomized to receive either IV infusion of autologous BM-MSC or suspension media. At 6 months, these treatments are switched between the two cohorts. The primary endpoints are to analyze the safety of MSC therapy in MS patients and to measure the reduction in the number and volume of new enhancing lesions over a 6-month period.

The IMSCTSG protocol has been adapted for use in multiple clinical trials with varying results. For example, Llufriu and colleagues completed a randomized placebo-controlled phase II trial with 9 RRMS patients who had failed conventional therapy [79]. At 6 months, patients treated with an IV infusion of BM-MSC had no statistical differences in clinical outcomes, brain MRI findings, and optical coherence tomography (OCT) measures. However, there was a trend towards a lower mean cumulative number of gadolinium-enhancing lesions on MRI. The authors concluded that BM-MSC are safe and may reduce inflammatory MRI parameters.

As mentioned previously, MSC may have a theoretical risk of malignant transformation. Therefore, recent studies have focused on investigating the feasibility of using autologous MSC-derived neuronal progenitors (MSC-NP) in lieu of BM-MSC to reduce pluripotency and to minimize the risk of ectopic differentiation after CNS transplantation [80,81]. A phase I open-label clinical trial showed that autologous IT transplantation of MSC-NP is safe and well tolerated. In addition, the authors reported an improved EDSS median in their cohort of 20 patients with progressive MS after treatment. Lastly, positive trends (e.g., muscle strength, bladder function) were more frequently observed in the subset of SPMS patients when compared to PPMS patients [82]. Other studies have shown similar results in the safety and efficacy of MSC-NP transplantation, demonstrating a potential therapeutic alternative [83]. However, further studies are needed to determine if transplantation of MSC-NP has better outcomes when compared to BM-MSC.

As noted above, MSC-CM has been investigated for its therapeutic potential in preclinical animal models. Recently, Danbour and colleagues assessed the safety and feasibility of IT treatment with BM-MSC followed by MSC-CM in patients with MS [84]. The study was conducted as an open-label prospective phase I/IIa clinical trial. No serious adverse effects were reported after the treatment. However, due to the small number and heterogeneity of enrolled patients, it was not possible to obtain statistically significant differences in the efficacy measurements (e.g., EDSS score, clinical, cognitive, ophthalmological, and radiological).

To date, cell therapy with MSC has been, overall, well tolerated and safe. Still, it is not known whether this treatment is capable of reducing inflammatory MS disease activity or promoting the regeneration of damaged areas in the CNS.

4. Other Stem Cells under Research

4.1. Neuronal Stem Cells (NSC)

In the last decade, there has been particular interest in utilizing NSC as a cellular therapy. Adult NSC are found mostly in two regions of the anterior brain: the subgranular zone (SGZ) within the hippocampal dentate gyrus and the subventricular zone (SVZ) lining the lateral ventricles [85,86]. NSC can give rise to neuronal progenitor cells (NPC) to produce neurons, astrocytes, and oligodendrocytes [87,88]. In EAE, NPC can be activated to migrate to inflammatory demyelinating tissue in the CNS, and differentiate into oligodendrocytes, thus having a potential for therapeutic benefits [10].

One major limitation is the limited number of endogenous NSC available to participate in repair mechanisms [89]. For this reason, therapeutic strategies in animal models are looking into the allogenic infusion of NSC. For example, IVT-transplanted NPC at the peak of EAE migrated exclusively into inflamed white matter and subsequently differentiated into oligodendrocytes; however, their direct implication in myelin repair remains unclear [90]. Additionally, other studies have demonstrated the presence of NPC in some chronically demyelinated lesions [91]. This finding suggests that the absence of NPC in pathological tissue is an unsatisfactory explanation for the clinical symptoms. An alternative proposition to explain this phenomenon is that the prevalent inflammatory setting in EAE produces a non-permissive environment for oligodendrocyte precursor cells (OPC) differentiation and function.

The current clinical trial using NPC comes from MSC-NP, as we previously described.

4.2. Human Embryonic Stem Cells (hESC)

hESC have been considered for cell therapy, owing to their capability to differentiate into all the germ layer derivatives. Specifically, the ability of hESC to differentiate into neural lineage has attracted scientific attention regarding the potential treatment of MS [92]. For example, transplanting hESC-derived neural progenitors into EAE mice led to diminished clinical symptoms. Histological studies revealed the presence of transplanted neural progenitors in mice brains, however, remyelination and the production of mature oligodendrocytes were not observed. The clinical improvement was hypothesized to result from immunosuppressive and neuroprotective mechanisms [12]. Further studies are required to better understand the mechanism of action of hESC in treating CNS demyelinating disease.

There have been a few published case reports using hESC to treat MS with limited data suggesting the safety of the therapy [93]. However, well-designed clinical trials are required to show the long-term efficacy and safety of hESC in the treatment of MS.

4.3. Induced Pluripotent Stem Cells (iPSC)

Lastly, iPSC are pluripotent cells that have been reprogrammed from somatic cells from skin and other tissues. These cells have the potential to become OPC, hence, they may constitute a suitable cellular therapy modality from an autologous source [94]. The therapeutic potential of iPSC is still under research, but some studies suggest that oligodendrocyte precursor-derived iPSC are capable of ameliorating the clinical and pathological features of EAE [95]. However, the therapeutic effect was found to be mostly due to a neuroprotective effect rather than remyelination. Moreover, the efficient differentiation of iPSC toward selected cell phenotypes could represent a great research challenge for directed disease therapy. Finally, recent studies suggest some caution for clinical development due to the potential for malignant transformation and immune rejection [96,97].

5. Conclusions

Immunoablative therapy followed by autologous hematopoietic stem cell transplantation should be considered in aggressive and treatment-refractory MS, since this treatment approach has shown increasing evidence of inducing long-term sustained remission and disability improvement. Further studies are needed to characterize which conditioning regimen should be used. On the other hand, MSC have emerged as a potentially powerful and safe cellular therapy for MS, but the dose, route of administration, and therapeutic effects need further exploration and quantification. Other novel forms of stem cell-based therapies for MS are, at this time, only in the early stages, including those based on hESC, iPSC, and NSC.

Funding: This research received no external funding.

Conflicts of Interest: The authors declare no conflict of interest.

References

1. Frischer, J.M.; Steiner, J.P.; Dal-Bianco, A.; Dal-Bianco, A.; Lucchinetti, C.F.; Rauschka, H.; Schmidbauer, M.; Laursen, H.; Sorensen, P.S.; Lassmann, H. The relation between inflammation and neurodegeneration in multiple sclerosis brains. *Brain* **2009**, *132*, 1175–1189. [CrossRef] [PubMed]
2. Reingold, S.C.; Steiner, J.P.; Polman, C.H.; Cohen, J.A.; Freedman, M.S.; Kappos, L.; Thompson, A.J.; Wolinsky, J.S. The challenge of follow-on biologics for treatment of multiple sclerosis. *Neurology* **2009**, *73*, 552–559. [CrossRef] [PubMed]
3. Wingerchuk, D.M.; Carter, J.L. Multiple sclerosis: Current and emerging disease-modifying therapies and treatment strategies. *Mayo Clin. Proc.* **2014**, *89*, 225–240. [CrossRef] [PubMed]
4. Freedman, M.S.; Selchen, D.; Arnold, D.L.; Prat, A.; Banwell, B.; Yeung, M.; Morgenthau, D.; Lapierre, Y. Treatment optimization in MS: Canadian MS Working Group updated recommendations. *Can. J. Neurol. Sci.* **2013**, *40*, 307–323. [CrossRef] [PubMed]
5. Sormani, M.P.; Li, D.K.; Bruzzi, P.; Stubinski, B.; Cornelisse, P.; Rocak, S.; De Stefano, N. Combined MRI lesions and relapses as a surrogate for disability in multiple sclerosis. *Neurology* **2011**, *77*, 1684–1690. [CrossRef] [PubMed]
6. Stem Cells in MS. Available online: https://www.nationalmssociety.org/Research/Research-News-Progress/Stem-Cells-in-MS (accessed on 11 January 2019).
7. Delemarre, E.M.; van den Broek, T.; Mijnheer, G.; Meerding, J.; Wehrens, E.J.; Olek, S.; Boes, M.; van Herwijnen, M.J.; Broere, F.; van Royen, A.; et al. Autologous stem cell transplantation aids autoimmune patients by functional renewal and TCR diversification of regulatory T cells. *Blood* **2016**, *12*, 91–101. [CrossRef] [PubMed]
8. Freedman, M.S.; Bar-Or, A.; Atkins, H.L.; Karussis, D.; Frassoni, F.; Lazarus, H.; Scolding, N.; Slavin, S.; Le Blanc, K.; Uccelli, A.; et al. The therapeutic potential of mesenchymal stem cell transplantation as a treatment for multiple sclerosis: Consensus report of the International MSCT Study Group. *Mult. Scler.* **2010**, *16*, 503–510. [CrossRef] [PubMed]
9. Seo, J.H.; Cho, S.R. Neurorestoration induced by mesenchymal stem cells. *Yonsei Med. J.* **2012**, *53*, 1059–1067. [CrossRef] [PubMed]
10. Picard-Riera, N.; Decker, L.; Delarasse, C.; Goude, K.; Nait-Oumesmar, B.; Liblau, R.; Pham-Dinh, D.; Baron-Van Evercooren, A. Experimental autoimmune encephalomyelitis mobilizes neural progenitors from the subventricular zone to undergo oligodendrogenesis in adult mice. *Proc. Natl. Acad. Sci. USA* **2002**, *99*, 13211–13216. [CrossRef] [PubMed]
11. Thiruvalluvan, A.; Czepiel, M.; Kap, Y.A.; Mantingh-Otter, I.; Vainchtein, I.; Kuipers, J.; Bijlard, M.; Baron, W.; Giepmans, B.; Brück, W.; et al. Survival and functionality of human induced pluripotent stem cell-derived oligodendrocytes in a nonhuman primate model for multiple sclerosis. *Stem Cells Transl. Med.* **2016**, *5*, 1550–1561. [CrossRef] [PubMed]
12. Aharonowiz, M.; Einstein, O.; Fainstein, N.; Lassmann, H.; Reubinoff, B.; Ben-Hur, T. Neuroprotective effect of transplanted human embryonic stem cell-derived neural precursors in an animal model of multiple sclerosis. *PLoS ONE* **2008**, *3*, e3145. [CrossRef] [PubMed]

13. Fassas, A.; Anagnostopoulos, A.; Kazis, A.; Kapinas, K.; Sakellari, I.; Kimiskidis, V.; Tsompanakou, A. Peripheral blood stem cell transplantation in the treatment of progressive multiple sclerosis: First results of a pilot study. *Bone Marrow Transplant.* **1997**, *20*, 631–638. [CrossRef] [PubMed]

14. Snowden, J.A.; Patton, W.N.; O'Donnell, J.L.; Hannah, E.E.; Hart, D.N. Prolonged remission of longstanding systemic lupus erythematous after autologous bone marrow transplant for non-Hodgkin's lymphoma. *Bone Marrow Transplant.* **1997**, *19*, 1247–1250. [CrossRef] [PubMed]

15. Van Gelder, M.; van Bekkum, D.W. Treatment of relapsing experimental autoimmune encephalomyelitis in rats with allogeneic bone marrow transplantation from a resistant strain. *Bone Marrow Transplant.* **1995**, *16*, 343–351. [PubMed]

16. Van Gelder, M.; Kinwel-Bohre, E.P.; van Bekkum, D.W. Treatment of experimental allergic encephalomyelitis in rats with total body irradiation and syngeneic BMT. *Bone Marrow Transplant.* **1993**, *11*, 233–241. [PubMed]

17. Van Gelder, M.; van Bekkum, D.W. Effective treatment of relapsing experimental autoimmune encephalomyelitis with pseudoautologous bone marrow transplantation. *Bone Marrow Transplant.* **1996**, *18*, 1029–1034. [PubMed]

18. Muraro, P.A.; Douek, D.C.; Packer, A.; Chung, K.; Guenaga, F.J.; Cassiani-Ingoni, R.; Campbell, C.; Memon, S.; Nagle, J.W.; Hakim, F.T.; et al. Thymic output generates a new and diverse TCR repertoire after autologous stem cell transplantation in multiple sclerosis patients. *J. Exp. Med.* **2005**, *201*, 805–816. [CrossRef] [PubMed]

19. Muraro, P.A.; Robins, H.; Malhotra, S.; Howell, M.; Phippard, D.; Desmarais, C.; de Paula Alves Sousa, A.; Griffith, L.M.; Lim, N.; Nash, R.A.; et al. T cell repertoire following autologous stem cell transplantation for multiple sclerosis. *J. Clin. Investig.* **2014**, *124*, 1168–1172. [CrossRef] [PubMed]

20. Glastone, D.E.; Peyster, R.; Baron, E.; Friedman-Urevich, S.; Sibony, P.; Melville, P.; Gottesman, M. High-dose cyclophosphamide for moderate to severe refractory multiple sclerosis. *Am. J. Ther.* **2011**, *18*, 23–30. [CrossRef] [PubMed]

21. Krishnan, C.; Kaplin, A.I.; Brodsky, R.A.; Drachman, D.B.; Jones, R.J.; Pham, D.L.; Richert, N.D.; Pardo, C.A.; Yousem, D.M.; Hammond, E.; et al. Reduction of disease activity and disability with high-dose cyclophosphamide in patients with aggressive multiple sclerosis. *Arch. Neurol.* **2008**, *65*, 1044–1051. [CrossRef] [PubMed]

22. Harrinson, D.M.; Gladstone, D.E.; Hammond, E.; Cheng, J.; Jones, R.J.; Brodsky, R.A.; Kerr, D.; McArthur, J.C.; Kaplin, A. Treatment of relapsing-remitting multiple sclerosis with high-dose cyclophosphamide infusion followed by glatimer acetate maintenance. *Mult. Scler. J.* **2012**, *18*, 202–209. [CrossRef] [PubMed]

23. Saccardi, R.; Freedman, M.S.; Sormani, M.P.; Atkins, H.; Farge, D.; Griffith, L.M.; Kraft, G.; Mancardi, G.L.; Nash, R.; Pasquini, M.; et al. A prospective, randomized, controlled trial of autologous haematopoietic stem cell transplantation for aggressive multiple sclerosis: A position paper. *Mult Scler. J.* **2012**, *18*, 825–834. [CrossRef]

24. Mancardi, G.; Saccardi, R. Autologous haematopoietic stem-cell transplantation in multiple sclerosis. *Lancet Neurol.* **2008**, *7*, 626–636. [CrossRef]

25. Openshaw, H.; Stuve, O.; Antel, J.P.; Nash, R.; Lund, B.T.; Weiner, L.P.; Kashyap, A.; McSweeney, P.; Forman, S. Multiple sclerosis flares associated with recombinant granulocyte colony-stimulating factor. *Neurology* **2000**, *54*, 2147–2150. [CrossRef]

26. Snowden, J.A.; Saccardi, R.; Allez, M.; Ardizzone, S.; Arnold, R.; Cervera, R.; Denton, C.; Hawkey, C.; Labopin, M.; Mancardi, G.; et al. Haematopoietic SCT in severe autoimmune diseases: Updated guidelines of the European Group for Blood and Marrow Transplantation. *Bone Marrow Transplant.* **2012**, *47*, 770–790. [CrossRef]

27. Saiz, A.; Blanco, Y.; Berenguer, J.; Gómez-Choco, M.; Carreras, E.; Arbizu, T.; Graus, F. Clinical outcome 6 years after autologous hematopoietic stem cell transplantation in multiple sclerosis. *Neurologia* **2008**, *23*, 405–407. [PubMed]

28. Shevchenko, J.; Kuznestsov, A.N.; Ionova, T.I.; Melnichenko, V.Y.; Fedorenko, D.A.; Kurbatova, K.A.; Gorodokin, G.I.; Novik, A.A. Long-term outcomes of autologous hematopoietic stem cell transplantation with reduced-intensity conditioning in multiple sclerosis: physician's and patient's perspectives. *Ann. Hematol.* **2015**, *94*, 1149–1157. [CrossRef] [PubMed]

29. Bacigalupo, A.; Ballen, K.; Giralt, S.; Lazarus, H.; Ho, V.; Apperley, J.; Slavin, S.; Pasquini, M.; Sandmaier, B.M.; Barrett, J.; et al. Defining the intensity of conditioning regimens: Working definitions. *Biol. Blood Marrow Transplant.* **2009**, *15*, 1628–1633. [CrossRef] [PubMed]

30. Gratwohl, A.; Passweg, J.; Bocelli-Tyndall, C.; Fassas, A.; van Laar, J.M.; Farge, D.; Andolina, M.; Arnold, R.; Carreras, E.; Finke, J.; et al. Autologous hematopoietic stem cell transplantation for autoimmune diseases. *Bone Marrow Transplant.* **2005**, *35*, 869–879. [CrossRef]

31. Saccardi, R.; Kozak, T.; Bocelli-Tyndall, C.; Fassas, A.; Kazis, A.; Havrdova, E.; Carreras, E.; Saiz, A.; Löwenberg, B.; te Boekhorst, P.A.; et al. Autologous stem cell transplantation for progressive multiple sclerosis: Update of the European Group for Blood and Marrow Transplantation autoimmune diseases working party database. *Mult. Scler. J.* **2006**, *12*, 814–823. [CrossRef] [PubMed]

32. Samjin, J.P.; te Boekhorst, P.A.; Mondria, T.; van Doorn, P.A.; Flach, H.Z.; van der Meché, F.G.A.; Cornelissen, J.; Hop, W.C.; Löwenberg, B.; Hintzen, R.Q. Intense T cell depletion followed by autologous bone marrow transplantation for severe multiple sclerosis. *J. Neurol. Neurosurg. Psychiatry* **2006**, *77*, 46–50. [CrossRef] [PubMed]

33. Nash, R.A.; Dansey, R.; Storek, J.; Georges, G.E.; Bowen, J.D.; Holmberg, L.A.; Kraft, G.H.; Mayes, M.D.; McDonagh, K.T.; Chen, C.S.; et al. Epstein-Barr virus-associated posttransplantation lymphoproliferative disorder after high-dose immunosuppressive therapy and autologous CD34-selected hematopoietic stem cell transplantation for severe autoimmune diseases. *Biol. Blood Marrow Transplant.* **2003**, *9*, 583–591. [CrossRef]

34. Mancardi, G.L.; Sormani, M.P.; Di Gioia, M.; Vuolo, L.; Gualandi, F.; Amato, M.P.; Capello, E.; Currò, D.; Uccelli, A.; Bertolotto, A.; et al. Autologous haematopoietic stem cell transplantation with an intermediate intensity conditioning regimen in multiple sclerosis: The Italian multi-centre experience. *Mult. Scler. J.* **2012**, *18*, 835–842. [CrossRef] [PubMed]

35. Curro', D.; Vuolo, L.; Gualandi, F.; Bacigalupo, A.; Roccatagliata, L.; Capello, E.; Uccelli, A.; Saccardi, R.; Mancardi, G. Low intensity lympho-ablative regimen followed by autologous hematopoietic stem cell transplantation in severe forms of multiple sclerosis: A MRI-based clinical study. *Mult. Scler. J.* **2015**, *11*, 1423–1430. [CrossRef] [PubMed]

36. Burt, R.K.; Loh, Y.; Cohen, B.; Stefoski, D.; Balabanov, R.; Katsamakis, G.; Oyama, Y.; Russell, E.J.; Stern, J.; Muraro, P.; et al. Autologous non-myeloablative haemopoeitic stem cell transplantation in relapsing-remitting multiple sclerosis: A phase I/II study. *Lancet Neurol.* **2009**, *201*, 805–816. [CrossRef]

37. Hammerschlak, N.; Rodrigues, M.; Moraes, D.A.; Oliveira, M.C.; Stracieri, A.B.; Pieroni, F.; Barros, G.M.; Madeira, M.I.; Simões, B.P.; Barreira, A.A.; et al. Brazilian experience with two conditioning regimens in patients with multiple sclerosis: BEAM/horse ATG and CY/rabbit ATG. *Bone Marrow Transplant.* **2006**, *45*, 239–248. [CrossRef] [PubMed]

38. Muraro, P.A.; Martin, R.; Mancardi, G.L.; Nicholas, R.; Sormani, M.P.; Saccardi, R. Autologous haematopoietic stem cell transplantation for treatment of multiple sclerosis. *Nat. Rev. Neurol.* **2017**, *13*, 391–405. [CrossRef] [PubMed]

39. Arruda, L.C.; de Azevedo, J.T.; de Oliveira, G.L.V.; Scortegagna, G.T.; Rogrigues, E.S.; Palma, P.V.B.; Brum, D.G.; Guerreiro, C.T.; Marques, V.D.; Barreira, A.A.; et al. Immunological correlates of favorable long-term clinical outcome in multiple sclerosis patients after autologous hematopoietic stem cell transplantation. *Clin. Immunol.* **2016**, *169*, 47–57. [CrossRef] [PubMed]

40. Fassas, A.; Kazis, A. High-dose immunosuppression and autologous hematopoietic stem cell rescue for severe multiple sclerosis. *J. Hematother. Stem Cell Res.* **2003**, *12*, 701–711. [CrossRef]

41. Sun, W.; Uday, P.; Hutton, G.J.; Zang, Y.C.; Krance, R.; Carrum, G.; Land, G.A.; Heslop, H.; Brenner, M.; Zhang, J.Z. Characteristics of T-cell receptor repertoire and myelin-reactive T cells reconstituted from autologous haematopoietic stem-cell grafts in multiple sclerosis. *Brain* **2004**, *127*, 996–1008. [CrossRef] [PubMed]

42. Darlington, P.J.; Touil, T.; Doucet, J.S.; Gaucher, D.; Zeidan, J.; Gauchat, D.; Corsini, R.; Kim, H.J.; Duddy, M.; Jalili, F.; et al. Diminished Th17 (not Th1) responses underlie multiple sclerosis disease abrogation after hematopoietic stem cell transplantation. *Ann. Neurol.* **2013**, *73*, 341–354. [CrossRef]

43. Gosselin, D.; Rivest, S. Immune mechanisms underlying the beneficial effects of autologous hematopoietic stem cell transplantation in multiple sclerosis. *Neurotherapeutics* **2011**, *8*, 643–649. [CrossRef]

44. Bowen, J.D.; Kraft, G.H.; Wundes, A.; Guan, Q.; Maravilla, K.R.; Gooley, T.A.; McSweeney, P.A.; Pavletic, S.Z.; Openshaw, H.; Storb, R.; et al. Autologous hematopoietic cell transplantation following high-dose immunosuppressive therapy for advanced multiple sclerosis: Long-term results. *Bone Marrow Transplant.* **2012**, *47*, 946–951. [CrossRef] [PubMed]

45. Muraro, P.A.; Pasquini, M.; Atkins, H.L.; Bowen, J.D.; Farge, D.; Fassas, D.; Freedman, M.S.; Georges, G.E.; Gualandi, F.; Hamerschlak, N.; et al. Long-term outcomes after autologous hematopoietic stem cell transplantation for multiple sclerosis. *JAMA Neurol.* **2017**, *74*, 459–469. [CrossRef] [PubMed]

46. Krasulová, E.; Trneny, M.; Kozak, T.; Vacková, B.; Pohlreich, D.; Kemlink, D.; Kobylka, P.; Kovárová, I.; Lhtáková, P.; Havrdov, E. High-dose immunoablation with autologous haematopoietic stem cell transplantation in aggressive multiple sclerosis: A single centre 10-year experience. *Mult. Scler. J.* **2010**, *16*, 685–693. [CrossRef]

47. Fassas, A.; Kimiskidis, V.K.; Sakellari, I.; Kapinas, K.; Anagnostopoulos, A.; Tsimourtou, V.; Kazis, A. Long-term results of stem transplantation for MS: A single-center experience. *Neurology* **2011**, *76*, 1066–1070. [CrossRef] [PubMed]

48. Cassanova, B.; Jarque, I.; Gascón, F.; Hernández-Boluda, J.C.; Pérez-Miralles, F.; de la Rubia, J.; Alcalá, C.; Sanz, J.; Mallada, J.; Cervelló, A.; et al. Autologous hematopoietic stem cell transplantation in relapsing-remitting multiple sclerosis: Comparison with secondary progressive multiple sclerosis. *Neurol. Sci.* **2017**, *38*, 1213–1221. [CrossRef] [PubMed]

49. Nash, R.A.; Hutton, G.J.; Racke, M.K.; Popat, U.; Devine, S.M.; Steinmiller, K.C.; Griffith, L.M.; Muraro, P.A.; Openshaw, H.; Sayre, P.H.; et al. High-dose immunosuppressive therapy and autologous HCT for relapsing-remitting MS. *Neurology* **2017**, *88*, 842–852. [CrossRef] [PubMed]

50. Nash, R.A.; Hutton, G.J.; Racke, M.K.; Popat, U.; Devine, S.M.; Griffith, L.M.; Muraro, P.A.; Openshaw, H.; Sayre, P.H.; Stüve, O.; et al. High-dose immunosuppressive therapy and autologous hematopoietic cell transplantation for relapsing-remitting multiple sclerosis (HALT-MS): A 3-year interim report. *JAMA Neurol.* **2015**, *72*, 159–169. [CrossRef] [PubMed]

51. Atkins, H.L.; Bowman, M.; Allan, D.; Anstee, G.; Arnold, D.L.; Bar-Or, A.; Bence-Bruckler, I.; Birch, P.; Bredeson, C.; Chen, J.; et al. Immunoablation and autologous haemopoietic stem-cell transplantation for aggressive multiple sclerosis: A multicentre single-group phase 2 trial. *Lancet* **2016**, *388*, 576–585. [CrossRef]

52. Burt, R.K.; Balabanov, R.; Sharrack, B.; Morgan, A.; Quigley, K.; Yaung, K.; Helenowski, I.B.; Jovanovic, B.; Spahovic, D.; Arnautovic, I.; et al. Association of nonmyeloablative hematopoietic stem cell transplantation with neurological disability in patients with relapsing-remitting multiple sclerosis. *JAMA* **2015**, *313*, 275–284. [CrossRef] [PubMed]

53. Sormani, M.P.; Muraro, P.; Schiavetti, I.; Signori, A.; Laroni, A.; Saccardi, R.; Mancardi, G.L. Autologous hematopoietic stem cell transplantation in multiple sclerosis: A meta-analysis. *Neurology* **2017**, *13*, 391–405. [CrossRef] [PubMed]

54. Uccelli, A.; Laroni, A.; Freedman, M.S. Mesenchymal stem cells for the treatment of multiple sclerosis and other neurological diseases. *Lancet Neurol.* **2011**, *10*, 649–656. [CrossRef]

55. Rice, C.M.; Kemp, K.; Wilkins, A.; Scolding, N.J. Cell therapy for multiple sclerosis: An evolving concept with implications for other neurodegenerative diseases. *Lancet* **2013**, *382*, 1204–1213. [CrossRef]

56. Pittenger, M.F.; Mackay, A.M.; Beck, S.C.; Jaiswal, R.K.; Douglas, R.; Mosca, J.D.; Moorman, M.A.; Simonetti, D.W.; Craig, S.; Marshak, D.R. Multilineage potential of adult human mesenchymal stem cells. *Science* **1999**, *284*, 143–147. [CrossRef] [PubMed]

57. Zhang, X.; Bowles, A.C.; Semon, J.A.; Scruggs, B.A.; Zhang, S.; Strong, A.L.; Gimble, J.M.; Bunnell, B.A. Transplantation of autologous adipose stem cells lacks therapeutic efficacy in the experimental autoimmune encephalomyelitis model. *PLoS ONE* **2014**, *9*, e85007. [CrossRef] [PubMed]

58. Li, D.; Chai, J.; Shen, C.; Han, Y.; Sun, T. Human umbilical cord-derived mesenchymal stem cells differentiate into epidermal-like cells using a novel co-culture technique. *Cytotechnology* **2014**, *66*, 699–708. [CrossRef]

59. Bai, L.; Lennon, D.P.; Maier, K.; Caplan, A.L.; Miller, S.D.; Miller, R.H. Human bone marrow-derived mesenchymal stem cells induce Th2 polarized immune response and promote endogenous repair in animal models of multiple sclerosis. *Glia* **2009**, *57*, 1192–1203. [CrossRef] [PubMed]

60. Zappia, E.; Casazza, S.; Pedemonte, E.; Benvenuto, F.; Bonanni, I.; Gerdoni, E.; Giunti, D.; Ceravolo, A.; Cazzanti, F.; Frassnoni, F.; et al. Mesenchymal stem cells ameliorate experimental autoimmune encephalomyelitis inducing T-cell anergy. *Blood* **2005**, *106*, 1755–1761. [CrossRef] [PubMed]

61. Zhang, J.; Li, Y.; Chen, Y.; Cui, Y.; Lu, M.; Elias, S.B.; Mitchell, J.B.; Hammill, L.; Vanguri, P.; Chopp, M. Human bone marrow stromal cell treatment improves neurological functional recovery in EAE mice. *Exp. Neurol.* **2005**, *195*, 16–26. [CrossRef] [PubMed]

62. Gerdoni, E.; Gallo, B.; Casazza, S.; Musio, S.; Bonanni, I.; Pedemonte, E.; Mantegazza, R.; Frassoni, F.; Mancardi, G.; Pedotti, R.; et al. Mesenchymal stem cells effectively modulate pathogenic immune response in experimental autoimmune encephalomyelitis. *Ann. Neurol.* **2007**, *61*, 219–227. [CrossRef] [PubMed]

63. Kemp, K.; Hares, K.; Mallam, E.; Heesom, K.J.; Scolding, N.; Wilkins, A. Mesenchymal stem cell-secreted superoxide dismutase promotes cerebellar neuronal survival. *J. Neurochem.* **2010**, *114*, 1569–1580. [CrossRef] [PubMed]

64. Wilkins, A.; Kemp, K.; Ginty, M.; Hares, K.; Mallam, E.; Scolding, N. Human bone marrow derived mesenchymal stem cells secrete brain-derived neurotrophic factor which promotes neuronal survival in vitro. *Stem Cell Res.* **2009**, *3*, 63–70. [CrossRef] [PubMed]

65. Krishnamoorthy, G.; Wekerle, H. EAE: An immunologist's magic eye. *Eur. Immunol.* **2009**, *39*, 2031–2035. [CrossRef] [PubMed]

66. Gordon, D.; Pavlovska, G.; Glover, C.P.; Uney, J.B.; Wraith, D.; Scolding, N.J. Human mesenchymal stem cells abrogate experimental allergic encephalomyelitis after intraperitoneal injection, and with sparse CNS infiltration. *Neurosci. Lett.* **2008**, *448*, 71–73. [CrossRef] [PubMed]

67. Kassis, I.; Grigoriadis, N.; Gowda-Kurkalli, B.; Mizrachi-Kol, R.; Ben-Hur, T.; Slavin, S.; Abramsky, O.; Karussis, D. Neuroprotection and immunomodulation with mesenchymal stem cells in chronic experimental autoimmune encephalitis. *Arch. Neurol.* **2008**, *65*, 753–761. [CrossRef] [PubMed]

68. Bai, L.; Lennon, D.P.; Caplan, A.I.; DeChant, A.; Hecker, J.; Kranso, J.; Zaremba, A.; Miller, R.H. Hepatocyte growth factor mediates mesenchymal stem cell-induced recovery in multiple sclerosis models. *Nat. Neurosci.* **2012**, *15*, 862–870. [CrossRef] [PubMed]

69. Karussis, D.; Kassis, I. Use of stem cells for the treatment of multiple sclerosis. *Expert Rev. Neurother.* **2007**, *7*, 1189–1201. [CrossRef] [PubMed]

70. Rivera, F.J.; Couillard-Despres, D.; Pedre, X.; Ploetz, S.; Caioni, M.; Lois, C.; Bogdahn, U.; Aigner, L. Mesenchymal stem cells instruct oligodendrogenic fate decision on adult neural stem cells. *Stem Cells* **2006**, *24*, 2209–2219. [CrossRef] [PubMed]

71. Glenn, J.D.; Smith, M.D.; Calabresi, P.A.; Whartenby, K.A. Mesenchymal stem cells differentially modulate effector CD8+ T cell subsets and exacerbate experimental autoimmune encephalomyelitis. *Stem Cells* **2014**, *32*, 2744–2755. [CrossRef]

72. Grigoriadis, N.; Lourbopoulos, A.; Lagoudaki, R.; Frischer, J.M.; Polyzoidou, E.; Touloumi, O.; Simeonidou, C.; Deretzi, G.; Kountouras, J.; Spandou, E. Variable behavior and complications of autologous bone marrow mesenchymal stem cells transplanted in experimental autoimmune encephalomyelitis. *Exp. Neurol.* **2011**, *230*, 78–89. [CrossRef] [PubMed]

73. von Bahr, L.; Batsis, I.; Moll, G.; Häqq, M.; Szakos, A.; Sunberg, B.; Uzunel, M.; Ringden, O.; Le Blanc, K. Analysis of tissues following mesenchymal stromal cell therapy in humans indicate limited long-term engraftment and no ectopic tissue formation. *Stem Cells* **2012**, *30*, 557–564. [CrossRef] [PubMed]

74. Riordan, N.H.; Ichim, T.E.; Min, W.P.; Wang, H.; Solano, F.; Lara, F.; Alfaro, M.; Rodriguez, J.P.; Harman, R.J.; Patel, A.N.; et al. Non-expanded adipose stromal vascular fraction cell therapy for multiple sclerosis. *J. Transl. Med.* **2009**, *7*, 29. [CrossRef] [PubMed]

75. Mohyeddin Bonab, M.; Yazdanbakhsh, S.; Loftfi, J.; Alimoghaddom, K.; Talebian, F.; Hooshmand, F.; Ghavamzadeh, A.; Nikbin, B. Does mesenchymal stem cell therapy help multiple sclerosis patients? Report of a pilot study. *Iran. J. Immunol.* **2007**, *4*, 50–57.

76. Karussis, D.; Karageorgiou, C.; Vaknin-Dembinsky, A.; Gowda-Kurkalli, B.; Gomori, J.M.; Kassis, I.; Bulte, J.W.; Petrou, P.; Ben-Hur, T.; Abramsky, O.; et al. Safety and immunological effects of mesenchymal stem cell transplantation in patients with multiple sclerosis and amyotrophic lateral sclerosis. *Arch. Neurol.* **2010**, *67*, 1187–1194. [CrossRef] [PubMed]

77. Yamout, B.; Hourani, R.; Salti, H.; Barada, W.; El-Hajj, T.; Al-Kutoubi, A.; Herlopian, A.; Baz, E.K.; Mahfouz, R.; Khalil-Hamdan, R.; et al. Bone marrow mesenchymal stem cell transplantation in patients with multiple sclerosis: A pilot study. *J. Neuroimmunol.* **2010**, *227*, 185–189. [CrossRef] [PubMed]

78. Bonab, M.M.; Sahraian, M.A.; Aghsaie, A.; Karvigh, S.A.; Hosseinian, S.M.; Nikbin, B.; Lotfi, J.; Khorramnia, S.; Motamed, M.R.; Togha, M.; et al. Autologous mesenchymal stem cell therapy in progressive multiple sclerosis: An open label study. *Curr. Stem Cell Res. Ther.* **2012**, *7*, 407–414. [CrossRef] [PubMed]

79. Llufriu, S.; Sepulveda, M.; Blanco, Y.; Marín, P.; Moreno, B.; Berenguer, J.; Gabilondo, I.; Martínez-Heras, E.; Sola-Valls, N.; Arnaiz, J.A.; et al. Randomized placebo-controlled phase II trial of autologous mesenchymal stem cells in multiple sclerosis. *PLoS ONE* **2014**, *9*, e113936. [CrossRef] [PubMed]

80. Harris, V.K.; Yan, Q.J.; Vyshkina, T.; Sahabi, S.; Liu, X.; Sadiq, S.A. Clinical and pathological effects of intrathecal injection of mesenchymal stem cell-derived neural progenitors in an experimental model of multiple sclerosis. *J. Neurol. Sci.* **2012**, *313*, 167–177. [CrossRef]

81. Harris, V.K.; Faroqui, R.; Vyshkina, T.; Sadiq, S.A. Characterization of autologous mesenchymal stem cell-derived neural progenitors as a feasible source of stem cells for central nervous system applications in multiple sclerosis. *Stem Cells Transl. Med.* **2012**, *1*, 536–547. [CrossRef] [PubMed]

82. Harris, V.K.; Stark, J.; Vyshkina, T.; Blackshear, L.; Joo, G.; Stefanova, V.; Sara, G.; Sadiq, S.A. Phase I trial of intrathecal mesenchymal stem cell-derived neural progenitors in progressive multiple sclerosis. *eBioMedicine* **2018**, *29*, 23–30. [CrossRef] [PubMed]

83. Harris, V.K.; Vyshkina, T.; Sadiq, S.A. Clinical safety of intrathecal administration of mesenchymal stromal cell-derived neural progenitors in multiple sclerosis. *Cytotherapy* **2016**, *18*, 1476–1482. [CrossRef] [PubMed]

84. Dahbour, S.; Jamali, F.; Alhattab, D.; Al-Radaideh, A.; Ababneh, O.; Al-Ryalat, N.; Al-Bdour, M.; Hourani, B.; Msallam, M.; Rasheed, M.; et al. Mesenchymal stem cells and conditioned media in the treatment of multiple sclerosis patients: Clinical, ophthalmological and radiological assessments of safety and efficacy. *CNS Neurosci. Ther.* **2017**, *2*, 866–874. [CrossRef] [PubMed]

85. Weiss, S.; Dunne, C.; Hewson, J.; Wohl, C.; Wheatley, M.; Peterson, A.C.; Reynolds, B.A. Multipotent CNS stem cells are present in the adult mammalian spinal cord and ventricular neuroaxis. *J. Neurosci.* **1996**, *16*, 7599–7609. [CrossRef]

86. Morshead, C.M.; Reynolds, B.A.; Craig, C.G.; McBurney, M.W.; Staines, W.A.; Morassutti, D.; Weiss, S.; van der Koou, D. Neural stem cells in the adult mammalian forebrain: A relatively quiescent subpopulation of subependymal cells. *Neuron* **1994**, *13*, 1071–1082. [CrossRef]

87. Ming, G.L.; Song, H. Adult Neurogenesis in the Mammalian Brain: Significant Answers and Significant Questions. *Neuron* **2012**, *70*, 687–702. [CrossRef] [PubMed]

88. Bakemore, W.F.; Hans, S.K. The origin of remyelinating cells in the central nervous system. *J. Neuroimm.* **1999**, *98*, 69–76. [CrossRef]

89. Armstrong, R.C.; Le, Q.T.; Flint, N.C.; Vana, A.C.; Zhou, Y.X. Endogenous cell repair of chronic demyelination. *J. Neuropathol. Exp. Neurol.* **2006**, *65*, 245–256. [CrossRef] [PubMed]

90. Ben-Hur, T.; Einstein, O.; Mizrachi-Kol, R.; Ben-Menachem, O.; Reinhartz, E.; Karussis, D.; Abramsky, O. Transplanted multipotential neural precursor cells migrate into the inflamed white matter in response to experimental autoimmune encephalomyelitis. *Glia* **2003**, *41*, 73–80. [CrossRef] [PubMed]

91. Chang, A.; Tourtellotte, W.W.; Rudick, R.A.; Trapp, B.D. Premyelinating oligodendrocytes in chronic lesions of multiple sclerosis. *N. Engl. J. Med.* **2002**, *346*, 165–173. [CrossRef]

92. Izrael, M.; Zhang, P.; Kaufman, R.; Shinder, V.; Ella, R.; Amit, M.; Itskovitz-Eldor, J.; Chebath, J.; Revel, M. Human oligodendrocytes derived from embryonic stem cells: Effect of noggin on phenotypic differentiation in vitro and on myelination in vivo. *Mol. Cell Neurosci.* **2007**, *34*, 310–323. [CrossRef] [PubMed]

93. Shroff, G. Human embryonic stem cells for the treatment of multiple sclerosis: A case report. *Case Rep. Int.* **2015**, *4*, 38–42. [CrossRef]

94. Czepiel, M.; Balasubramaniyan, V.; Schaafsma, W.; Stancic, M.; Mikkers, H.; Hiusman, C.; Boddeke, E.; Copray, S. Differentiation of induced pluripotent stem cells into functional oligodendrocytes. *Glia* **2011**, *59*, 882–892. [CrossRef] [PubMed]

95. Laterza, C.; Merlini, A.; De Feo, D.; Ruffini, F.; Menon, R.; Onorati, M.; Fredickx, E.; Muzio, L.; Lombardo, A.; Comi, G.; et al. iPSC-derived neural precursors exert a neuroprotective role in immune-mediated demyelination via the secretion of LIF. *Nat. Commun.* **2013**, *4*, 2597. [CrossRef] [PubMed]

96. Zhao, T.; Zhang, Z.N.; Rong, Z.; Xu, Y. Immunogenicity of induced pluripotent stem cells. *Nature* **2011**, *474*, 212–215. [CrossRef] [PubMed]

97. Okano, H.; Nakamura, M.; Yoshida, K.; Okada, Y.; Tsuji, O.; Nori, S.; Ikeda, E.; Yamanaka, S.; Miura, K. Steps toward safe cell therapy using induced pluripotent stem cells. *Circ. Res.* **2013**, *112*, 523–533. [CrossRef] [PubMed]

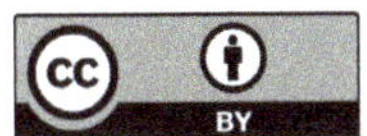

MDPI

St. Alban-Anlage 66

4052 Basel

Switzerland

Tel. +41 61 683 77 34

Fax +41 61 302 89 18

www.mdpi.com

Biomedicines Editorial Office

E-mail: biomedicines@mdpi.com

www.mdpi.com/journal/biomedicines